Series in BioEngineering

The Series in Bioengineering serves as an information source for a professional audience in science and technology as well as for advanced students. It covers all applications of the physical sciences and technology to medicine and the life sciences. Its scope ranges from bioengineering, biomedical and clinical engineering to biophysics, biomechanics, biomaterials, and bioinformatics.

More information about this series at http://www.springer.com/series/10358

Spyretta Golemati · Konstantina S. Nikita
Editors

Cardiovascular Computing—Methodologies and Clinical Applications

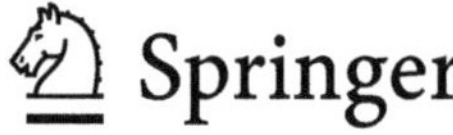

Editors
Spyretta Golemati
Medical School
National Kapodistrian
University of Athens
Athens, Greece

Konstantina S. Nikita
Biomedical Simulations
and Imaging Laboratory
National Technical University
of Athens
Athens, Greece

ISSN 2196-8861 ISSN 2196-887X (electronic)
Series in BioEngineering
ISBN 978-981-10-5091-6 ISBN 978-981-10-5092-3 (eBook)
https://doi.org/10.1007/978-981-10-5092-3

Library of Congress Control Number: 2018950815

This Springer imprint is published by the registered company Springer Nature Singapore Pte Ltd.
The registered company address is: 152 Beach Road, #21-01/04 Gateway East, Singapore 189721, Singapore

To my father Vassilios and my mother Polyniki

Spyretta Golemati

To my late father Spilios and my mother Kostoula

Konstantina S. Nikita

Preface

Cardiovascular computing is an interdisciplinary field aiming to deploy the principles and advances in computing and engineering to address current clinical challenges and provide new opportunities in cardiovascular science. This rapidly evolving scientific field has produced important new knowledge and has markedly improved our understanding of normal cardiovascular function as well as of pathophysiology, diagnosis and treatment of disorders like coronary artery disease, carotid atherosclerosis, heart rhythm abnormalities.

The book was envisioned as a comprehensive state-of-the-art description of the variety of advanced methodologies and applications of computing in cardiovascular research and clinical practice. The field of cardiovascular computing has encountered tremendous development in the last decades, spanning a wide range of different sub-areas, including among others sophisticated analysis of signals and images, modelling of complex physiological procedures and informatics approaches. This volume provides a collection of representative works of different disciplines covered by cardiovascular computing, reflecting the large diversity in this field. The intention of this project is to disseminate new insights into cardiovascular computing obtained by innovative methods of measuring, analysing and modelling cardiovascular data. For this purpose, the contributions included herein are written by leading scientists actively involved at the interface between cardiovascular science and computing engineering and technology.

The book is structured into six parts. In part I, the basic principles of cardiovascular anatomy and physiology are outlined, and a description is provided of current and emerging technologies for cardiovascular imaging. Parts II and III present methodologies for analysis of cardiovascular signals and images, respectively. Part IV discusses approaches for mathematical and computational modelling of cardiovascular data. Part V describes informatics methods, including artificial intelligence, data mining and big data analytics. Finally, part VI is dedicated to specific examples of cardiovascular computing in clinical practice, like stroke prediction, management of atrial fibrillation and applications in the intensive care unit.

The book is intended for a broad readership of various levels, from advanced undergraduate and postgraduate students to researchers and clinicians interested and/or involved in the science and practice of cardiovascular medicine and its interaction with computing technology.

We wish to thank the authors of all chapters for their commitment, valuable time and efforts towards providing high-quality contributions. We would also like to express our gratitude to Springer team members for their understanding, patience and support for materialising this project.

We hope that the book will serve as a useful reference to the readers and that it will stimulate intellectual excitement.

Athens, Greece

Spyretta Golemati
Konstantina S. Nikita

Contents

Part I
Cardiovascular Physiology: Basic Principles and Measurement

Cardiovascular Anatomy and Physiology: Basic Principles and Challenges

Aimilia Varela and Constantinos H. Davos

Abstract The cardiovascular system has several characteristics that makes it unique and amazingly complicated. The goal of cardiovascular anatomy and physiology is to describe and explain the anatomical and physical elements that are responsible for the origin, development and function of this particular system. This chapter will, mainly, focus on the basic principles of anatomy and physiology giving insights to the cardiac function and circulatory control. Considering the importance of cardiovascular system for the human body and that cardiovascular disease is the main cause of significant morbidity and mortality worldwide, the authors will also try to describe, within this chapter, the most important challenges for modern cardiology in the 21st century.

1 Basic Principles of Cardiovascular Anatomy and Physiology

The cardiovascular system consists of the heart, blood vessels and lymphatics maintaining the adequate circulation of oxygenated blood around the vascular network during normal activity, at rest and periods of exercise or stress. The normal heart lies in the centre of the cardiothoracic cavity under the breast bone and is rotated about 30° to the left lateral in front of the lungs. It is formed by the folding of the primitive vascular tube, at about the third week of gestation, which appears in the splanchnic mesodermal tissue near the pericardial cavity. The layers of the heart wall, inside to outside, are the endocardium, the myocardium, the epicardium and the pericardium. Briefly, the endocardium forms the inner layer which is directly connected to all the

A. Varela · C. H. Davos (✉)
Cardiovascular Research Laboratory, Clinical, Experimental Surgery and Translational Research Center, Biomedical Research Foundation, Academy of Athens, 4 Soranou Ephessiou Street, 11527 Athens, Greece
e-mail: cdavos@bioacademy.gr

A. Varela
e-mail: evarela@bioacademy.gr

S. Golemati and K. S. Nikita (eds.), *Cardiovascular Computing—Methodologies and Clinical Applications*, Series in BioEngineering,
https://doi.org/10.1007/978-981-10-5092-3_1

cardiac appendages; the four valves, the chordae tendineae and the papillary muscles. The myocardium is the middle muscular layer and it functions by assisting in the contraction and relaxation of the cardiac walls. The muscular layer which covers the external surfaces of the heart is called epicardium. It is directly fused with the myocardium internally and is in contact with the serous layer of the pericardium. The latter is a fibrous connective tissue membrane that covers entirely the heart and the roots of the great vessels. It has an inner and an outer layer which form the pericardial sac [1].

The basic heart muscle cell is a part of a syncytium (atrial and ventricular syncytium) in which the individual cells are held together with fibrous tissue and possesses inherent rythmicity. The areas crossing the cardiac muscle fibers are called intercalated discs; they are actually cell membranes that separate individual cardiac muscle cells from one another. The basic muscle unit is the sarcomere and every cell contains a nucleus and numerous mitochondria. Gap junctions allow all cardiac muscle cells to be linked electrochemically, so that activation of a small group of cells spreads like a wave throughout the entire heart. The electrical activity triggering the contraction of each sarcomere leads to a wave of depolarization and contraction across the myocardium [2, 3].

The heart, as shown in Fig. 1, is divided into a left and right side by a muscular wall called the septum and has four chambers: the right atrium, the right ventricle, the left atrium and the left ventricle and four valves. The tricuspid valve in the right and the mitral valve in the left heart separate each atrium from its associated ventricle (atrioventricular valves). They are attached to fibrous rings that encircle each valve annulus prohibiting backward flow during forceful contractions of the ventricles. The pulmonary valve lies between the right ventricle and the pulmonary artery and the aortic valve between the left ventricle and the aorta (semilunar valves); both ensuring unidirectional flow to the artery. Pressure gradients across the valves are the major determinants of opening and closure [2, 3].

The cardiac cycle involves a sequence of electrical, mechanical, hemodynamic and molecular activities of the heart through one complete heart beat. The cardiac cycle is repeated approximately 70–80 times per minute and includes the systolic (contraction) and diastolic (relaxation) activities of the atria and ventricles. The heart rate (HR) and rhythm are regulated by the conduction system that is controlled by a specialized group of cells localized in the sinoatrial node in the right atrium muscle near the superior vena cava orifice. These pacemaker cells have three unique characteristics; automaticity, conductivity and contractility. Briefly, the mechanism of pacemaker potential begins with K^+ exit from the cell through potassium channels and the slow leak of Na^+ into the cell which causes membrane potential to slowly drift up to a threshold that triggers Ca^{++} influx from outside (−40 mV).When this threshold for voltage-gated Ca^{++} channels is reached, fast calcium channels open, permitting explosive entry of Ca^{++} thus causing a sharp rise in the depolarization level. The time that peak depolarization is achieved, voltage-gated K^+ channels open causing repolarization to the initial "unstable resting potential". The action potential recorded in a ventricular muscle fiber, averages about 105 mV, which means that the intracellular potential rises from a very negative value, about −85 mV, between beats

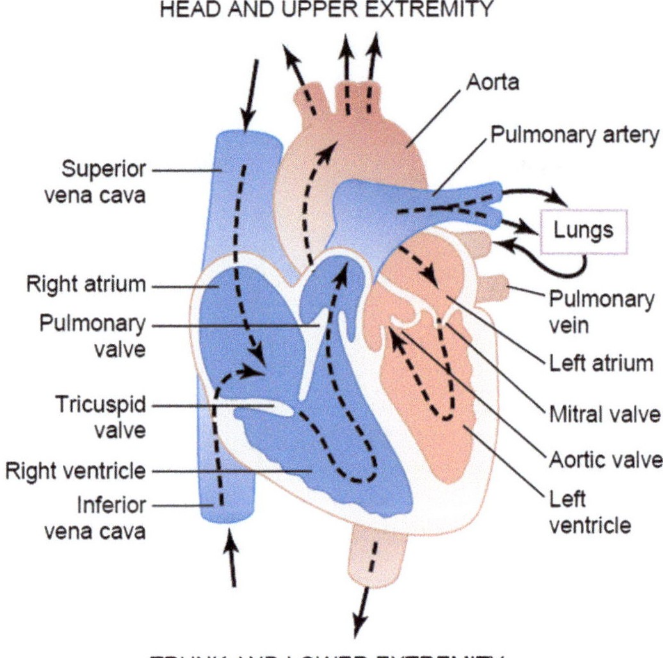

Fig. 1 Structure of the heart and course of blood flow through chambers and heart valves. (Reprinted from [2] with permission by Elsevier Saunders Inc)

to a slightly positive value, about +20 mV, during each beat. After the initial spike, the membrane remains depolarized for about 0.2 s, exhibiting a plateau as shown in Fig. 2, followed at the end of the plateau by abrupt repolarization. The presence of this plateau in the action potential causes ventricular contraction [2–5].

The impulses spread across the two atria as the impulses from the sinoatrial node reach the atrioventricular node in the right atrium, near the tricuspid valve. Then, the cells of the bundle of His in the septum are activated and the impulse passes via the right and left bundle branches (which are splitting into anterior and posterior divisions) reaching the Purkinje fibers thus activating the ventricles. A pulse is defined as a wave of distension of an artery allowing the contraction of the left ventricle. The coordinated repetitive electrical consequences of atrium and ventricular depolarization and repolarization can be displayed as an electrocardiographic signal [5].

Following electrical stimulation, mechanical events occur in the proper sequence and degree to provide adequate blood flow. These events are the two phases of the cardiac cycle; diastole and systole. Atrial diastole begins as blood fills the atria. Ventricular diastole describes the isovolumetric ventricular relaxation period during which the ventricular pressure rapidly falls below the pressure in the aorta, the volume remains unchanged and the four valves are closed. Then, the aortic valve opens and

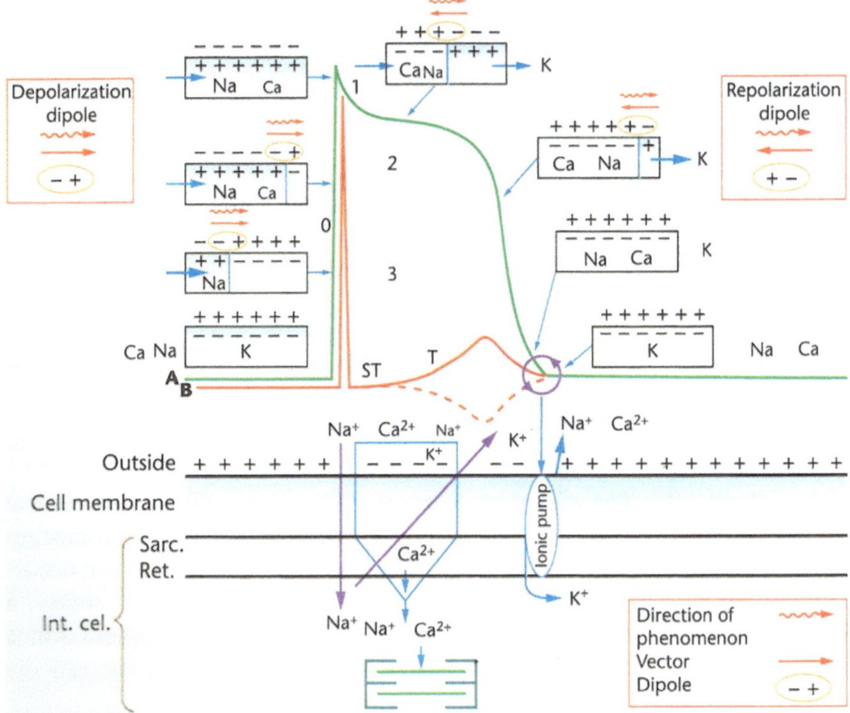

Fig. 2 Electro-ionic changes that occur in the cellular depolarization and repolarization in the contractile myocardium. A presents the action potential curve and B the curve of the electrogram of a single cell (repolarization with a dotted line) or left ventricle (normal ECG curve with a positive continuous line). (Reprinted from [4] with authors' permission)

a rapid ventricular filling occurs. Ventricular diastasis is a slower filling event since the most of the ventricular volume is already occupied by blood. Atrial systole or kick occurs and forces the remaining volume of the blood from the atria into the ventricles. At the end of this interval, as shown in Fig. 3, the blood volume is the end-diastolic volume and the ventricular pressure is the end-diastolic pressure, [2, 3].

The isovolumetric contraction occurs due to the increased tension in the ventricles as the action potential enters (ventricular depolarization). The aortic valve remains closed during the entire phase. Ventricular ejection occurs as the ventricle pressure exceeds aortic and pulmonary arterial pressure; the semilunar valves open and the blood is forced out. This interval ends when the semilunar valves close and the ventricles begin to relax. The closing causes a small increase in blood pressure (BP) visible as the dicrotic notch on a plot of BP against time. The amount of blood remaining in the ventricles at this time is called end-systolic volume while the amount of blood ejected is called stroke volume and equals the difference between the end-diastolic and end-systolic volume. Cardiac output refers to the amount of

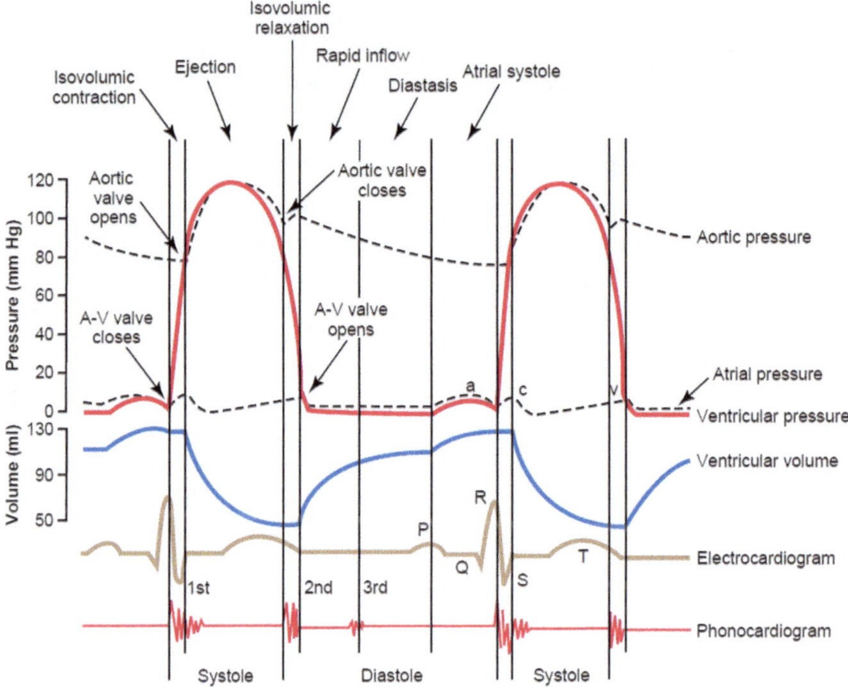

Fig. 3 Events of the cardiac cycle showing changes in left atrial pressure, left ventricular pressure, aortic pressure, ventricular volume, the electrocardiogram and the phonogram during systole and diastole. (Reprinted from [3] with permission by Elsevier Saunders Inc)

blood the heart pumps in one minute and is equal to HR multiplied by the stroke volume. The pumping effectiveness of the heart is controlled by the sympathetic and parasympathetic cardiac autonomic nervous system. Activation of sympathetic nerves increases HR (positive chronotropy), contractility (positive inotropy), rate of relaxation (increased lusitropy) and conduction velocity (positive dromotropy) while parasympathetic effects are opposite. The sympathetic system generally down-regulates parasympathetic activity, and vice versa. Sympathetic activation constricts arteries and arterioles increasing vascular resistance while sympathetic-induced constriction of veins (capacitance vessels) decreases venous compliance and blood volume thus increasing venous pressure [6].

The cardiovascular system is made up of two major circulatory systems, acting together. The pulmonary circulation, where the right side of the heart pumps deoxygenated blood to the lungs through the pulmonary artery and then returns oxygenated blood to the left atrium through the pulmonary veins. The systemic circulation, where the left side of the heart pumps the oxygenated blood to the rest of the body through the aorta, arteries, arterioles, systemic capillaries and then returns the deoxygenated blood with waste products to the right atrium through the venules and great veins [1].

The major vessels that carry blood to and from the heart are the inferior and superior vena cava which convey deoxygenated blood from the lower and upper extremities of the body, respectively, and the aorta which conveys oxygenated blood away from the heart to the entire organism. Arteries have thick, muscular, elastic walls to accommodate the blood flow (oxygen and nutrients) at high speeds and pressure. Capillaries are very small vessels that facilitate the transport of oxygen and nutrients into the cells and carbon dioxide and waste products away from them, respectively. Veins have thinner muscular walls and one-way valves that help move the blood that is low in oxygen and high in carbon dioxide back to the heart. The heart has its own blood supply; the coronary circulation, an essential determinant of myocardial performance. The volume of coronary blood flow under normal conditions is largely regulated by myocardial oxygen demands. There are two main coronary arteries, the left and the right. The coronary arteries originate from the aorta and form many branches which terminate in arterioles supplying a vast capillary network. The left coronary artery originates as main left coronary artery and then splits into two main branches; the left anterior descending and the circumflex coronary artery. Cardiac veins remove the deoxygenated blood from the heart muscle which is then delivered to the right atrium [1, 6].

The cardiovascular system is controlled by the autonomic nervous system which regulates cardiac output, systemic vascular resistance and local organ blood flow to ensure maintenance of optimal arterial pressure. Blood pressure is the amount of force exerted against the arterial wall by the blood and is measured in millimeters of mercury (mmHg). The maximum BP achieved during the contraction of the heart is called systolic blood pressure (SBP). Systolic blood pressure relates to the contraction strength of the cardiac muscle and the cardiac output, the systemic vascular resistance and the viscosity of the blood. The following simplified equation present this relationship:

$$\begin{aligned} Blood\ Pressure\ (BP) &= Cardiac\ Output\ (CO) \\ &\quad \times\ Systemic\ Vascular\ Resistance\ (SVR) \\ Cardiac\ Output &= Heart\ Rate \times Stroke\ Volume \end{aligned}$$

After the contraction, the aortic valves close and pressure difference between peripheral circulation and aortic arch causes blood to flow towards the peripheral arteries. Due to this flow, BP decreases until the heart beats again and the minimum BP just before next contraction is called diastolic blood pressure (DBP). These measures of BP undergo natural variations throughout the day (in a circadian rhythm); they also change in response to stress, nutritional factors, drugs or disease. Cardiac performance is determined by oxygen and energy consumption, BP and cardiac output (mean arterial blood flow) depending on four fundamental factors; preload, afterload, ventricular contractility and HR. Preload is the stretching of muscle fibers just before the onset of ventricular systole. According to Starling's law, the more the heart muscles stretch during diastole, the more forcefully they contract during systole. Afterload refers to the pressure that ventricular myocytes must generate to overcome the higher aorta pressure and eject blood. Contractility is the inherent ability of the cardiac muscle to contract normally, independent of external conditions [2, 3, 6].

2 Challenges in Cardiovascular Medicine

Considering that cardiovascular system is one of the most important systems in the organism, the first to function with an embryo, and that cardiovascular disease (CVD) is causative of significant morbidity and mortality expanding in developed and developing countries, this unit will focus to the challenges in cardiovascular medicine at the 21st century.

By the end of the 1950s the National Heart, Lung and Blood Institute Framingham Heart Study, had defined the major clinical risk factors namely, elevated serum cholesterol, high BP and smoking with the additional contributions of physical inactivity, obesity, and diabetes to be esteemed the following decades. However, the total burden of CVD and its risk factors will continue to increase with a prediction to reach 36% of all deaths in 2020 [7–9]. The major complexities focused to the lack of established coronary risk factors in a large group of patients with CVD and that a very substantial portion of the population is not yet receiving the adequate preventive or therapeutic treatment because their clinical application may be limited by ethical, political or economic factors. On the other hand, in the majority of patients who receive the optimal therapy in the most successful clinical trials the course of CVD remains unchanged and the number of high risk individuals will continue to expand due to the current improved technologies [9].

Furthermore, there are also two emerging epidemics of CVD; atrial fibrillation and heart failure. Atrial fibrillation is independently associated with increased risk of all-cause mortality [10, 11] and the latter has become the single most frequent cause of hospitalization in individuals 65 years of age or older [12]. Long term use of cardiovascular drugs, especially in the elderly is another important issue since not enough evidence exists to justify their use beyond 5–10 years. [13] The population of older adults is expanding rapidly and geriatric cardiology should meld cardiovascular perspectives with multimorbidity, polypharmacy, cognitive decline and other clinical, social, financial, and psychological dimensions of aging [14, 15].

Another important issue is the functional and anatomical imaging. Imaging is critical to modern health care systems particularly in the management of patients with CVD [16]. However, there is a large evidence gap between the feasibility of its performance, its contribution to improve patient outcomes and economic efficiency [17–19]. As the national health care environment becomes more demanding in financial resources, there will be a greater need for research-based health care decisions by providing evidence of the effectiveness of different treatment options [20], identification of clinical needs and their translation into innovation and technology development [21, 22].

Primary prevention of CVD is also of highest importance. Two complementary strategies are usually advocated; the “population” and the “high-risk” approach. The former aims at reducing the disease burden in the whole community, while the latter focuses on the most vulnerable individuals. The main target is to prevent the development of CVD through changes in legislation or social policies at the society level and through risk factor modifications taking into account genetic susceptibility, social, economic, cultural factors and the use of evidence based treatments at individual level. Regarding secondary CVD prevention, clinical trials have contributed substantially to documenting the importance of modifying risk factors (i.e. cholesterol or BP levels) or applying novel medication in reducing morbidity and mortality of CVD patients [7, 8].

Additionally, cardiovascular epidemiology has revealed as an ever more powerful science and new coronary risk factors have been identified, principally through population-based methods. In patients who have already clinical disease, the identification of the responsible genes will allow elucidation of the responsible mechanisms, and this in turn should lead to more effective therapies [9]. Systems biology approach to CVD risk stratification maybe employed for improving risk-estimating algorithms through addition of new derived biomarkers. In addition, modeling of personalized benefit-of-treatment may help in guiding choice of intervention [23]. Finally, well-organized trials relevant to public health needs by adequate support from both government and industry will be also very promising [15]. In conclusion, it seems that the early diagnosis procedures and better disease management tools in everyday life care are the most significant challenges for medical community in order to support the cardiovascular system through life time, effectively.

References

1. Kahle W, Leonhardt H, Platzer W (1985) Color atlas and textbook of human anatomy. Inner organs. Circulatory system. The Heart, vol 2, Greek edn. Copyright © 1985 Litsas Company
2. Guyton, AC, Hall JE (2006) The Heart. Unit 3. Chapter 9. Textbook of medical Physiology, 11th edn. Copyright © 2006 Elsevier Saunders Inc
3. Guyton AC, Hall JE (2006) The normal electrocardiogram. Unit 3. Chapter 9. Textbook of medical Physiology, 11th edn. Copyright © 2006 Elsevier Saunders Inc
4. de Luna AB, Batchvarov VN, Malik M (2006) The morphology of the Electrocardiogram. Chapter 1. The ESC textbook of cardiovascular medicine. Copyright © 2006 European Society of Cardiology
5. Goldschlager N (2000) Electrocardiography. Chapter 42, Part VII. Cecil textbook of medicine, 21st edn. Copyright © 2000 W B Saunders Company
6. Burkhoff D, Weisfeldt ML (2000) Cardiac function and circulatory control. Chapter 40, Part VII. Cecil textbook of medicine. 21st edn. Copyright © 2000 W B Saunders Company
7. Tzoulaki I, Elliott P, Kontis V, Ezzati M (2016) Worldwide exposures to cardiovascular risk factors and associated health effects: current knowledge and data gaps. Circulation 133(23):2314–2333. https://doi.org/10.1161/CIRCULATIONAHA.115.008718
8. McAloon CJ, Boylan LM, Hamborg T, Stallard N, Osman F, Lim PB, Hayat SA (2016) The changing face of cardiovascular disease 2000–2012: an analysis of the world health organisation global health estimates data. Int J Cardiol 224:256–264. https://doi.org/10.1016/j.ijcard.2016.09.026
9. Braunwald E (1997) Shattuck lecture–cardiovascular medicine at the turn of the millennium: triumphs, concerns, and opportunities. N Engl J Med 337(19):1360–1369 PMID: 9358131

10. Kirchhof P, Benussi S, Kotecha D et al. (2016) ESC Guidelines for the management of atrial fibrillation developed in collaboration with EACTS: the task force for the management of atrial fibrillation of the European society of cardiology (ESC)Developed with the special contribution of the European heart rhythm association (EHRA) of the ESCEndorsed by the European stroke organisation (ESO). Eur Heart J 2016:27. pii: ehw210 PMID: 27567408
11. Colilla S (2013) Estimates of current and future incidence and prevalence of atrial fibrillation in the U.S. adult population. Am J Cardiol 112:1142–1147
12. Ponikowski P, Voors AA, Anker SD et al (2016) ESC Guidelines for the diagnosis and treatment of acute and chronic heart failure: the task force for the diagnosis and treatment of acute and chronic heart failure of the European Society of Cardiology (ESC). Developed with the special contribution of the heart failure association (HFA) of the ESC. Eur J Heart Fail 18(8):891–975. https://doi.org/10.1002/ejhf.592 PMID:27207191
13. Rossello X, Pocock SJ, Julian DG (2015) Long-Term use of cardiovascular drugs: challenges for research and for patient care. J Am Coll Cardiol 66(11):1273–1285. https://doi.org/10.1016/j.jacc.2015.07.018
14. Bell SP, Orr NM, Dodson JA, Rich MW, Wenger NK, Blum K, Harold JG, Tinetti ME, Maurer MS, Forman DE (2015) What to Expect From the Evolving Field of Geriatric Cardiology. J Am Coll Cardiol 66(11):1286–1299. https://doi.org/10.1016/j.jacc.2015.07.048
15. Yusuf S (1999) Randomised controlled trials in cardiovascular medicine: past achievements, future challenges. BMJ 319(7209):564–568 PMID:10463903
16. Lancellotti P, Płońska-Gościniak E, Garbi M et al (2015) Cardiovascular imaging practice in Europe: a report from the European Association of Cardiovascular Imaging. Eur Heart J Cardiovasc Imaging 16(7):697–702. https://doi.org/10.1093/ehjci/jev116
17. Shaw LJ, Narula J (2008) Cardiovascular imaging quality-more than a pretty picture! JACC Cardiovasc Imaging 1(2):266–269. https://doi.org/10.1016/j.jcmg.2008.01.005
18. Douglas PS, Cerqueira MD, Berman DS et al (2016) The future of cardiac imaging: report of a think tank convened by the American college of cardiology. JACC Cardiovasc Imaging 9(10):1211–1223. https://doi.org/10.1016/j.jcmg.2016.02.027
19. Hendel RC, Patel MR, Allen JM et al (2013) Appropriate use of cardiovascular technology: 2013 ACCF appropriate use criteria methodology update: a report of the American College of Cardiology Foundation appropriate use criteria task force. J Am Coll Cardiol 61(12):1305–1317. https://doi.org/10.1016/j.jacc.2013.01.025
20. Wiener DH (2014) Achieving high-value cardiac imaging: challenges and opportunities. J Am Soc Echocardiogr 27(1):1–7. https://doi.org/10.1016/j.echo.2013.08.027
21. Weissman NJ, Soman P, Shah DJ (2013) Multimodality imaging: opportunities and challenges. JACC Cardiovasc Imaging 6(9):1022–1023. https://doi.org/10.1016/j.jcmg.2013.07.003
22. Shinbane JS, Saxon LA (2016) Digital monitoring and care: virtual medicine. Trends Cardiovasc Med 26(8):722–730
23. Björnson E, Borén J, Mardinoglu A (2016) Personalized cardiovascular disease prediction and treatment-a review of existing strategies and novel systems medicine tools. Front Physiol 7:2. https://doi.org/10.3389/fphys.2016.00002

Current and Emerging Technologies for Cardiovascular Imaging

Erik Hedström, Ellen Ostenfeld, Marcus Carlsson, Per M. Arvidsson, Christos G. Xanthis, Kostas Haris, Einar Heiberg and Anthony H. Aletras

Abstract Cardiovascular disease is the leading cause of death in the western world. With the application of theoretical physics to the clinic, a variety of imaging technologies are available to the physician for diagnosing and accurately quantifying disease progression. These tools can influence how therapies are applied and impact patient outcome. Radiographic methods based on x-rays are used for diagnosis (Computed Tomography) and therapy (catheterization suite). Nuclear medicine with Single Photon Emission Tomography (SPECT) and Positron Emission Tomography (PET) are routinely used for detecting irreversible and reversible ischemic injury. Ultrasound echocardiography is also routinely used for visualizing contractile function and quantifying blood velocities. Cardiac Magnetic Resonant Imaging allows for a one-stop-shop evaluation of the cardiovascular system including function, tissue perfusion and viability and well as edema visualization, extracellular volume imaging, iron overload, etc. The emergence of new technologies for acquiring data with existing techniques, such as sparse undersampling, and radically new approaches, such as Optical Coherence Tomography and Near Infrared Spectroscopy, open uncharted domains and promise even better diagnostics in the future.

1 Introduction

The main disease in the cardiovascular system is atherosclerosis causing plaques that limit blood flow and cause imbalance between supply and demand of oxygen, so called ischemia. The plaques can rupture and cause a local blood clot i.e. thrombosis,

E. Hedström · E. Ostenfeld · M. Carlsson · P. M. Arvidsson · C. G. Xanthis · K. Haris · E. Heiberg
A. H. Aletras (✉)
Faculty of Clinical Sciences, Department of Clinical Physiology and Nuclear Medicine, Lund University and Skåne University Hospital, Lund, Sweden
e-mail: Aletras@hotmail.com

C. G. Xanthis · K. Haris · A. H. Aletras
Laboratory of Computing, Medical Informatics and Biomedical – Imaging Technologies, Faculty of Health Sciences, School of Medicine, Aristotle University of Thessaloniki, Thessaloniki, Greece

S. Golemati and K. S. Nikita (eds.), *Cardiovascular Computing—Methodologies and Clinical Applications*, Series in BioEngineering,
https://doi.org/10.1007/978-981-10-5092-3_2

called thrombosis. This results in an acute and severe decrease in blood flow where the ischemia, if not relieved, causes cell death i.e. infarction. Infarction results in loss of contractile function in the heart muscle potentially leading to heart failure and arrhythmia. These effects of ischemia are the reason why myocardial infarction is the main killer in the world. The study of blood flow to the heart is therefore of great clinical interest.

With the advent of electronics, theoretical physics were applied to diagnostic medicine. Diagnostic imaging techniques have become essential for patient evaluation and treatment. This chapter will first focus on current imaging technologies used in diagnosing cardiovascular disease i.e. x-rays, ultrasonic imaging, computed tomography (CT), nuclear imaging and magnetic resonance imaging (MRI) [1, 2]. Last, emerging technologies will be presented. The reader is encouraged to further reading via the references presented herein. The physics of medical imaging may well be complemented by more in-depth medical physics literature.

2 Conventional Radiography (X-Ray) Applications in Cardiovascular Imaging and Intervention

Conventional chest x-ray and invasive angiography have generally been replaced with CT and MRI for accurate first-line diagnosis, with the exception of cases where intervention is expected in the same session, as with diagnostic invasive angiography. However, as chest x-ray imaging is widely available and still performed on a routine screening basis, as part of clinical work-up or as a follow-up examination, incidental findings indicative of vascular pathology may be identified. In those cases further imaging is, to an increasing extent, advocated for diagnosis or severity scoring. Conventional invasive angiography combined with endovascular intervention, with its limited invasiveness and reduced overall risk, has increased in use as a replacement for open surgery.

2.1 X-Rays: Basic Physics

In their most basic form, as applied for chest x-ray imaging, x-ray images are 2-dimensional representations of 3-dimensional objects (Fig. 1). A difference should be noted between overall image quality and diagnostic quality, where the latter is more important as the experienced reading physician usually sees beyond noise, poor resolution and artifacts. Exams should be performed with adequate image quality without excessive radiation. The radiation dose is the amount of energy deposited to the mass of tissue (J/kg = Gy) and can also be expressed in radiography as the dose-area product (DAP) by multiplying the dose by the exposed area (mGy $\times$ cm^2).

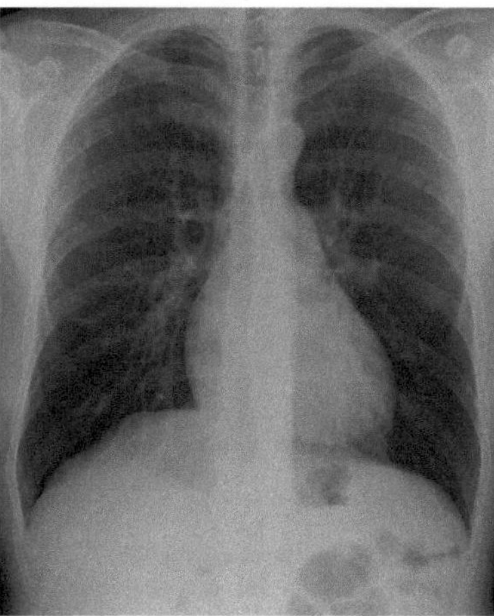

Fig. 1 Chest x-ray imaging. A standard inhaled frontal chest x-ray acquired with the patient standing. Tissue where more photons have passed through the body is darker in the image, such as the lungs, and tissue where a larger extent of photons is attenuated is brighter, such as the heart, soft tissue, skeletal structures and abdominal organs. With a single projection, a particular structure's exact position in space cannot be known, which is why a second projection 90° to the first is usually assessed (c.f. Fig. 3 top left)

X-rays are photons produced in a tube where electrons are let to collide with an anode in vacuum, dependent on current (mA) and voltage (kV) during a certain exposure time (s). Whereas the current gives the number of released electrons, the voltage affects the velocity of those electrons, thereby also determining the energy of produced photons. As low-energy photons are almost completely absorbed by tissue without adding information to the image, filtration is performed as a means of radiation protection. Moreover, collimators are used to decrease the area being irradiated resulting in decreased radiation and reduced scatter, thus improving image quality. With digital systems and so-called automatic exposure, control dose optimization can be performed, for example, with increased voltage and automatically reduced current and/or exposure duration (mA × s product), although at a slight cost in increased scatter but with overall high diagnostic image quality.

Image contrast refers to differences in x-ray penetration between different tissues. The two main interactions between diagnostic x-ray photons and tissue are the photoelectric effect (absorption) and the Compton effect (partial absorption and scatter). The photoelectric effect is the main contributor to differences in x-ray attenuation and image information together with photons that have passed through the object without interaction, whereas scattered photons reaching the detector contribute to background and noise, as their location of initial tissue interaction is not known. Scatter can be reduced by applying a grid consisting of linear lead (Pb) septa allowing only photons coming directly from the tube to reach the detector, however, also in part reducing the number of those primary photons. The overall effect is that

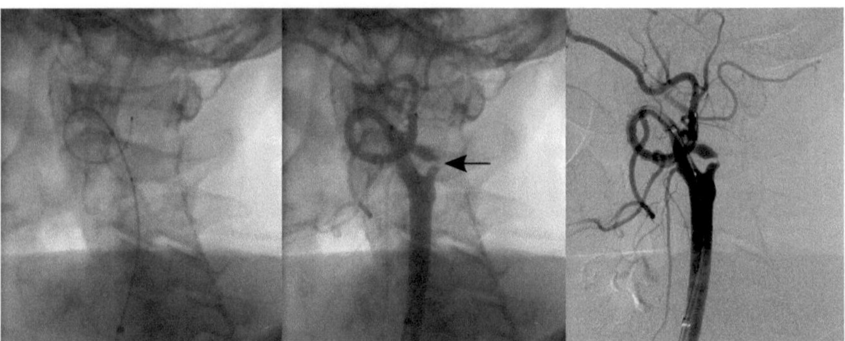

Fig. 2 Contrast agent is needed/DSA. Conventional angiography with the carotid artery catheterized, shown without *(left)* and with *(middle)* a high-attenuation property contrast agent, indicating the need of a contrast agent to visualize the vasculature and in this particular case a stenosis in the internal carotid artery (arrow). Note that the image gray scale has been inverted compared with static x-ray images, such as shown in Fig. 1. Digital subtraction angiography (DSA; right). The subtraction of an initial mask of background structures from the acquired images with contrast agent improves vasculature depiction in comparison with the standard conventional angiography with contrast agent as shown in the middle panel

the current-time product needs to be increased for adequate image quality with an increase in patient dose.

For angiography, a contrast agent is needed to visualize the vasculature as blood has similar attenuation properties as surrounding tissue (Fig. 2, left and middle). Contrast agents with high attenuation properties, such as iodinated contrast agents, are routinely used. Also, carbon dioxide is used since it acts as a negative contrast agent allowing more photons to pass without attenuation. Carbon dioxide does not have the limitations of nephrotoxicity or allergic reactions associated with standard iodinated contrast agents; however, it should preferably not be used superior to the diaphragm for arterial angiography due to risk of gas embolization. Digital subtraction angiography (DSA), where an initial mask of background structures is subtracted from the later acquired images with contrast agent, improves vasculature depiction and also allows blood flow to be visualized more clearly as a function of time (Fig. 2, right). As two images are subtracted the resulting image has a higher degree of noise. Therefore, DSA images are acquired at higher doses than standard, indicating the importance of limiting the duration of imaging and treatment in order to reduce patient radiation dose.

2.2 X-Rays: Heart and Thoracic Aorta

As noted, conventional 2D chest x-ray imaging is not necessarily a primary tool for diagnosis of cardiovascular disorders, but is still used as a general routine screening tool and for follow-up. Signs of cardiovascular pathophysiology can be such as an enlarged cardiac silhouette (Fig. 3, top left, top middle, top right), widening of the mediastinum or pulmonary vessel enlargement and tapering (Fig. 3, bottom left). The aorta may show elongation or pathological widening indicative of aortic aneurysm (Fig. 3, bottom right) and displaced calcified plaques may be suggestive of aortic dissection. For congenital aortic disease, coarctatio aortae may show signs of a prominent ascending aorta, absence of proximal descending aortic arch, a "3" sign as indentation at the site of coarctatio, and costal notching due to dilated collateral vessels. Signs may be unspecific and further examinations may be needed for accurate diagnosis. However, conventional invasive aortography may be added in the few cases where computed tomography or magnetic resonance imaging are inconclusive or when endovascular intervention is planned (Fig. 4).

2.3 X-Rays: Coronary Arteries

Conventional invasive coronary angiography is increasingly replaced with widely available computed tomography contrast angiography with calcium scoring or magnetic resonance angiography with or without contrast agent, including for diagnosis of variations in coronary artery anatomy and anomalies. However, conventional angiography yields the opportunity of simultaneous therapy with balloon expansion of a stenosis, extraction of thrombus material and stenting, so-called percutaneous coronary intervention (PCI) (Fig. 5). Conventional coronary angiography is advocated in suspected coronary artery disease with severe symptoms and in patients with high-risk features and acute coronary symptoms. Moreover, the spatial resolution is higher for conventional angiography and depicts both smaller branches and the more distal parts of the coronary tree when compared with computed tomography and magnetic resonance angiography.

Conventional coronary angiography is performed under local anesthesia with catheter- and guide wire-based access to the coronary arteries through either the femoral or radial artery. An iodinated contrast agent is selectively injected into the left and right coronary, respectively. Angiography depicts the lumen of epicardial large vessels and does not give direct information about vessel wall changes or myocardial perfusion. Additional methods such as intra-vascular ultrasound (IVUS) showing plaque composition and thus differentiation of soft plaques from fibrotic lesions, and assessment of myocardial blush grade indicating perfusion of the myocardium, can be used. While IVUS has been used for decades, the value of IVUS for guiding therapy is still debated. New methods have evolved for intra-coronary plaque assessment. Optical coherence tomography (OCT) is an established medical imaging technique in ophthalmology and has been applied to invasive assessment to help diagnose coronary artery disease. With near-infrared wavelength light it has higher resolution and is suited for assessing the endothelial surface of coronary plaques. Near-infrared spectroscopy (NIRS) is another new technique, based on so-called molecular over-

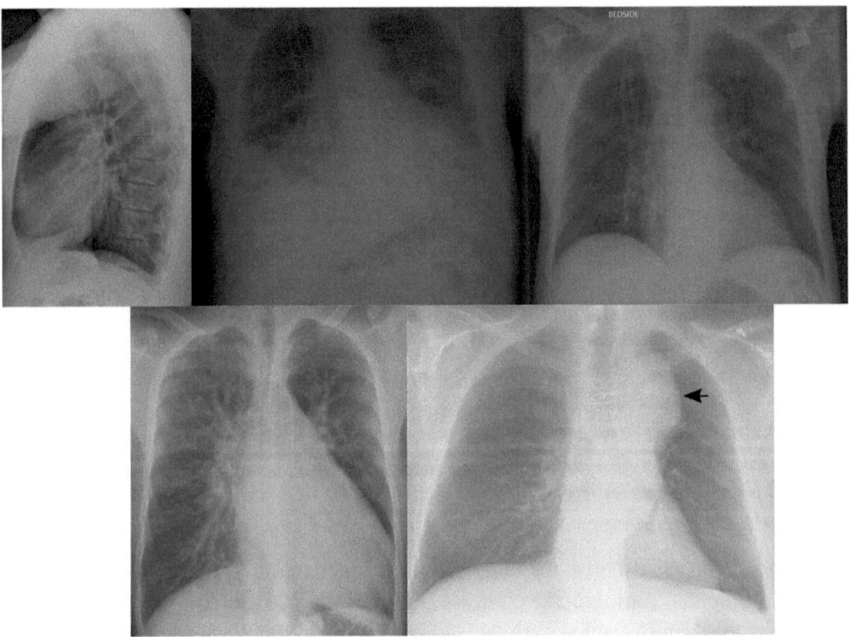

Fig. 3 x-ray cardiovascular pathophysiology. **Top left:** A standard inhaled lateral chest x-ray with the patient in standing position (c.f. Figure XR1). The cardiac silhouette may be considered enlarged and rounded, suspicious of, but not necessarily diagnostic of, pericardial fluid. This suggested diagnosis was confirmed by echocardiography, **Top middle and top right:** A bedside frontal chest x-ray with the patient in the supine position before (top middle) and after (top right) treatment. Initially (top middle), an enlarged cardiac silhouette, pronounced pulmonary vessels and bilateral pleural effusion are found, suggestive of the primary diagnosis being cardiac failure. After treatment (top right) with diuretics, the cardiac silhouette is more towards its normal size albeit still slightly large, the pulmonary vessels almost normalized and the pleural effusion no longer visualized and the diaphragm clearly marked. It is important to note, however, that pleural effusion may still exist as fluid in a supine chest x-ray may amount to quite a large volume without major image changes as the fluid accumulates posteriorly and thus gives a general density increase without a sharp border. **Bottom left:** A standard inhaled frontal chest x-ray acquired with the patient standing. A markedly enlarged cardiac silhouette combined with widened proximal pulmonary arteries and tapering of pulmonary vessels to the periphery are indicative of pulmonary hypertension. **Bottom right:** A standard inhaled frontal chest x-ray acquired with the patient standing. In this case the cardiac silhouette and pulmonary vessels are normal whereas the aorta is tortuous and markedly enlarged at the level of the aortic arch (arrow), indicative of an aortic aneurysm

tone and combination of vibration, yielding information on, for instance, coronary lipid content.

Fractional flow reserve (FFR) with invasive coronary angiography is quite commonly used to determine hemodynamic significance of coronary artery disease, as angiography in itself cannot determine the functional severity of a stenotic lesion. The pressure ratio across a stenosis under maximum hyperemia (e.g. during adenosine administration) is measured invasively. A normal coronary artery without stenosis

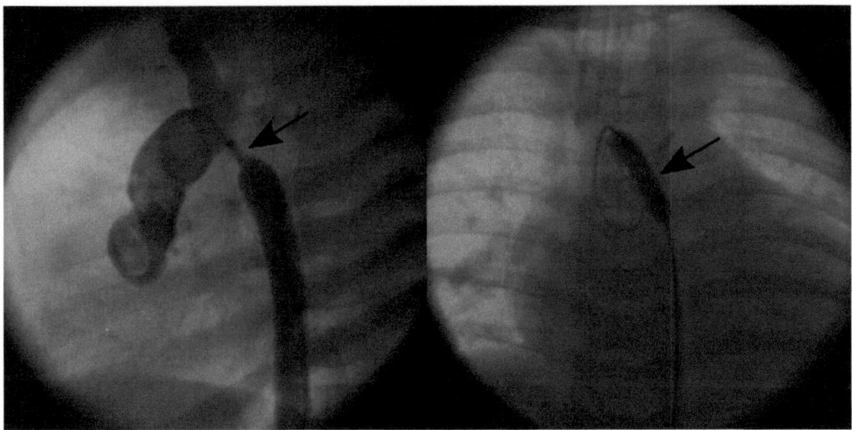

Fig. 4 A conventional angiography with contrast agent showing a severe coarctation of the aorta (left; arrow). An intervention with balloon expansion was performed (right; arrow). Invasive pressure measurements over the stenosis were performed before and after treatment, and indicated successful treatment

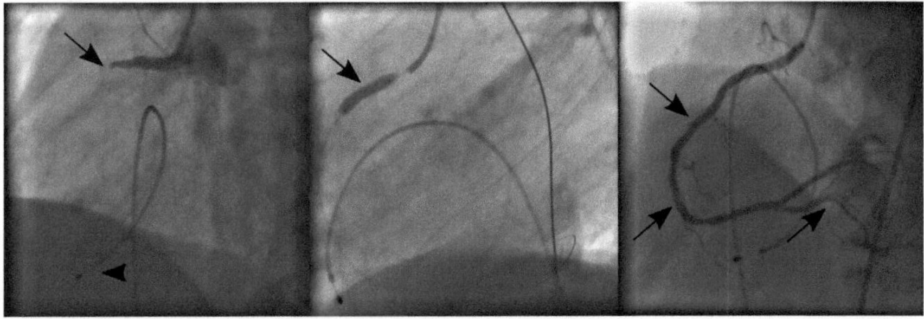

Fig. 5 PCI. Coronary angiography in a previously healthy 84-year old male, with sudden chest pain and bradycardia, suggestive of a proximal right coronary artery stenosis. A temporary pacemaker lead (left; arrowhead) was placed due to bradycardia. Angiography showed a proximal occlusion (left; arrow) of the right coronary artery, which was treated with balloon expansion and stenting (middle; arrow) resulting in normalized blood flow and the complete right coronary artery visible after treatment (right; arrow)

has no significant drop in pressure and the FFR is close to 1. An FFR value <0.75 is indicative of a stenosis causing myocardial ischemia, while FFR >0.80 rarely is associated with ischemia and there is no need for revascularization. FFR values between 0.75 and 0.80 are considered a 'grey zone', where other clinical information is added for determination of whether the patient receives revascularization therapy or not. FFR guided intervention has shown improved outcome [3]. A more recent method, instantaneous wave-free ratio (iFR), independent of adenosine, shows promising results for guiding intervention, but is as of yet not as widely applied [4].

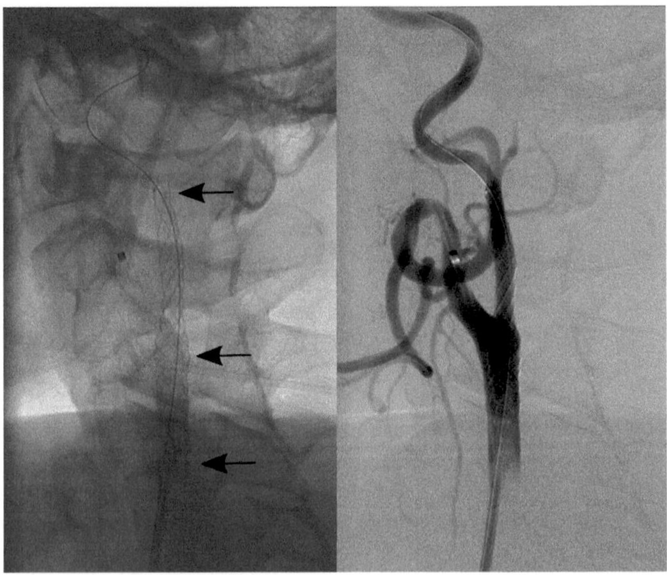

Fig. 6 Carotid angio. Conventional carotid artery angiography showing endovascular intervention with treatment of a stenosis in the internal carotid artery by placement of a stent (left; arrows) and normalized blood flow after treatment (right). The left image is a standard acquisition without contrast agent, whereas the right image is a DSA image with contrast agent

2.4 X-Rays: Carotid Arteries

Conventional carotid artery angiography is not commonly performed in asymptomatic stenosis, and is generally only applied as endovascular intervention in patients with previous surgery or radiation to the region (Fig. 6). Otherwise, open surgery is performed as studies so far indicate that this method is superior to endovascular intervention in the carotid arteries.

3 Computed Tomography—CT

Cardiovascular computed tomography (CT) is well established for the assessment of the heart, large vessels and coronary arteries with calcium detection and plaque characterization [1, 2, 5, 6].

Cardiovascular CT requires high spatial and temporal resolution [7] and therefore CT scanners with at least 64 simultaneous detectors (rows) with short gantry rotation times, thin-slice collimation, and ECG for gating and triggering of image acquisition, are preferred. By increasing the number of detector rows image quality, radiation dose and diagnostic accuracy are also improved [8].

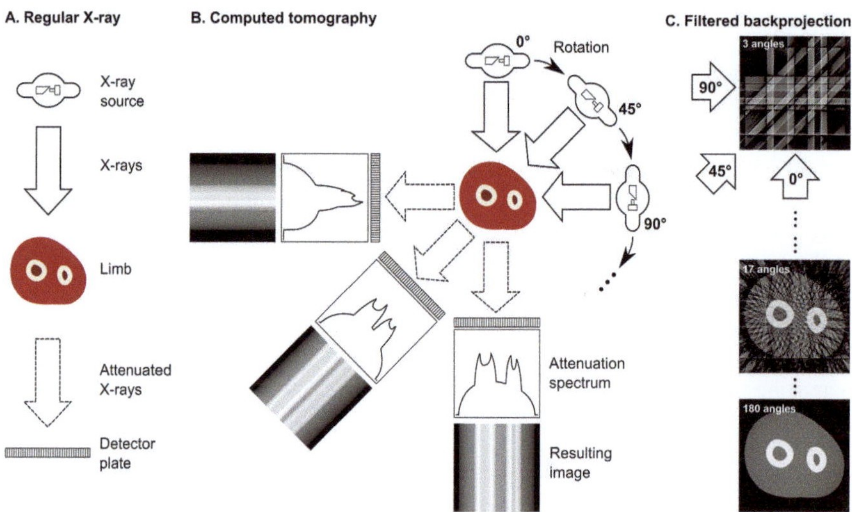

Fig. 7 CT Basic Physics. Schematic illustration of computed tomography (CT). **a** Shows the results of an image from one x-ray source from only one angle. **b** Shows one x-ray transmitter and detector rotating around the volume of interest with resulting back projections, here from three different angles. Modern CT-scanner can have several detectors and dual-sources. **c** The projections from all angles are filtered and merged into one filtered back projection. A long rotation time would increase the temporal resolution. Though, this increases the risk of motion artifacts causing blurring of the image. A short rotation time is therefore preferred and this requires a low pitch factor to maintain a good temporal resolution

3.1 CT: Basic Physics

Compared with 2D x-ray, computed tomography is the transmission and registration of x-rays in a large number of projection angles (Fig. 7). With multiple slices transmitted and detected simultaneously a section of the volume of interest is scanned. Thus multi-planar image reconstruction in three dimensions is also feasible after signal acquisition. Four factors affect the image quality in cardiac CT: Temporal resolution, spatial resolution, low contrast resolution and ECG monitoring.

3.2 CT: Temporal Resolution

The acquisition time depends on the number of rows, the gantry rotation time and beam pitch. The beam pitch is the patient displacement, or table feed, per 360° gantry rotation divided by the detector width. Thus, a short rotation time is preferred to avoid blurring of the image due to motion artifacts (such as those arising from the beating heart) combined with a very small pitch factor.

3.3 CT: Spatial Resolution

Spatial resolution refers to the ability to clearly distinguish small objects in an image. The detector width, slice collimation and data sampling are related to spatial resolution so that more simultaneous detector rows inherently yield higher spatial resolution. The typical voxel size is 0.4 mm × 0.4 mm × 0.4–2 mm with the two in-plane dimensions depending on the size of the field of view and the depth depending on the acquisition configuration and the reconstruction. This is sufficient to assess atherosclerotic plaques, dissections and to some extent stents in the coronary arteries as well as in the larger arteries. Administration of nitroglycerin just prior to a scan of the coronary arteries is the clinical standard and dilates the vessels, thereby increasing the number of pixels viewed per vessel.

3.4 CT: Low Contrast Resolution

Attenuation coefficients of different tissues are referenced to the attenuation of water within the voxel and are referred to as Hounsfield units (HU). Water is defined as 0 HU and air as −1000 HU. Some characteristics of tissues are fat with −50 to 0 HU, low density non-calcified plaque <30 HU and calcifications well above 130 HU. Contrast resolution refers to the ability to distinguish objects with different attenuation from one another. There is a direct relationship of low contrast resolution with radiation dose and image noise. Image noise is the main limitation, when structures exhibit low contrast resolution. Image noise may be reduced by increased current (mAs) at the cost of increased radiation dose or by increased slice thickness at the cost of spatial resolution. Further, iodinated contrast agents can be used to enhance the signal-to-noise ratio between the vessel lumen and wall.

3.5 CT: ECG Monitoring

Electrocardiogram monitoring is necessary for CT of the coronary arteries and the aortic root (Fig. 8). The scan is synchronized to the R-waves of the ECG to avoid motion artifacts. Image quality and radiation dose is related to the heart rate. For improved image quality the scan is triggered to the diastolic phase of the heart cycle, which is prolonged by administering heart rate lowering agents (beta blockers and sinus node blockers). An acquisition is generally either based on retrospective cardiac phase selection throughout the whole heart cycle allowing for reconstruction of any cardiac phase at the cost of a high radiation dose, or with prospective ECG triggering to scan during a fraction of the heart cycle, preferably during end-diastole. The advantage of prospective ECG triggering is the lower radiation dose, whereas a

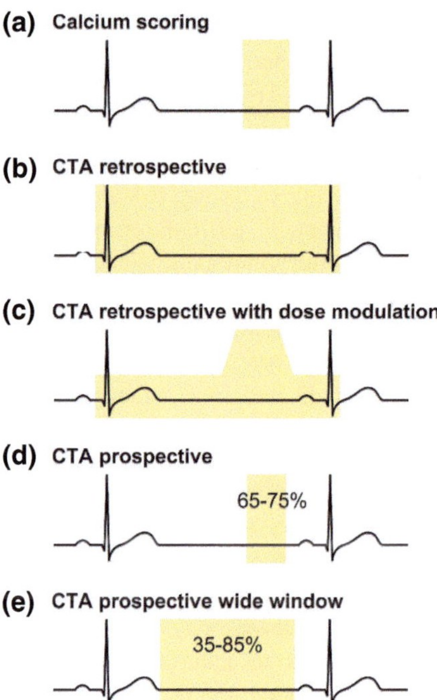

Fig. 8 ECG-gated and triggered CT scan. Illustrations of different types of ECG-gated and ECG-triggered computed tomography angiographic (CTA) examinations. The coronary arteries and aortic root are moving the least in the end-diastolic and end-systolic phase of the heart cycle. Diastole is longer at low compared to high heart rate. Image quality increases when the scan is triggered to the longer diastolic phase of the heart cycle in patients with low heart rate. **a** Non-contrast calcium score scanned in diastole. **b** Retrospective ECG-gated CTA is a helical acquisition during a complete heart cycle. Tube current remains constant during the heart cycle. **c** Retrospective ECG-gated CTA with dose modulation. Tube current is modulated during a helical acquisition with high dose when good image quality for coronary arteries are expected. **d** Prospective ECG-triggered CTA acquisition in diastole, preferably 65–75% into the RR-interval. **e** Prospective ECG-triggered CTA acquisition with a longer time window. In patients with high heart rate, more heart phases could be included in the scan, preferably during both end-diastole and end-systole (e.g. from 35 to 85% of the RR-interval). The advantage of prospective ECG-triggering is lower radiation dose compared to helical/retrospective ECG-gated

disadvantage is the presence of so-called stitching artifacts between subvolumes in sequential scans (Fig. 9b, d), especially in arrhythmia and high heart rates.

3.6 CT: Coronary Artery Disease

Coronary artery disease (CAD) is caused by formation of atheromatous plaques in the arteries. Acute myocardial infarction results from acutely restricted coronary flow to the myocardium mainly due to atherosclerotic obstructing lesions in the coronary arteries. Obstruction of blood flow to the myocardium causes myocardial cell death, necrosis, which is replaced by fibrotic scar tissue. In some cases, infarcted myocardium may contain calcifications and fatty infiltration (Fig. 12a) [1].

Multidetector CT contrast-enhanced angiography (CTA) can assess calcified plaques including calcium scoring (a strong risk marker of CAD), non-calcified plaques with fatty or fibrous content, positive remodeling of the vessel wall and lumen stenosis, and coronary artery anomalies. It can also detect the presence of decreased perfusion in the ischemic or infarcted myocardium, of ventricular dilatation and of subendocardial calcification and fatty replacement (Fig. 12a). In cases of diagnosis of coronary artery by-pass graft patency where invasive coronary angiography is non-diagnostic or contraindicated, ECG-triggered CTA has incremental value.

For calcium scoring, volumes of more than 3 mm^3 with attenuation density $\geq$130 HU at 3 mm slice thickness are automatically marked by dedicated software. A particular strength of CTA is the high sensitivity, specificity and especially the high negative predictive value (97–100%) for obstructive stenosis in patients with low to intermediate pretest likelihood for CAD [2, 9]. Thus, it can rule out the presence of CAD in patients with chest pain or suspected CAD. All vessels greater than 1.5 mm should be graded for stenosis severity. Further, some plaque characteristics are independently associated with future acute coronary ischemic events. These high-risk features include low-density plaque, spotty calcification, positive remodeling and signet ring sign (Fig. 9a–c).

Stent patency is a challenge to assess due to metal artifacts and highly dependent on stent type, metal composition, size, orientation, and surrounding tissue. Dedicated reconstruction kernels in the newer high-end CT scanners can optimize images; however, there is still a variable success for evaluation of patency of the lumen within the stent (Fig. 9b, d).

3.7 CT: Cardiac Morphology

Accurate assessment of cardiovascular morphology by CTA is simplified by multiplanar reconstruction, maximum intensity projection (Fig. 10) and 3D volume rendering. Pericardial structural features such as pericardial thickening, calcification, effusion and masses are easily detected. However, pericardial effusion with high protein content can be difficult to differentiate from thickened pericardium. Valvular disease and cardiac function ECG-gated dynamic 3D reconstructions of the heart valves or chambers open the possibility to functional assessment of the valves and the myocardium, however at a cost of relatively increased radiation as images are acquired throughout the cardiac cycle.

In patients with elevated pulmonary arterial pressure or a volume-overloaded right ventricle, CT can show enlargement of the main pulmonary artery, dilatation and hypertrophy of the right ventricle (Fig. 10), enlargement of the right atrium, flattening of the interventricular septum, reflux of contrast agent into the inferior

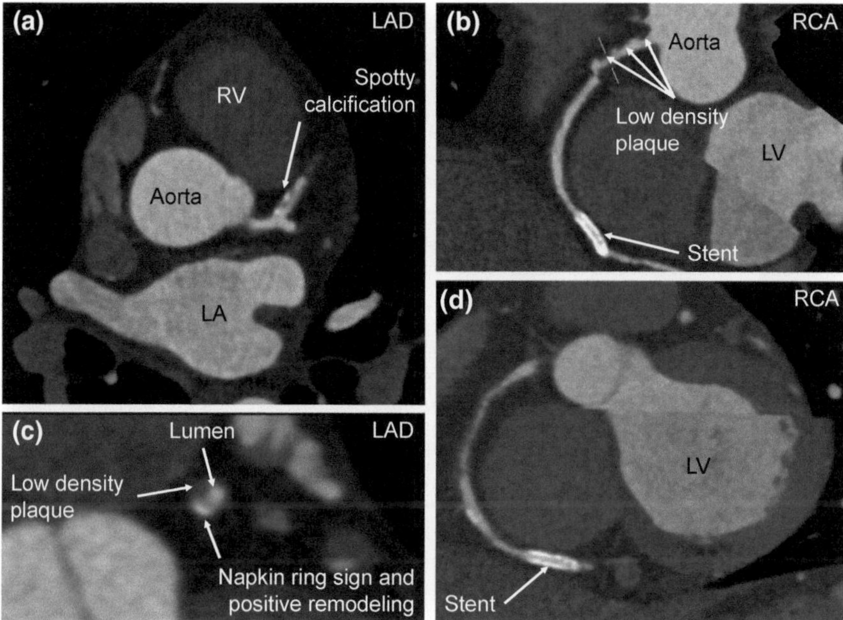

Fig. 9 Coronary artery disease. Example of a patient with chest pain examined for coronary artery disease. **a** Spotty calcification in left anterior descending artery (*LAD*). **b** Low density plaques in the proximal part and stent in the distal part of right coronary artery (*RCA*). **c** Signet ring sign, positive remodeling and low density component of the plaque. **d** Stents are a challenge to examine for in-stent stenosis due to metal artefact. Note the non-aligned steps of the scans in (**b**) and (**d**), also known as stitching artifacts. *LA*, Left atrium; *LV*, Left ventricle; *RV*, Right ventricle

vena cava and pericardial effusion. Before electrophysiological ablation in patients with atrial fibrillation CTA (or MRI) is used to assess left atrial and pulmonary vein anatomy (Fig. 10c) to guide intervention.

3.8 CT: Aorta, Pulmonary Artery and Carotid Artery

Although the aorta can be assessed with high sensitivity and specificity by CTA [10], the aortic root and ascending aorta show significant motion artifacts in a majority of non-ECG-triggered CTA examinations. Therefore, ECG triggering is recommended when imaging these proximal aortic structures, so that CTA can provide detailed 3D depiction with high spatial resolution.

Computed tomography angiography can be used for diagnosis and follow-up of aneurysms (segmental dilatation; Fig. 11b) or dissection (tearing of the inner vessel wall layer; Fig. 11d) of the aorta. In cases of dissection, the complete extent of vascular involvement with intimal tear and flap, potential aortic root and coronary

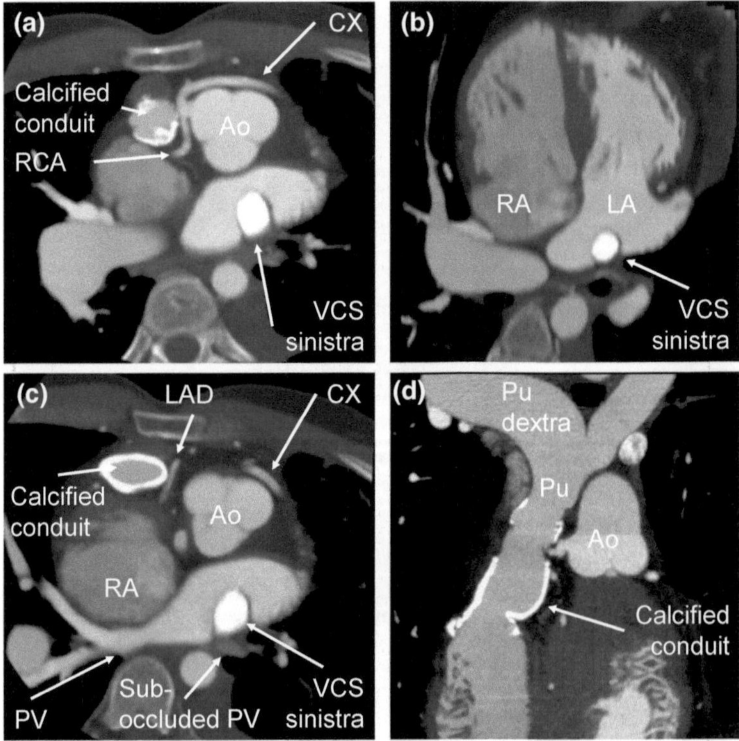

Fig. 10 Congenital heart disease, pulmonary artery and veins. Example of a patient with congenital heart disease with coronary anomaly and persistent left superior vena cava **a**, transposition with morphologic left ventricle connected to the pulmonary circulation and morphologic right ventricle connected to systemic circulation **b**, occluded left pulmonary vein **c** and calcified conduit in the right sided outflow tract with dilated pulmonary artery **d**. *Ao*, Aorta; *CX*, Left circumflex artery; *LA*, Left atrium; *LAD*, Left anterior descending artery; *PU*, Pulmonary artery; *PV*, Pulmonary vein; *RA*, Right atrium; *RCA*, Right coronary artery; *VCS*, Superior vena cava

artery involvement, pericardial or pleural effusion and delayed contrast agent delivery to organs are assessed with the same scan.

Acute pulmonary artery embolism or chronic thromboembolic pulmonary hypertension can be demonstrated by filling defects in the pulmonary arteries in non-ECG-triggered CT pulmonary angiogram. Compared with the gold standard, ventilation/perfusion single photon emission computed tomography, assessment of anatomy and potential differential diagnoses is simplified.

Stroke is, in a majority of cases, caused by carotid atherosclerotic disease and the risk of stroke is also correlated with the degree of carotid stenosis. The two main reasons to ischemic brain disease by carotid atherosclerosis are embolization and reduced blood flow with impaired collateral circulation and/or impaired vasoreactivity. With non-ECG-triggered CTA, stenosis and plaque burden as well as

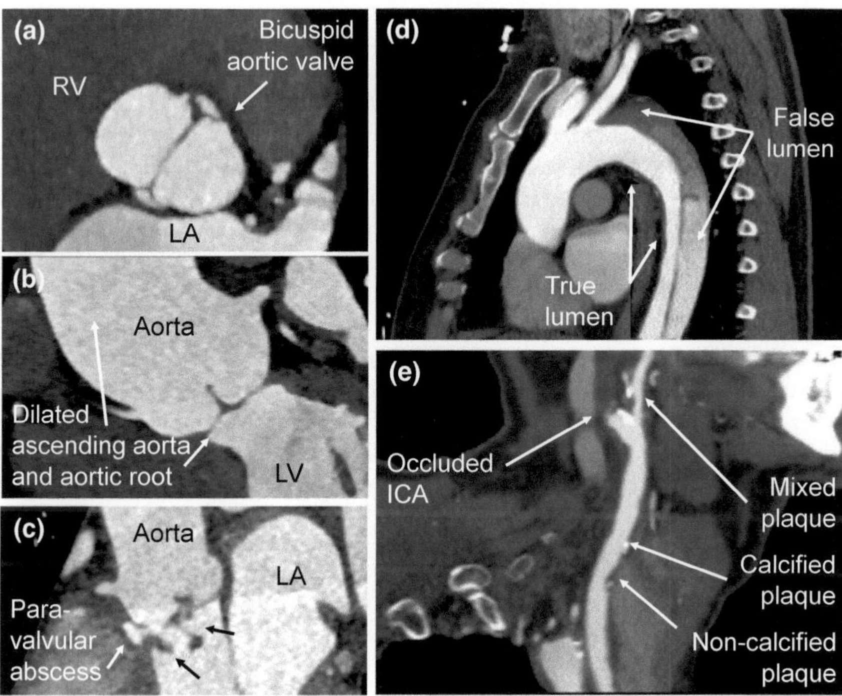

Fig. 11 Aortic valve, aorta and carotid artery. Example of a patient with bicuspid aortic valve (**a**) and dilatation of the aortic root and ascending aorta (**b**). **c** Example of a patient with infective endocarditis on the aortic valve. **1.** Example of large vegetations with thickening of the cusps and flail of one cusp causing acute severe aortic regurgitation. **2.** Example of presence of a paravalvular abscess that was not visualized by echocardiography, neither by transthoracic nor by transesophageal. **d** Example of a patients with aortic dissection in the arcus and descending thoracic aorta. True lumen is smaller than the false lumen. In the proximal part the false lumen is not fully filled with contrast due to low flow. CTA can also disclose the complete extent of vascular involvement with intimal tear and flap, aneurysm, aortic valve involvement, coronary artery compression or dissection, pericardial or pleural effusion and visceral artery involvement. CTA yield good information for planning treatment with high sensitivity and specificity. **e** Example of maximum intensity projection showing an occlusion of the internal carotid artery (ICA) proximally, calcified and low-density non-calcified plaque in the common carotid artery and mixed plaque in the proximal part of the external carotid artery. *LA*, Left atrium; *LV*, Left ventricle; *RV*, Right ventricle

plaque composition (Fig. 11e) can be assessed, with low-density lipid-rich plaques with a thin cap being high-risk markers.

3.9 CT: Evolving Applications

Perfusion examination of the heart at rest and at stress can delineate a potential myocardial ischemic region. Coronary CTA can assess irreversible myocardial damage. Presence of mural thrombus as well as subendocardial calcifications and fat in the left ventricle (Fig. 12b) imply prior infarction in the area. CT perfusion is a promising tool for the future handling of patients with coronary heart disease [11].

CT FFR is a non-invasive variant of fractional flow reserve (FFR) computed from standard imaging of coronary CTA. CT FFR is computed from a patient-specific generated anatomical model of the aortic root and coronary arteries, from a physiological model of vessel response to a simulated condition of hyperemia including ventricular mass calculation and from the application of computational fluid dynamics on the coronary arteries. Pressure and flow is calculated simultaneously at all points in the coronary arteries (Fig. 12c). CT FFR relates closely to invasive FFR and appears to be a potential method to defer unnecessary invasive examination in patients with chest pain [11].

4 Nuclear Medicine

Nuclear medicine techniques are widely used for studying perfusion [12]. The most common method is myocardial perfusion single photon emission computed tomography (SPECT) but perfusion imaging with positron emission tomography (PET) has gained more attention. The principles for SPECT and PET are similar but the two methods use different scanners and SPECT is a cheaper method whereas PET still is costly and limited to dedicated centers. Both techniques can detect, localize and quantify the degree of ischemic myocardium. The degree of ischemia is related to the prognostic outcome of cardiac events, i.e. myocardial infarction and death. Therefore, SPECT and PET can be used to guide treatment in patients with angina as well as after infarction.

4.1 Nuclear Medicine: Radionuclides

A radioactive perfusion tracer is injected in a peripheral vein to image blood flow. The uptake of the perfusion tracer is related to tissue blood flow, and therefore a small amount (3%) of the radioactivity will be in the heart. The photons from the radioactive decay of the radionuclide are registered with a SPECT or PET scanner. The detectors register photons from the 3-dimensional volume of the thorax including the heart and automated image reconstruction generates 2-dimensional slices of the left ventricle. In SPECT the most commonly used radionuclide is 99 m-Technetium (Tc) which has a gamma decay with photons of 140 keV. PET uses positron emitting

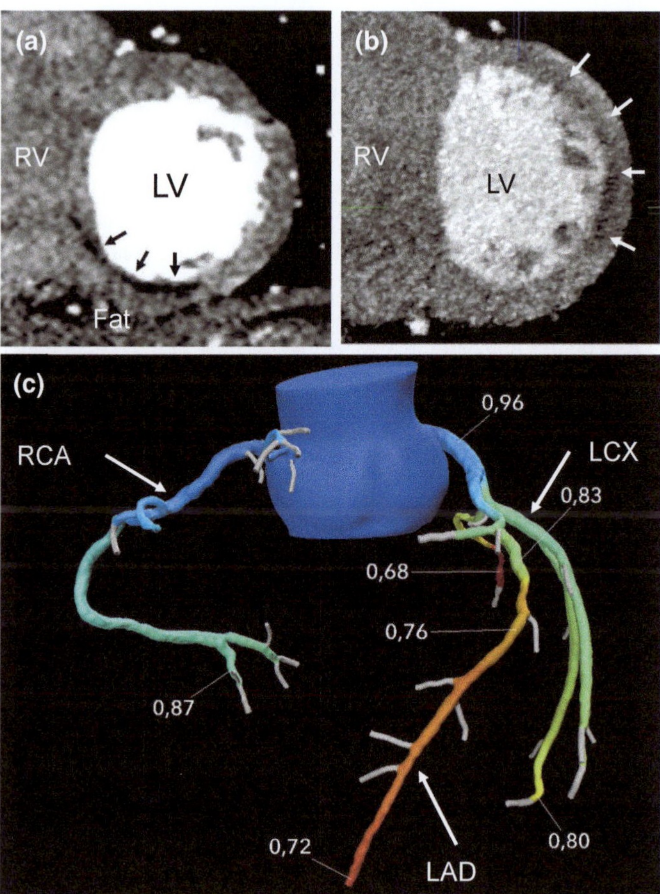

Fig. 12 Lipomatous metaplasia, perfusion and CT FFR. **a** Example of a patient with a right coronary artery infarction visualized in a short-axis view with subendocardial lipomatous metaplasia of the myocardium in the inferior and inferoseptal wall is seen low Hounsfield units below 0 indicating high fat content (black small arrows). This is a sign of an old infarction. **b** Computed tomography angiography (CTA) perfusion provides functional assessment by evaluating contrast filling of the myocardium at rest as a complement to standard assessment of coronary anatomy. The image shows an example of perfusion with CTA in a short-axis image. The subendocardial dark areas with lower contrast filling of the myocardium represent hypoperfusion (white small arrows), in this case due to stenosis of a marginal branch. With courtesy of Klaus Kofoed and Mathias Sørgaard, Rigshospitalet, Copenhagen, Denmark. **c** Example of a patient fraction flow reserve (FFR) measured with computed tomography (CT_{FFR}). CT_{FFR} is computed from a patient-specific generated anatomical model of the aortic root and coronary arteries, from a physiological model of vessel response to a simulated condition of hyperemia including ventricular mass calculation and from application of computational fluid dynamics on the coronary arteries. Pressure and flow is calculated simultaneously at all points in the coronary arteries. The image was analyzed off-site and with courtesy of Jesper Møller Jensen, Aarhus University Hospital, Denmark. *LCX*, Left circumflex artery; *LAD*, left anterior descending artery; *RCA*, Right coronary artery, *LA*, Left atrium; *LV*, Left ventricle; *RV*, Right ventricle

tracers that result in annihilation of an electron resulting in two photons in each direction with 511 keV. As a result of the lower keV, the photons in SPECT are more attenuated on their way from the site of decay to the detector when compared to PET. Therefore, PET has superior image quality and performs better especially in large patients. Moreover, the spatial resolution is higher in PET compared to SPECT. The injected radionuclide can be a perfusion tracer in itself, for example nitrogen-13 ammonia [13NH$_3$] in PET, meaning that the radionuclide distributes in the body in proportion to blood flow. Thallium 201 (201Tl) was the major perfusion tracer previously for SPECT and is also both a perfusion tracer and radionuclide. Thallium is less commonly used for SPECT today due to a lower kEV compared to Tc and therefore poorer image quality as well as because of the longer half-life higher radiation dose to the patient. Technetium-99 m needs to be coupled to a perfusion tracer before injection to the patient and the two most common are sestamibi and tetrofosmin. These compounds bind to the mitochondria in the cells and therefore the resulting perfusion maps are a composite of both perfusion as well as of the number of living cells. A perfusion defect can therefore be explained by decreased perfusion and myocyte loss due to an infarction. The half-life of the isotopes used in SPECT (Technetium 6 h and Thallium 73 h) are much longer compared to those used in PET (e.g. 82-Rubidium 76 s and 13-N-ammonia 10 min). This means that there must be a cyclotron in proximity to the PET scanner to do 13-N-ammonia or Oxygen 15–labeled water perfusion scans. However, 82-Rubidium, can be obtained from commercial generators.

The injection of the radionuclide is done during peak stress, induced either by exercise or by means of a pharmacological agent that causes vasodilatation. If the perfusion images from the scanner show homogenous uptake of the radionuclide, the examination is normal and no further imaging is needed. However, if a perfusion defect is seen, a resting injection is needed to be able to compare with the perfusion at rest. A perfusion defect that is unchanged between rest and stress indicates irreversible myocardial damage most often caused by infarction (Fig. 13) and a perfusion defect that is only present at stress signifies stress-induced ischemia (Fig. 14).

4.2 Nuclear Medicine: Attenuation Correction

Another reason for an unchanged perfusion defect can be attenuation of the photons due to tissues between the heart and the detector. To untangle this problem, attenuation correction is used, using an acquired map of the body attenuation properties and mathematically compensating for the attenuation in the SPECT images. Nowadays this is often done using computed tomography (CT) built into the SPECT system. The emitted photons are used for the SPECT images and the transmitted X-rays generate an attenuation map to correct the SPECT images. If a SPECT-CT system is not available, a simple solution is to repeat the SPECT acquisition with the patient lying on the stomach (prone). A defect is understood to be caused by attenuation if

Fig. 13 If low signal is detected both during rest and stress then the area depicts infarcted myocardium

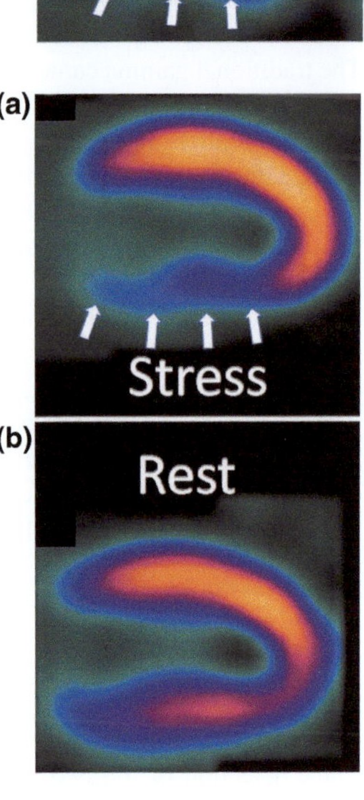

Fig. 14 If low signal is detected only during stress but not during rest than the myocardium is ischemic but viable

the defect is present when lying on the back and moves or disappears when lying prone.

4.3 Nuclear Medicine: Gated Images and ECG Triggering

ECG-triggering or "gating" is routinely used during the SPECT and PET and the recorded data are organized into images at different points during the heart cycle based on the ECG. This enables functional studies of the left ventricle as the perfusion images of the myocardium can be put into a video (CINE loop). This enables studies of global and regional left ventricular function. Automated processing software provides endocardial contours and thus left ventricular volumes throughout the heart cycle. Therefore, the end-diastolic volume (EDV) and end-systolic volume (ESV) the ejection fraction (EF) can be obtained.

4.4 Nuclear Medicine: The SPECT Scanner

The traditional gamma camera in a SPECT scanner uses the generation of flashes of light when photons collide with a sodium iodide crystal. This faint light is detected by photo-multipliers and digitally processed. A collimator ensures that only photons in a straight line from the object to the crystal passes through to the detector. Traditionally two detectors are placed at a 90° angle and move in a half-circle around the patient to obtain information from the object at different angles so as to reconstruct the image in 3D-space.

Developments in SPECT techniques have resulted in digital detectors instead of photo-multiplier tubes, use of cadmium-zinc telluride crystals with higher sensitivity, and improved reconstruction algorithms. These changes have resulted in more photons being detected and less information needed for reconstruction. Thus, scanning time and injected radioactive dose can be significantly decreased. Another recent development involves using focused collimator techniques that enable acquisition of the entire 3D-volume without movement of the detector.

4.5 Nuclear Medicine: The PET Scanner

In PET scanners, the collimator and detector are placed on a ring around the patient. Thus, detection of the two photons generated by the annihilation of the electron by the positron is detected at two places of the detector simultaneously, so called coincident detection. If the photons are not detected in pairs, the signal is ignored. The detector design is similar to SPECT with a flash of light being produced by a crystal and converted to an electric signal. However, the PET scanner has higher spatial resolution and higher detection efficiency compared to SPECT.

5 Ultrasound

Ultrasound of the heart (echocardiography) and the greater vessels, including the carotid arteries, is an integral part of cardiovascular diagnosis and clinical management. It is by far the most used non-invasive modality for assessment of cardiac structures and of vessel characteristics [1].

5.1 *Ultrasound: Basic Physics*

Sound waves are caused by vibrating sources (piezoelectric elements) and propagated, attenuated, scattered and reflected differently depending on tissue, producing echoes from tissue interfaces. The ultrasound transducer is both the source and detector of reflections of ultrasound beams. Ultrasound is described in terms of frequency in hertz (Hz) or wavelength in millimeters (mm), amplitude in decibels (dB) and propagation velocity (m/s) (Fig. 15). Image resolution is no greater than 1–2 wavelengths and penetration depth into the body is directly associated to wavelength with longer wavelengths penetrating deeper.

The spatial resolution is considered in all three dimensions: the axial (depth), the lateral (width) and the elevational (thickness) resolution (Fig. 15D). The focal zone of the ultrasound beams is where the ultrasound beams are the closest, providing the best spatial resolution. These principles also apply to 3-dimensional ultrasound for which several adjacent scan planes are acquired simultaneously.

Transducers are either linear, curvilinear or phased arrays. The linear array utilizes parallel beam lines whereas the curvilinear and phased arrays have fan-shaped beamlines. The narrower beamline used in phased arrays is useful for echocardiography as it fits between the ribs. The linear and curvilinear arrays are generally used for peripheral and deeper vasculature, respectively.

5.2 *Ultrasound: Doppler Imaging*

Doppler imaging is based on the detection of a frequency change of the transmitted wave due to reflection from a moving object (e.g. blood cells or myocardium; Fig. 16a). The object's velocity can be calculated from the frequency shift and the angle between the object's moving direction and the ultrasound beam (Doppler equation). Either continuous-wave or pulsed Doppler is applied where continuous-wave Doppler transmits and receives ultrasound continuously along the entire length of an ultrasound beam. The advantage is that high-frequency shifts (velocities) can be measured continuously and pressure can be calculated from the velocity-pressure relationship over a flow-limiting area (e.g. valve or stenosis) by the modified Bernoulli equation, $P = 4 \times V^2$; P is pressure change and V is velocity across the area. Pulsed

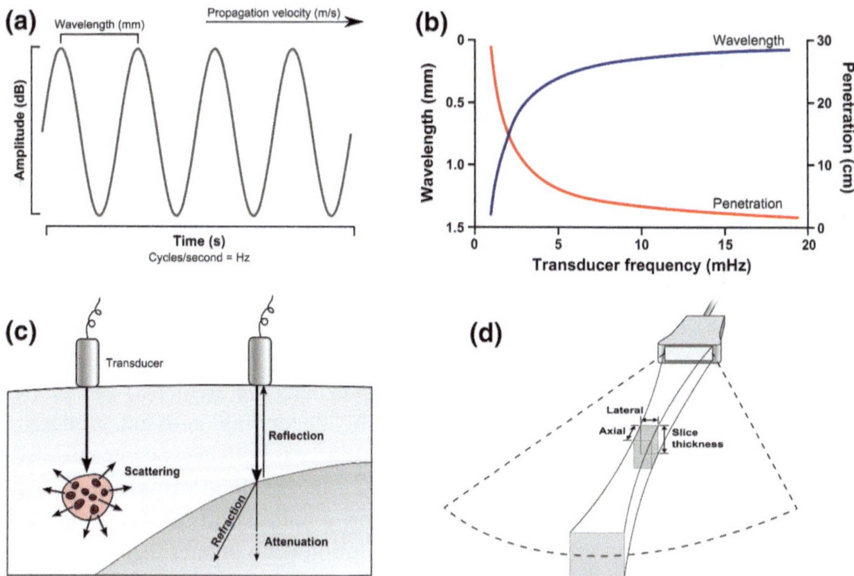

Fig. 15 Ultrasound physics. **a** Schematic diagram of a sound wave. Sound propagation velocity is dependent of the transmitted medium properties and not so much on frequency or amplitude. As an example, bone including calcifications does not allow propagation of the medical frequencies and air has the lowest propagation velocity. These tissues are therefore not penetrable and can limit the acoustic window. **b** Graphic illustration of frequency and wave length as well as penetration of the ultrasound wave in the tissue. With increasing frequency, the resolution increases and the penetration decreases. The penetration depth is limited to around 200 wave lengths, which translates to a penetration depth of approximately 30 cm for a transducer with 1 MHz, 10 cm for 3 MHz, 6 cm for 5 MHz and 3.75 cm for 8 MHz. **c** Schematic illustration of interactions of ultrasound waves and tissue. Reflection is the ultrasound waves coming back from the tissue interface with the same frequency to the probe. Scattering is the ultrasound changing in all directions by small inhomogeneities in the tissue or moving particles, such as blood cells, changing the frequency. Refraction is a change of direction of the ultrasound resulting in image artifacts. Attenuation is the intensity decrease and absorption of the ultrasound waves, which limits the penetration depths. **d** Schematic illustration of beam geometry with the spatial resolution dependent on the converging ultrasound beams in axial (depth), lateral (width) and elevational (thickness) level. The focal zone is where the ultrasound beams are converging the most. A sample volume with pulsed Doppler should e.g. be in the focal zone for best spatial resolution

Doppler discriminates Doppler signals from different depths allowing detection of moving objects in sample volumes along the axis of the ultrasound beam. The advantage is that it enables measurements in specific samples or positions along the beam (Fig. 16).

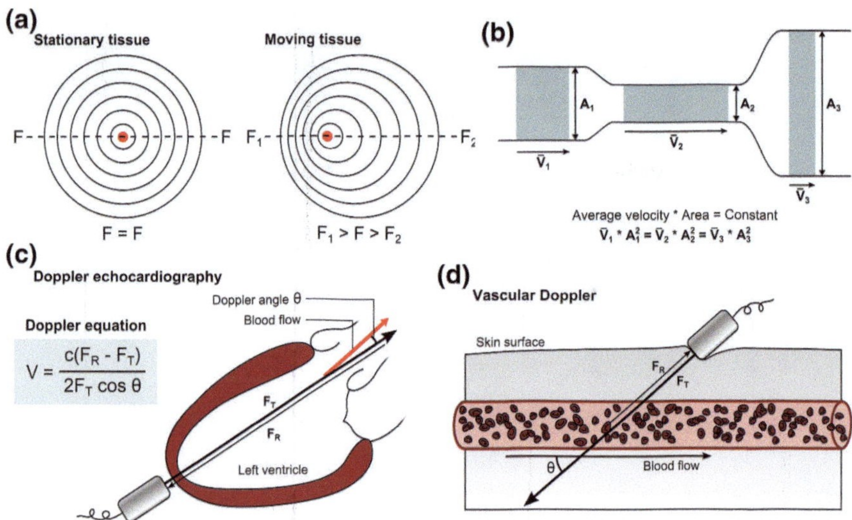

Fig. 16 Doppler imaging. **a** Schematic illustration of the Doppler effect. A stationary tissue reflects the ultrasound with the same wavelength and frequency F as transmitted. A moving tissue reflects the ultrasound beam with a higher frequency F_2 when the tissue is moving towards the transducer and with a lower frequency F_1 when moving away from the transducer; $F_1 > F > F_2$. **b** Illustration of the principle of conservation of mass. The amount of blood flowing (stroke volume) remains constant in all part of a closed tube (e.g. vessel). Volume is the product of blood flow V and area A in each part of the vessel. Stroke volume can therefore be calculated as the cross-sectional area times the velocity time integral of the Doppler signal from a pulse wave in the vessel or heart. Since stroke volume is the same in the stenotic part (2) and proximal to the stenosis (1), area in the stenotic part A_2 equals $(A1 \times V_1)/V_2$. **c** Illustration of the Doppler equation. The Doppler signals from e.g. blood can be calculated into flow and velocities from speed of sound in blood c, transducer frequency F_T, received backscattered frequency F_R and the cosine of the angle Θ between the direction of motion and the beam axis. In echocardiography, the beam direction is aimed to minimize the influence of the Doppler angle. In vascular ultrasound (**d**), the beam direction is frequently not aligned with the motion direction and the Doppler angle is important to include in the velocity calculation

5.3 *Ultrasound: Clinical Examination*

The core elements of an ultrasound examination of the heart (echocardiography) and the large vessels are dimensions, thickness, wall abnormalities, function, stenosis or leakage and estimation of pressures [13–15]. Echocardiographic images are preferably acquired ECG triggered and with the patient in the left lateral decubitus position. Ultrasound of the large vessels is acquired in the supine position and ECG triggering is not necessary.

Echocardiography can detect ventricular dilatation and dysfunction and on a regional level hypokinesia (decreased contractility), akinesia (no contractility), dyskinesia (contractility in the wrong direction) or hyperkinesia (hyperdynamic contractions). A mural thrombus can be detected and verified with opacification of the left ventricular lumen by intravenously administered ultrasound contrast agents, and

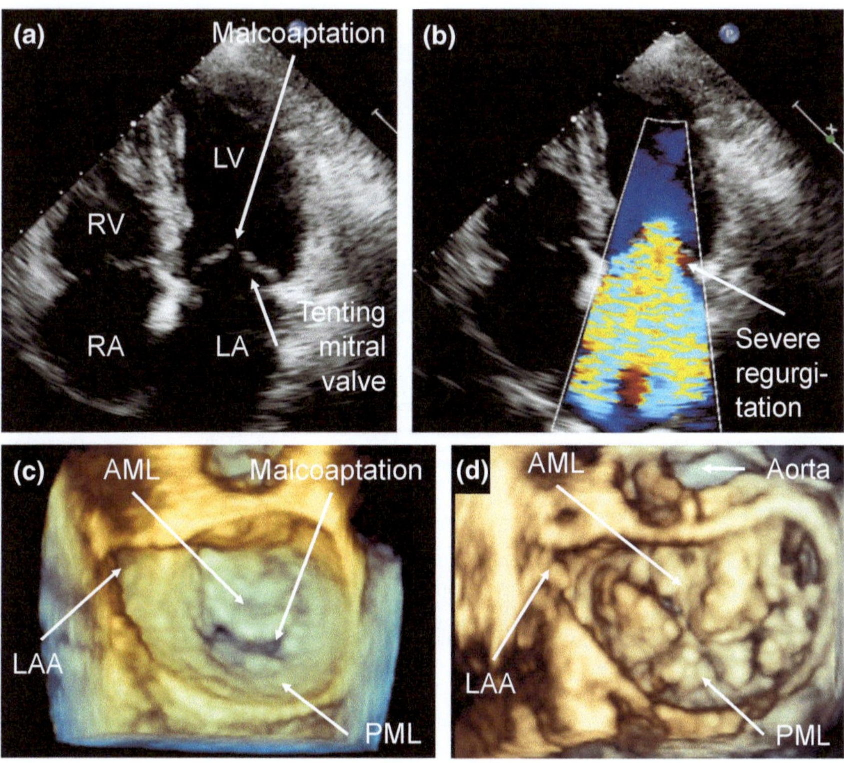

Fig. 17 Ischemic heart disease and mitral valve regurgitation. **a–c** Example of a patient with ischemic heart disease. **a** 4-chamber view with a dilated left ventricle and left atrium. Tethering of the cordae causes tenting of the leaflets above the atrio-ventricular plane and the leaflets do not meet causing malcoaptation of the mitral valve as well as mitral valve regurgitation. **b** Color Doppler image illustrating central severe mitral valve regurgitation (yellow/light blue), secondary to dilatation, filling out most of the enlarged left atrium. **c** Three-dimensional transesophageal echocardiography looking at the mitral valve from the atrial side show the leaflet do not meet. **d** Example of patient with mitral valve regurgitation due to mitral valve prolapse. Three-dimensional image of a patient with multiple prolapses of both anterior and posterior leaflet (Barlow's disease) looking from the atrial side towards the mitral valve. With courtesy from Carl Meurling, Dept of Cardiology, Skåne University Hospital, Lund University, Sweden. *AML*, Anterior mitral valve leaflet, *LA*, Left atrium; *LAA*, Left atrial appendage; *LV*, Left ventricle; *PML*, Posterior mitral valve leaflet; *RA*, Right atrium; *RV*, Right ventricle

chronic congestion can be shown as pulmonary vein dilatation and backward failure to the right side of the heart.

Acute heart failure can be shown by echocardiography (and other modalities) as dilated chambers, hypertrophy, impaired ventricular function, valvular dysfunction, pericardial effusion, and dilatation of the pulmonary artery or inferior vena cava (Fig. 17). In cases of chronic heart failure, typical findings are dilatation of atria as well as ventricles, LV hypertrophy, scars and aneurysms, diastolic as well as systolic dysfunction, valvular dysfunction and pericardial effusion.

Obstruction of the outflow tract (Fig. 18) is shown as calcification and/or fibrosis of the valve with decreased opening and doming of the leaflets. The pressure gradient and valve orifice area can be estimated from Doppler imaging by the Bernoulli and continuity equation (Figs. 18 and 19) and from planimetry of the opening area. Valvular regurgitation and its severity can be assessed by regurgitant jet estimation by color Doppler and by semi-quantitative measurements from Doppler (Fig. 19). Evidence of reversal flow in the aorta (aortic valve insufficiency), pulmonary veins (mitral valve insufficiency/stenosis) and hepatic veins (tricuspid valve insufficiency) can be suggestive of grade of severity. In infectious endocarditis the valvular vegetation and dysfunction can be shown, and destruction of the affected valve and surrounding structures are indicated by paravalvular leakage and abscess formation [16].

Structural heart disease such as cardiomyopathy and congenital heart disease may be investigated using echocardiography including anatomy, flow and function [13, 17, 18]. Pericardial disease can be diagnosed using ultrasound but evaluation of pericardial morphology may be limited. In pulmonary hypertension echocardiography may differentiate between pressure-loaded and volume-loaded right ventricles [19].

The aorta can be assessed by ultrasound [20], with grading of an aneurysm and for follow-up of potential progression. Depending on the aneurysm location and acoustic windows, additional imaging by CTA or MRA may however be needed for adequate determination of severity. Although ultrasound can detect aortic dissection, the absence of such on echocardiography should be interpreted cautiously and should be assessed by CTA.

Carotid artery ultrasound can assess calcified and non-calcified atherosclerotic plaques. A low-density plaque with a thin cap and ulcerations are more prone to cause ischemic events. Ultrasound can characterize intimal wall thickening, narrowing of the artery lumen and plaque composition. Color Doppler can visualize flow acceleration and pulsed Doppler is used for velocity measurements for grading of hemodynamic significant stenosis (Fig. 20).

5.4 Ultrasound: Evolving Applications

Speckle tracking echocardiography measures strain deformation of the myocardium, which may refer to linear deformation relative to baseline length. The Lagrangian strain is $\varepsilon = \Delta L/L_0$ of which L_0 is the baseline length and ΔL is the difference in length at a specific time. A positive strain is lengthening or stretching and a negative strain is shortening or compression. The faster the length difference occurs, the higher the strain rate. All cardiac chambers are accessible to deformation analysis. Deformation can be assessed longitudinally (a high negative global longitudinal ventricular strain value is a good prognostic marker), radially (a high positive radial strain value is a good marker) and circumferentially (a high negative circumferential strain value

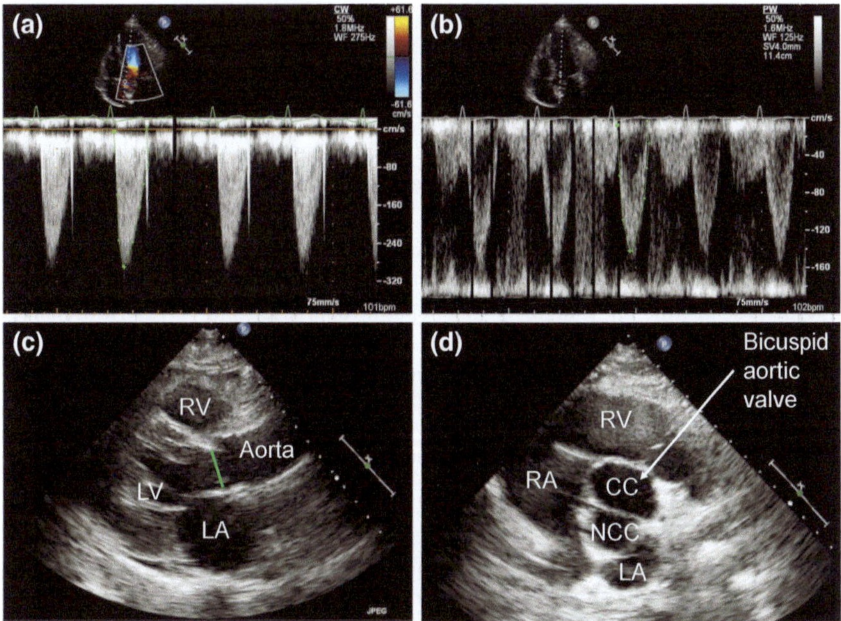

Fig. 18 Aortic valvular disease. **a–c** Example of a patient with aortic valve stenosis. The aortic valve area is 1 cm^2, calculated according to the principle of conservation of mass from (**a**) velocity time integral of the continuous-wave Doppler across the aortic valve (green line with dots) of 51 cm with a maximum velocity 2.9 m/s (equals maximum gradient of 33 mmHg using modified Bernoulli equation), from (**b**) velocity time integral of the pulsed Doppler in the left ventricular outflow tract (green line with dots) of 25 cm and from (**c**) the diameter (green straight line) in the left ventricular outflow tract of 2 cm from the parasternal long-axis view. (**d**) Example of a patient with aortic valve regurgitation. Short axis view shows a bicuspid aortic with a non-coronary cusp (*NCC*) and fusion of the left and right coronary cups (*CC*). With courtesy from Carl Meurling, Dept of Cardiology, Skåne University Hospital, Lund University, Sweden. *LA*, Left atrium; *LV*, Left ventricle; *RA*, Right atrium; *RV*, Right ventricle

is a good marker). Strain assessment is a promising tool for the future handling of patients with heart disease [13].

6 MRI: Physics

Magnetic Resonance Imaging (MRI) is a medical imaging technique that, since its invention in the early 1970s, has matured to become one of the most active areas in medicine and biomedical technology. Unfolding the underlying basic principles of MRI can be performed in many different ways. In this chapter, basic MR physics are introduced in a simple descriptive manner in order to give readers an overview of how an MR system operates. In order to do so, the term "Magnetic Resonance

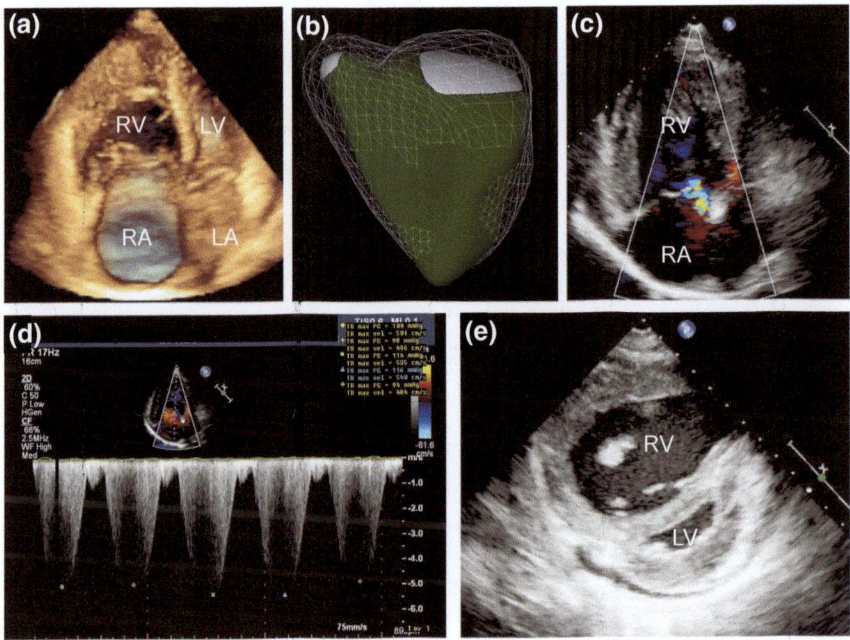

Fig. 19 Right ventricular disease. Example of a patient with tricuspid valve regurgitation due to pulmonary arterial hypertension. **a** Three-dimensional image of a dilated right ventricle and atrium in 4-chamber view. **b** Three-dimensional echocardiographic endocardial volume rendering of the right ventricle. Green is at and-systole and the mesh is at end-diastole. The tricuspid valve is the white area to the upper right and the pulmonary valve is the white area to the upper left in the image. Apex is downwards and the septum is bulging out in systole. **c** Color Doppler in the 4-chamber view shows a regurgitant jet across the tricuspid valve (yellow/light blue) and **d** the maximum velocity from continuous-waved Doppler (green and blue markings) is in average 5.1 m/s, which equals a trans-tricuspid gradient of 104 mmHg. **e** In the short-axis view, the septum is converging into the small left ventricle due to high right ventricular pressure and an underfilled left ventricle. *LA*, Left atrium; *LV*, Left ventricle; *RV*, Right ventricle

Imaging" is broken down in its components and each one of them is described in a separate section.

7 MRI: Physics—Magnetic

Clinical MRI is based on receiving signals emitted by the hydrogen atoms, which are abundant in the human body in water and other molecules. The hydrogen atom consists of a nucleus with a single positively charged proton, which has a magnetic moment. This magnetic moment has a magnitude and a direction and can be considered as a small magnet that spins along its axis. In its simplest representation, each magnet can be represented as a 3D vector, which is called spin.

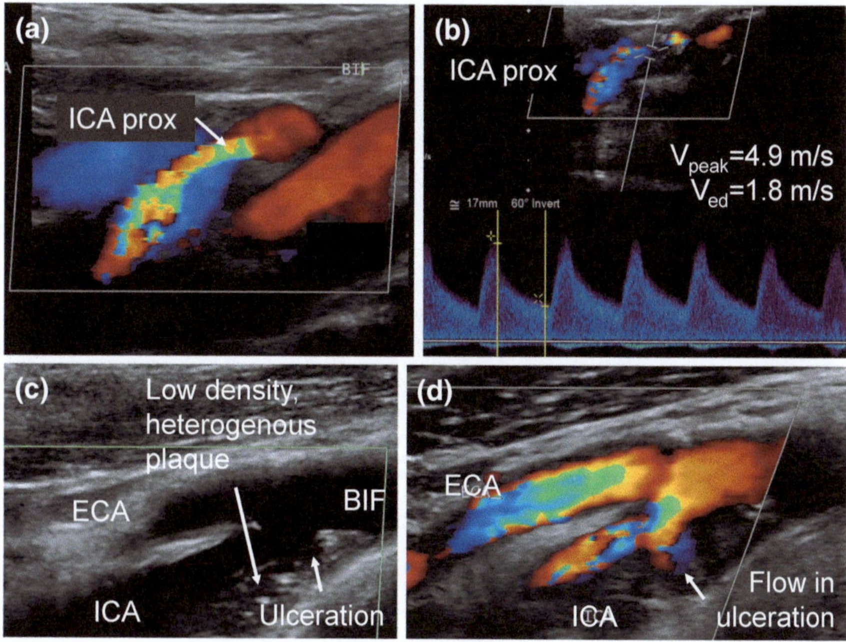

Fig. 20 Carotid artery disease. Example of two patients with right internal carotid artery stenosis of 95-99% (**a–b**) and of 65% (**c–d**). **a** Color Doppler in the proximal internal carotid artery is not laminar but highly turbulent (green/orange) and **b** pulsed Doppler with the sample volume in the turbulent area shows increased peak systolic velocity of 4.9 m/s and end-diastolic velocity of 1.8 m/s. **c** Example of a patient with an ulceration of a plaque in the right internal carotid artery with low-density and heterogenous plaque from the right carotid bifurcation 2 cm into the internal carotid artery. **d** The color Doppler shows turbulent flow across the stenosis and swirling flow into the ulceration (red and blue colors). *BIF*, Carotid bifurcation; *ECA*, External carotid artery; *ICA*, Internal carotid artery

The main component of an MRI system is a large magnet that forms a strong static magnetic field around the area to be imaged. The external magnetic field is denoted by B_0 and its strength is measured in Tesla (T). A typical clinical scanner has a magnetic field strength of 1.5–3.0 T. Figure 21 illustrates the magnet and the other components of an MR system. It can be seen that inside the MRI scanner there are the gradient-coils and the radiofrequency-coils. Gradient coils are oriented along the three orthogonal directions and are mounted just inside the bore (i.e. opening) of the magnet. They are used in MRI in order to create small linear variations to the magnetic field by adding to or subtracting from the main magnetic field B_0. The radiofrequency (RF) coils are part of a transmitter and a receiver system. The transmit RF coil is used to send RF pulses that excite the spins, whereas the receiver RF coil is used to receive the resulting signal from the patient's spins. The same RF coil can be utilized for both transmission and reception.

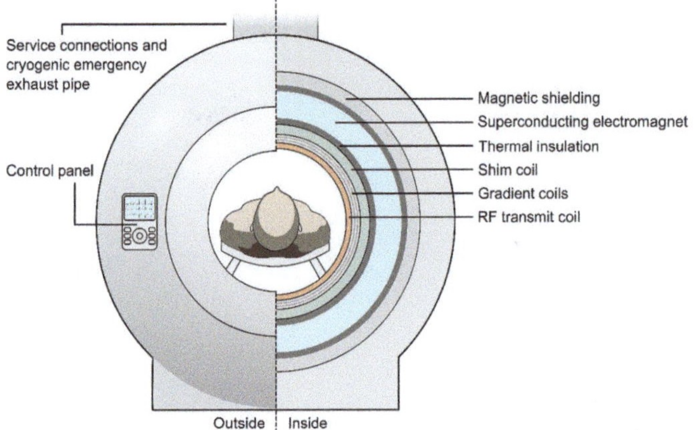

Fig. 21 Typical arrangement of an MRI scanner

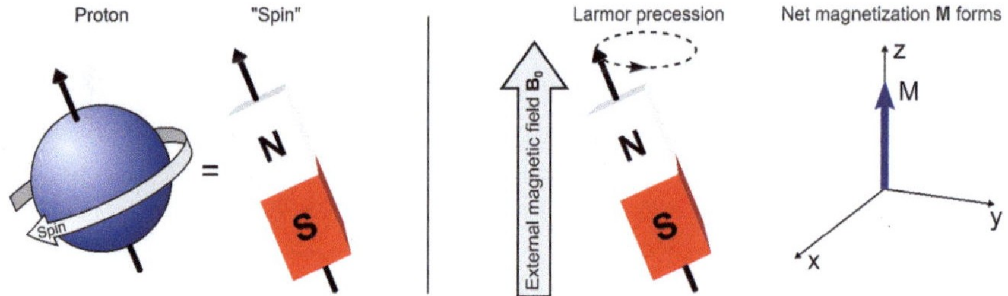

Fig. 22 Left: The proton behaves as a spinning magnet dipole. Right: Spin alignment inside an external magnetic field. The net magnetization vector is the sum of all spins and it is aligned with the z-axis

Once spins are placed in a strong magnetic field, a force is exerted on them causing them to align mostly parallel to the external magnetic field and precess (i.e. spin like a spinning top) about it (Fig. 22). The frequency of precession (in Hz) of the spins about the external magnetic field depends on the type of nucleus involved and is also linearly proportional to the strength of the magnetic field. The frequency of precession is defined by the Larmor equation:

$$\omega = \gamma B_0$$

where γ is the so-called gyromagnetic ratio, which is a property of the nucleus involved and it is equal to 42.56 MHz/T for hydrogen nuclei. For the hydrogen nucleus, the Larmor frequency is approximately 64 MHz for a typical clinical MRI scanner of 1.5 T.

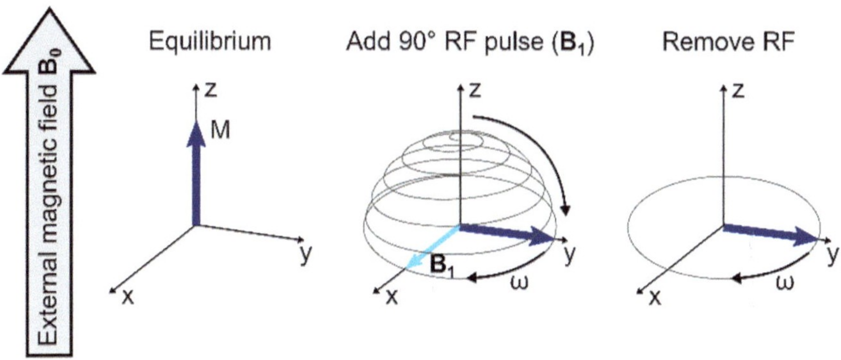

Fig. 23 The spins aligned with the z-axis (and the external magnetic field) and perturbed by the short duration RF pulse and are tipped onto the xy-plane. On the xy-plane the spins precess after the RF pulse has ended

8 MRI: Physics—Resonance

Up to this point the patient has been placed into the strong magnetic field of the MRI scanner and the spins of the patient's tissues have been aligned along B_0. The creation of the MR signal that provides the diagnostic information is based on forcing the spins away from the z-axis (which is aligned with B_0) down to the transverse xy plane (perpendicular to B_0), as illustrated in Fig. 23. This is accomplished by applying a secondary magnetic field through the transmission of a short radiofrequency (RF) pulse. The RF pulse contains a magnetic field B_1 which is perpendicular to B_0 and oscillates at the Larmor frequency. When the RF pulse and the spins have the same frequency, only then the spins can pick up RF energy and leave the equilibrium state. This phenomenon is called "resonance" and the B_1 is said to be on-resonance with the spins.

The path that the spins will follow, while the on-resonance condition is satisfied, is governed by the precession of the spins about the two magnetic fields B_1 and B_0. Once the spins have been moved away from the z-axis and the RF pulse is turned off, we can measure the spins by detecting the voltage they induce onto a loop of wire (Faraday's law of induction). This voltage is the signal recorded by the RF receive coil. This experiment is called the one-pulse experiment and the resulting signal is called the Free Induction Decay (FID) Fig. 24.

As soon as the RF excitation pulse is switched off, spins begin to relax back to their equilibrium state following two independent mechanisms: longitudinal relaxation and transverse relaxation. Longitudinal relaxation or spin-lattice relaxation refers to the realignment of the spins with the main magnetic field due to the loss of energy (which they absorbed from the RF pulse) to their surroundings. Transverse relaxation or spin-spin relaxation refers to the decay of the spins' signal due to an increase in entropy (disorder). The first process is characterized by the spin-lattice relaxation

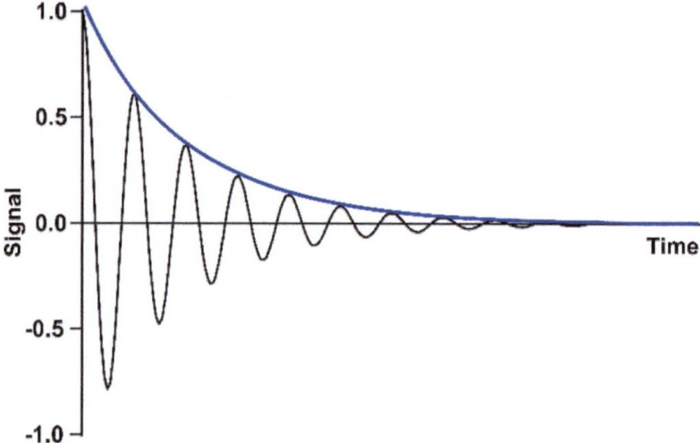

Fig. 24 The spinning magnetization on the xy-plane gives rise to the magnetic resonance signal i.e. the Free Induction Decay (FID)

time T_1 whereas the second process is characterized by the relaxation time constant T_2. When static field inhomogeneity affects the spins then T_2^* relaxation is observed.

9 MRI: Physics—Imaging

For the spatial localization of the origin of the MR signal within the body, i.e. in order to get an image, a series of events has to be executed by the MR system in a specific manner. This series of events is referred to as a pulse sequence and it is described by a pulse sequence diagram that shows how the RF coils and gradient coils are utilized during an MR session Fig. 25. Three distinct processes are used for MR imaging: slice selection, frequency encoding and phase encoding. Slice selection is the process where the origin of the MR signal is restricted spatially to a plane (slice) within the patient. This is achieved by concurrently activating the RF transmit-coil and the gradient-coils in order to excite only the spins that satisfy the on-resonance condition. Frequency encoding is the process where the MR signal from within the slice is encoded along one direction of the slice in order to determine its origin along that direction. This is accomplished by concurrently activating the RF receiver and the gradient-coils along that direction so that the frequency of the MR signal is modulated in proportion to the position of the spins along that direction. Phase encoding is the process that allows the encoding of the MR signal along the second direction of the slice by modulating its phase in proportion to the position of the spins along this second direction. This is achieved by turning on the gradient coil along the second direction for a short time after the RF pulse. Phase encoding must be repeated multiple times, each time with a different amount of phase modulation.

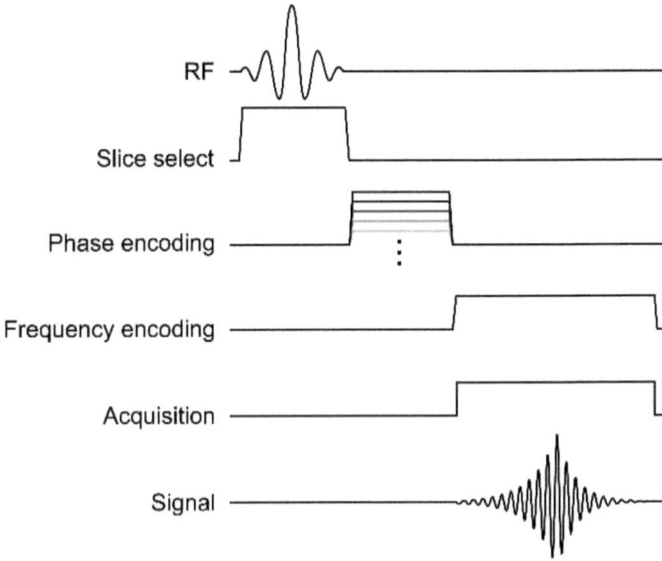

Fig. 25 The pulse sequence diagram of a simple imaging sequence

Once the MR signals from multiple phase-encoded experiments have been collected, they are placed in a matrix, called k-space. The 2D Fourier Transformation of k-space results in the anatomical image of the selected slice.

Depending on how the MR signal is formed, pulse sequences can be grouped into two categories: Spin-Echo and Gradient-Echo. These can produce images whose contrast is defined by the relaxation properties of the tissues (T1, T2). Image contrast may also get influenced by the amount of protons (Proton Density, PD) within a tissue and/or the homogeneity of the static magnetic field.

10 MRI: Cardiovascular Imaging

Cardiovascular magnetic resonance (CMR) imaging opens up a host of new possibilities, both clinically and in research. MRI differences in tissue signal intensity (i.e. contrast) arise from the magnetic relaxation properties of tissue, and are determined by how these properties are manipulated by the RF and gradient pulses. This enables three-dimensional, non-ionizing evaluation of 3D cardiac volumes and function, blood flow quantification, mapping of complex blood vessel anatomy, soft tissue characterization, as well as infarct and ischemia imaging. CMR examinations are typically tailored to the specific clinical question, but commonly include overview images for gross anatomy, time-resolved images of the heart in short-axis and long-axis projections, flow measurements in the great arteries, and contrast-

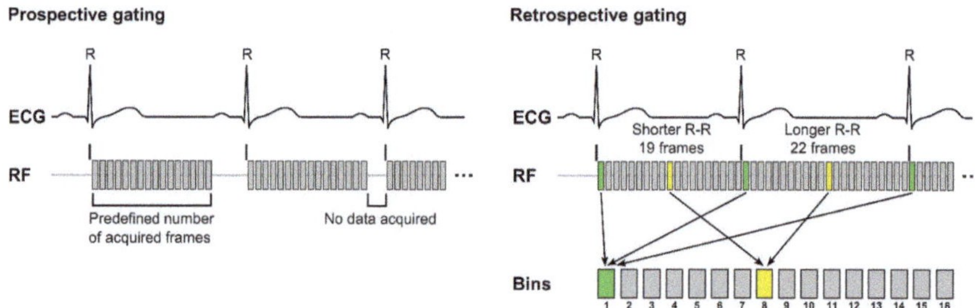

Fig. 26 ECG gating. Gating can be performed either prospectively (starting anew at each R wave) or retrospectively (continuous image acquisition with sorting afterwards). Prospective gating is mainly used for sequences that seek to minimize motion, for example tissue mapping; these sequences typically introduce a 400–600 ms delay from the ECG R wave to the RF readout, as the heart is almost immobile during mid-diastole. The main benefit of using retrospective gating is full coverage of the cardiac cycle without loss of acquisition efficiency

enhanced imaging for visualization of perfusion and myocardial scar. CMR imaging comes with some specific challenges that are mostly related to cardiac and respiratory motion. Implementation of sophisticated gating techniques and pulse sequences have addressed most of these problems.

Most CMR imaging utilizes electrocardiographic gating. To acquire time-resolved images of the heart, it is common practice to collect an electrocardiogram (ECG) from the patient during scanning. The ECG signal is then fed back into the scanner, filtered, and used to synchronize the MR acquisition to the cardiac phases [21]. The resulting images are sorted into bins according to their relative position in the cardiac cycle, a process known as gating (Fig. 26).

Respiratory motion can affect CMR image quality. In addition to cardiac motion, the entire intrathoracic cavity undergoes cyclic respiratory motion. The most common solution is to ask the patient hold their breath during image acquisition, which is feasible using short imaging sequences. However, this technique is inapplicable where scan duration becomes unbearably long, for example during certain flow measurements. Other methods include placing a bellows between the patient and receiver coil, which enables image acquisition during preset parts of the respiratory cycle, or tracking the motion of the diaphragm using a “navigator pre-pulse” that plays out before the main imaging sequence (Fig. 27).

Arrhythmias are also an issue. In severe cases of arrhythmia, e.g. atrial fibrillation or frequent ventricular extrasystoles, the aforementioned methods may be inadequate as the beat-to-beat variability in heart frequency becomes too great. In these cases, it is possible to employ “real-time imaging” [22], an imaging strategy where the entire image is read out in part of a single heartbeat, instead of the repeated sampling used to fill the image acquisition matrix (k-space) in gated images. Image readout is repeated in succession for each slice position until an adequate number of timeframes have been captured. The resulting images typically have lower spatial and/or temporal resolution and lower contrast compared to gated images (Fig. 28).

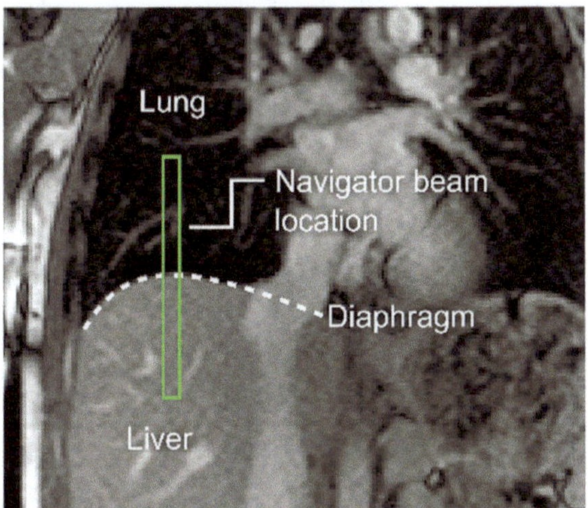

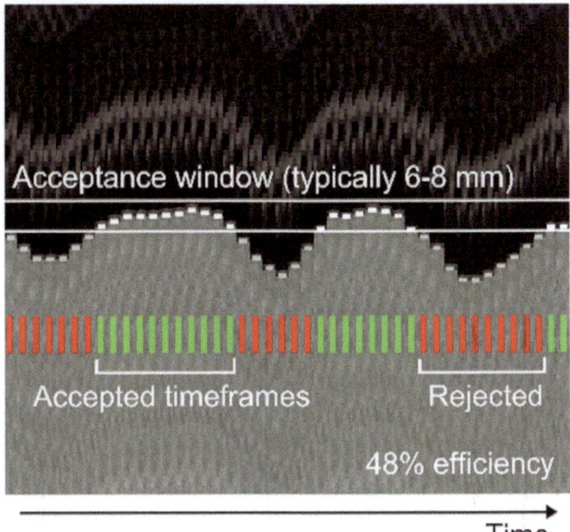

Fig. 27 Navigator gating can be utilized to compensate for diaphragmal respiratory motion. The top panel shows the location of the navigator beam, which will sample the lung/liver border at regular intervals to ascertain the current position of the diaphragm. Collected images are accepted for reconstruction if the diaphragm was inside the navigator window at the time of acquisition (bottom panel)

High static magnetic field strength can potentially improve image quality. Currently, the most common magnetic field (B_0) strength for CMR is 1.5 T; however, stronger magnets (3–7 T) are seeing increased use. Higher field strength increases the signal-to-noise ratio (i.e. a measure of how mush signal exists relative to the noise), which can be used to shorten scan times or improve image quality. However, imaging at higher fields puts higher demand on both gradient systems, RF amplifiers, and field homogeneiety requirements. Additionally, the stronger field induces artifacts on the ECG, and other gating methods may then be necessary. These include

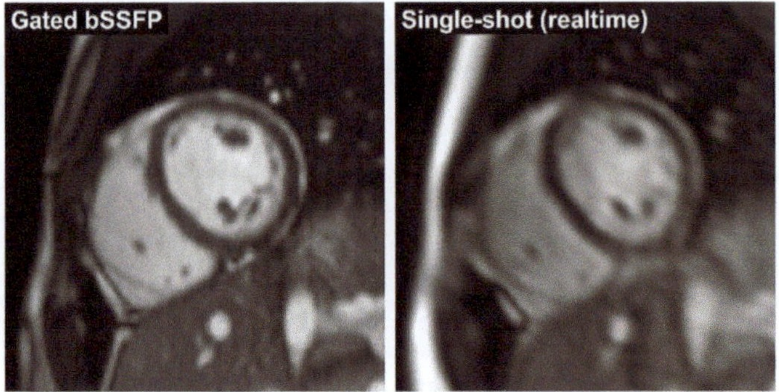

Fig. 28 Gated images are the standard approach (left panel). If gating is not applicable, e.g. during severe arrhythmia, single-shot imaging can be employed. Typically, such images have lower spatial and/or temporal resolution compared to gated cine images

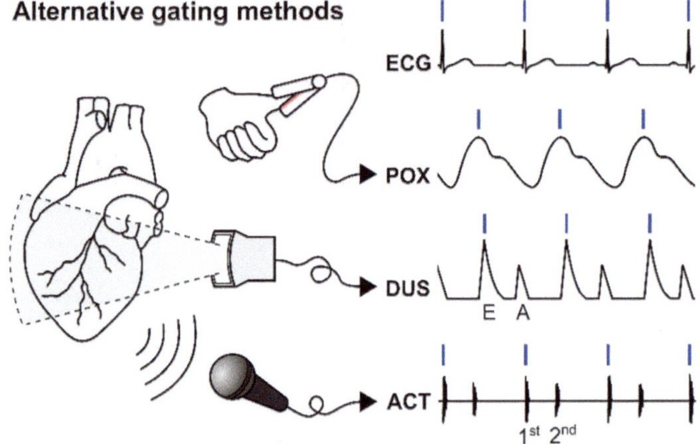

Fig. 29 Comparison of different cardiac gating methods. Pulse oximetry (POX) is typically performed using a finger clamp, and is less precise than ECG gating due to the smoothness of the saturation curve. Doppler ultrasound (DUS) can be analyzed in various ways; shown here is the transmitral E (early diastole) and A (atrial contraction) flow peaks. Cardiac sounds can also be sampled and filtered for acoustic cardiac triggering (ACT). Here, the first heart sound (resulting from closure of the aortic valve) is used for triggering. Note the triggering delay in pulse oximetry and ultrasound compared to the ECG and ACT

pulse oximetry gating using a clip on the fingertip, ultrasonic gating, acoustic gating using a microphone sampling the heart sounds (Fig. 29), and advanced self-gating techniques that utilize patterns in the raw image data (k-space) to sort image frames to their respective places in the cardiac cycle.

CMR can be used for the assessment of myocardial function. Global ventricular function is typically measured by manual or automatic segmentation of time-resolved anatomical images (Fig. 30), acquired using a sequence called balanced steady-state

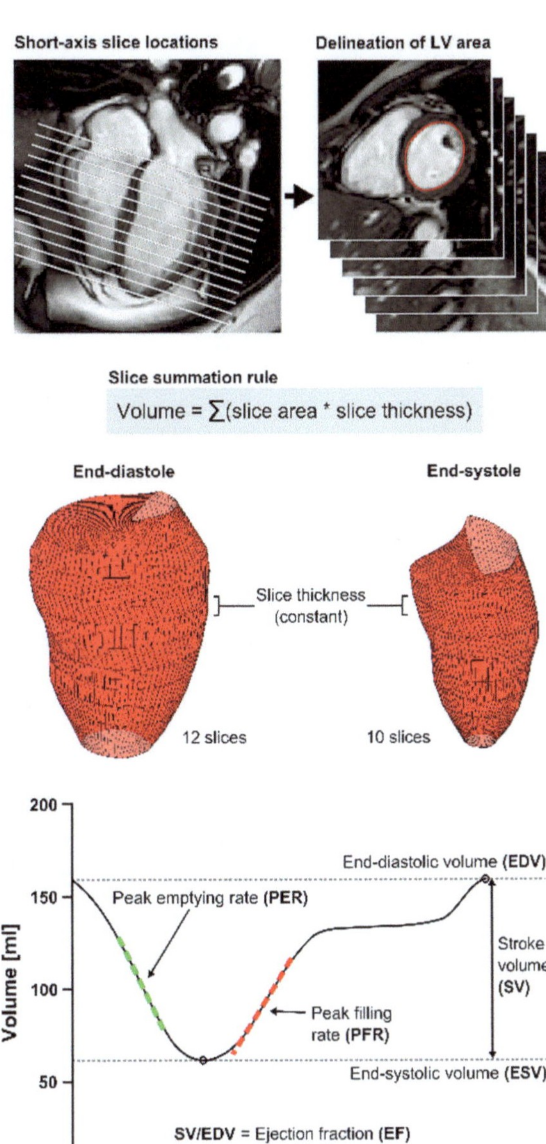

Fig. 30 Assessment of myocardial volumes, motion, global function and more using time-resolved bSSFP imaging. Top, the short-axis stack orientation is shown in relation to a long-axis (four-chamber) image. The left ventricle is delineated in all slices, and the total volume is calculated by summation of slice volumes. The slice thickness remains constant throughout the image acquisition but the number of slices varies over time due to longitudinal contraction of the ventricles. Bottom: the results can be plotted as a volume-time diagram, which contains functional and physiological information regarding the status of the ventricle

free precession (bSSFP) [23]. The main advantage of this imaging sequence is that it provides high contrast between the myocardium and its surroundings. Regional myocardial function is assessed using visual scoring or by strain analysis (regional myocardial shortening), which can be calculated using a number of imaging strategies (Fig. 31).

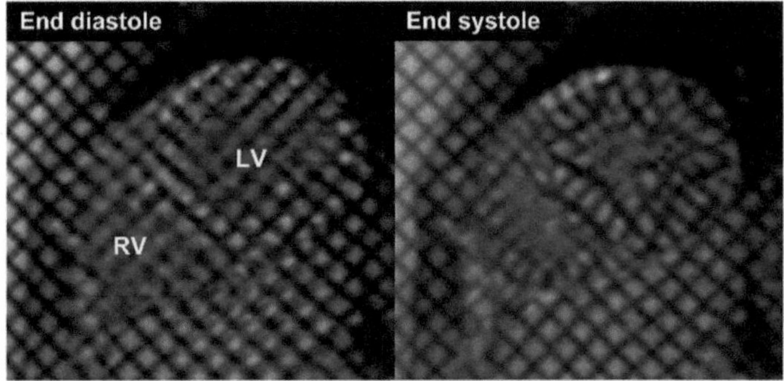

Fig. 31 Tagging enables analysis of regional wall deformation (strain). The left panel shows a midventricular slice where a "tagging" grid is applied by a RF pulse, which causes signal voids (black lines). The grid covering the myocardium is deformed as the ventricle contracts, showcasing the accumulated circumferential and radial strain. Also note that the grid pattern is no longer visible in the blood pool due to mixing of the blood. Quantitative analysis by grid tagging is time and labor intensive; other methods for strain analysis include phase contrast, *displacement encoding with stimulated echoes* (DENSE), *harmonic phase* (HARP), and *strain encoding* (SENC)

Flow measurements can also be made. Instead of using the magnitude of the net magnetization vector (which represents the sum of the spins), it is possible to use its phase (a.k.a. angle) to encode information regarding tissue velocity [24]. This method is called phase contrast (PC), and enables quantification of flow in the heart and blood vessels. PC-CMR is the most accurate way of measuring cardiac output, valvular insufficiencies, and shunt flows (Fig. 32). Velocity is measured within a predefined velocity encoding (VENC) window which should be set slightly higher than the expected peak flow velocity; if the VENC is exceeded, the signal "wraps around" and aliasing results (Fig. 33). Flow can be measured in any vessel of sufficient size; as a rule of thumb, 4–5 voxels across the vessel lumen are required to provide accurate measurements [25], which effectively makes scan time the limiting factor.

Exogenous agents can be introduced for obtaining contrast-enhanced imaging. Myocardium may be infarcted, hibernating, ischemic, edematous, or healthy, and CMR can differentiate between these by a combination of imaging sequences and contrast agents. Gadolinium-based contrast agents (Gd) distribute in the extracellular space and do not cross the membranes of viable cells; they shorten T1 and can be used in combination with different sequences and timings to evaluate the presence and extent of scar tissue, hypoperfusion, and edema (Fig. 34). Gadolinium agents are injected in a peripheral vein and imaging is then performed during the delivery of the contrast agent (first-pass perfusion), at baseline and during infusion with a vasodilator drug. Areas of myocardium with impaired perfusion have a slower rate of Gd uptake compared to healthy myocardium during vasodilation, resulting in a darker region in the image. After 10–20 min, Gd has dispersed evenly into the extracellular space in both healthy myocardium and infarcted areas (scar tissue). Since infarcted tissue has a larger proportion of extracellular space compared to normal, such areas will have a higher concentration of Gd and hence enhanced signal in a T1-weighted image.

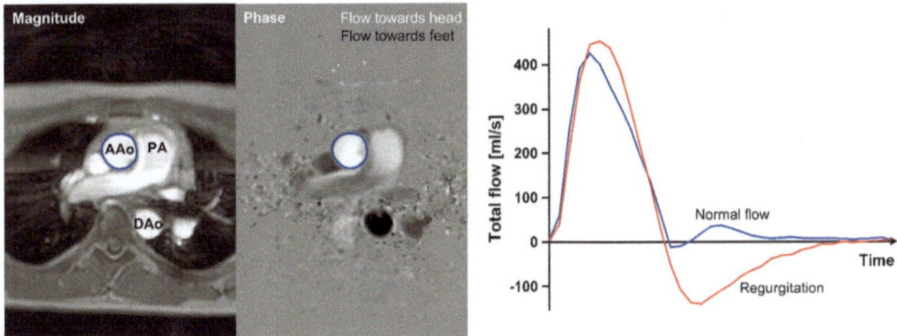

Fig. 32 Phase contrast imaging of flow. The left panel shows a transthoracic image slice through the ascending aorta (AAo), descending aorta (DAo). The image cuts obliquely through the pulmonary artery (PA). In the phase image, the grayscale represents velocity. The average velocity multiplied with a vessel area (blue ROI) enables flow quantification. Right: Normal versus regurgitant aortic flow as measured with phase contrast. The area under the curve is the effective stroke volume

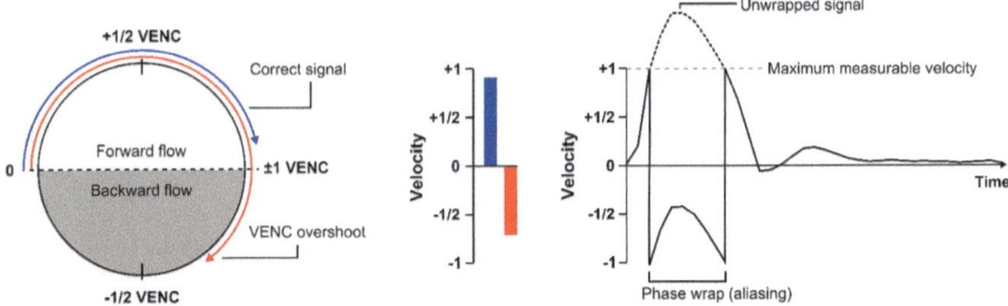

Fig. 33 Phase wraps occur when the velocity in a voxel exceeds the velocity encoding (VENC) envelope, resulting in "aliasing" or phase wraps (left panel). The red arrow indicates a spin with accumulated phase in excess of 1 VENC, which will be translated into backward flow (middle panel). In some circumstances, these can be corrected ("unwrapped", right panel)

This observed increase in signal is referred to as late gadolinium enhancement (LGE) [26]. During the waiting period from first-pass perfusion to LGE, it is possible to perform other scans with added benefit from the increased signal-to-noise ratio which results from Gd administration. This includes contrast-enhanced bSSFP [27], which measures the myocardium at risk in an acute myocardial ischemic injury, enabling evaluation of treatment efficacy.

Relaxation constants can be measured with mapping techniques. While LGE imaging is nowadays the clinical standard for assessment of focal myocardial lesions such as infarction and peri-myocarditis, it is not well suited for the evaluation of diffuse disease processes. To fill this gap, quantitative mapping techniques have been developed, including T1-, T2-, T2*-, and extracellular volume (ECV) mapping (Fig. 35). T1 and T2 are affected by edema – reflecting inflammation – but also by lipid deposition, hemorrhage, amyloid protein deposition, and several other processes. T1 mapping is often performed using the modified Look-Locker inversion recovery

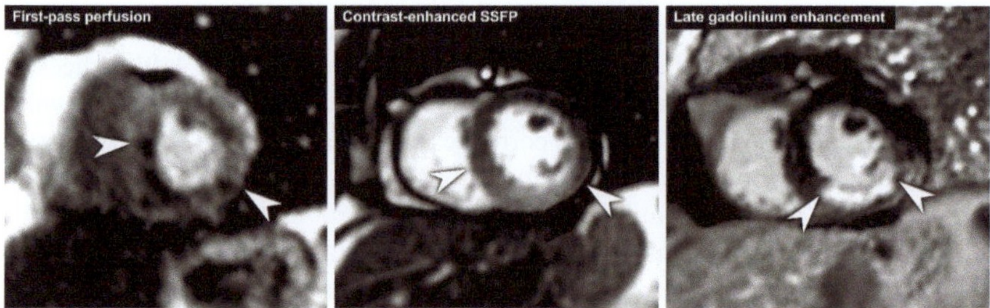

Fig. 34 This patient underwent imaging 3 days after having a myocardial infarction in the inferior wall. The first-pass perfusion reveals slower contrast uptake in the inferior wall and part of the septum. Contrast-enhanced SSFP shows the extent of the myocardium at risk, i.e. the part of the myocardium that was subjected to ischemia. Late gadolinium enhancement reveals that the final infarct did not encompass the entire myocardium at risk. The white area is the infarcted area, which was limited to the subendocardium. The difference between the myocardium at risk and the final infarct size is a measure of the treatment effect

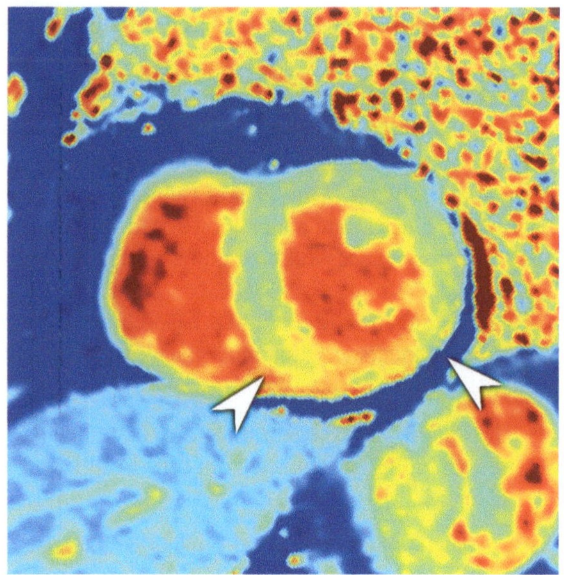

Fig. 35 T1 map of the same patient as in Figure **MRI_15**. Note the increased T1 values in the inferior part of the myocardium, reflecting edema which stems from the ischemic injury

(MOLLI) sequence [28], and can acquired with Gd or – importantly – without ("native T1"). If both T1 and native T1 maps are acquired, it is possible to compute the extracellular volume fraction (by co-registration of images and correction for the hematocrit [29]. T2-weighted imaging is commonly performed using turbo spin echo (TSE) sequences but can also be performed using bSSFP; while this sequence normally has both T1 and T2 contrast, a preparation pulse can be used to mitigate the T1 effects before acquisition [30]. Regardless of which method is used, it is crucial to perform proper validation of the measurements, to ensure that the quantitative values are both accurate and precise.

Iron load can also be measured with CMR. Certain diseases, such as thalassemia, can result in a build-up of iron deposits in the heart and liver. If left unchecked, this can lead to heart and/or liver failure. Iron has ferromagnetic properties which shortens T2*, and the tissue iron load correlates with T2* decay [31]. Consequently, patients depending on regular transfusions are followed up with T2* measurements of the heart and liver to optimize treatment.

In conclusion, CMR uniquely provides customizable image contrast which enables quantification of cardiovascular phenomena that are unreachable by other imaging modalities. The added cost of the CMR examination compared to e.g. ultrasound is potentially outweighed by the added information provided. Technical developments in image acquisition and signal post-processing are continuously opening up new applications for MR imaging in the cardiovascular system.

11 MRI: The Emergence of Sparse Imaging in Cardiovascular Disease Diagnostics

MRI offers both high spatial resolution and excellent soft-tissue contrast. For these reasons, it is recognized as the modality of choice for many common diseases. However, one major limitation is that the data acquisition is time consuming causing substantial problems if the patient cannot remain motionless. Therefore, the acceleration of the MRI data acquisition speed is one of the main research directions in MRI. The most successful techniques up to date are *Parallel Imaging* [32, 33] and *Compressed Sensing*.

Image acquisition acceleration based on compressed sensing [34, 35] relies on k-space data undersampling under the assumption that the following two conditions are satisfied:

(i) the image is **sparse** in a transform domain, and
(ii) the sampling pattern is **incoherent** resulting in incoherent and noise-like artifacts [5].

The idea behind compressed sensing is that sparse images, appropriately undersampled, can be recovered accurately despite the fact that the Nyquist sampling rate is violated. This undersampling results in remarkable acquisition acceleration. In the following, the essential meaning of sparsity and incoherence are explained. An image is sparse in a transform domain if its representation in that domain consists of a small number of non-zero coefficients while the rest are almost zero. Most images are not sparse in their native representation and, therefore, they must be transformed to become sparse. Finding the most appropriate "sparsifying" transform is a crucial step in applying compressed sensing. Commonly used sparsifying transforms are the wavelet transform and the finite differences. More recent advances towards this direction take into account dictionaries [36, 37]. In practice, incoherence of artifacts means that the linear reconstruction artifacts caused by k-space undersampling look like noise. Although undersampling k-space at random positions guarantees incoherency, the required rapid gradient switching causes eddy currents that severely downgrade the quality of the reconstructed images. Among the various sampling patterns that guarantee incoherency, the radial sampling is considered advantageous [38].

Next, according to compressed sensing theory, if a signal $\boldsymbol{d}$ is sparse and the undersampling scheme is incoherent, it can be accurately reconstructed by solving the following nonlinear optimization problem:

$$\min_{d} \|\boldsymbol{\Psi d}\|_0, \quad s.t. \boldsymbol{\Phi}_u \boldsymbol{d} = \boldsymbol{m}, \tag{1}$$

where $\|\boldsymbol{d}_0\|$ counts the nonzero elements of $\boldsymbol{d}$, $\boldsymbol{\Psi}$ represents the sparsifying transform, $\boldsymbol{\Phi}_u$ the measurement matrix and $\boldsymbol{m}$ the under-sampled data. The problem in Eq. (1) is NP-hard and, therefore, other computationally tractable formulations have been proposed [39]. One such alternative is to replace the $\boldsymbol{L}_0$ norm with the $\boldsymbol{L}_1$ norm:

$$\min_{d} \|\boldsymbol{\Psi d}\|_1, \quad s.t. \boldsymbol{\Phi}_u \boldsymbol{d} = \boldsymbol{m}. \tag{2}$$

The problem in Eq. (2) is referred to as *basis pursuit problem* and its solution coincides with the solution of the problem in Eq. (1) when it is sparse enough [35]. To take into account the measurement noise, the problem in Eq. (2) is modified as follows:

$$\min_{d} \|\boldsymbol{\Psi d}\|_1, \quad s.t. \|\boldsymbol{\Phi}_u \boldsymbol{d} - \boldsymbol{m}\|_2^2 < \varepsilon. \tag{3}$$

This problem, referred to as *basis pursuit denoising,* can be formulated as unconstrained optimization in the so called Lagrangian form [5]:

$$\min_{d} \|\boldsymbol{\Phi}_u \boldsymbol{d} - \boldsymbol{m}\|_2^2 + \lambda \|\boldsymbol{\Psi d}\|_1. \tag{4}$$

The optimization problem in the above equation can be solved by the nonlinear conjugate gradient with backtracking line search [40].

12 Emerging Technologies

Current cardiovascular imaging technologies such as MRI, CT, SPECT, and echocardiography, provide great capabilities to image general morphology and function. Emerging techniques typically focus on provide complementary information, typically by adding information on function on molecular level or plaque composition.

Several of the emerging techniques will likely not have a role in clinical daily routine, but are already today important imaging tools to study pre-clinical findings and how these can be translated into animal studies, and human clinical trials [41].

13 Emerging Technologies: Coronary Imaging

One of the main clinical cardiovascular challenges to determine if there are plaques in the coronary vessels, and if so how vulnerable they are. There are currently three emerging techniques for plaque imaging IVUS, OCT, and NIRS. All three technologies have the capability of detecting plaques and are all catheter based. Being catheter based is a major drawback as it is an invasive investigation, but on the other hand if something is detected then a catheter based intervention can be performed during the same session.

14 Emerging Technologies: Intravascular Ultrasound (IVUS)

During a cardiac catheterization a miniaturized ultrasound probe is placed in the tip of a catheter. Using high frequency ultrasound, between 30–50 MHz (producing an axial resolution of about 50 μm, and a lateral resolution of 250 μm) the technique allows to visualize fine structures such as blood-intima border, external elastic membrane [42]. Tissue penetration is about 4–8 mm. A two dimensional image is formed and as the catheter is pulled back during imaging a view of the coronary vessel can be obtained.

15 Emerging Technologies: Optical Coherence Tomography (OCT)

OCT uses light instead of sound and was first developed for use in ophthalmology. Subsequently it was used to study unsteady coronary plaque [43]. Used wavelength is typically 1250–1350 nm. Saline is injected to displace blood during imaging as blood must be completely removed to avoid significant signal attenuation.

16 Emerging Technologies: Near Infrared Spectroscopy (NIRS)

In NIRS light is also used and the system converts the reflected signal to a spectrum, which can, using trained algorithms, be classified as a chemogram and serve as a map. Used bandwidth is 800–2500 nm. Early adaptation in humans were performed by Gardner and co-workers [44].

For clinical use, IVUS and OCT have been shown to be useful to optimize stent placement [41]. NIRS has been shown to be able to localize lipid core burden, but its role is yet to be established. There are ongoing randomized trials for all three modalities to determine the utility of these emerging methods in clinical practice [41].

17 Emerging Technologies: Molecular Imaging

Another class of emerging cardiovascular imaging techniques are different methods to image specific molecular targets in the cardiovascular system. The attractiveness of molecular imaging is that the used contrast agents can highlight a wide range of functional information where the image molecules bind to desired channels, receptor molecules or antibodies. Below are two emerging techniques for molecular imaging that potentially could have cardiovascular utility.

18 Emerging Technologies: Fluorescence Tomography Imaging (FTI)

Fluorescence Tomography Imaging (FTI) uses near infrared radiation to obtain quantitative images of targeted activated fluorescent agents in soft tissue in vivo. Spatial resolution is on the order of 1–5 mm and imaging depth about 5–50 mm. FTI has been shown to be valuable in small animal imaging and holds a potential for clinical application, albeit with the limited depth as a major limitation.

19 Emerging Technologies: Magnetomotive Ultrasound (MMUS)

By applying a time varying magnetic field to a volume with superparamagnetic iron oxide (SPIO) nanoparticles the tissue can be set in motion which can be detected with ultrasound. The induced motion is in the order of micrometers and phase and frequency detection is required for detection of regions with nanoparticles [45]. The technique is currently being applied in pre-clinical animal setting and is far from being using in humans although the nanoparticles are approved as a contrast agent for MRI since many years.

References

1. Montalescot G, Sechtem U, Achenbach S, Andreotti F, Arden C, Budaj A, Bugiardini R, Crea F, Cuisset T, Di Mario C, Ferreira JR, Gersh BJ, Gitt AK, Hulot JS, Marx N, Opie LH, Pfisterer M, Prescott E, Ruschitzka F, Sabaté M, Senior R, Taggart DP, van der Wall EE, Vrints CJ; ESC Committee for Practice Guidelines, Zamorano JL, Achenbach S, Baumgartner H, Bax JJ, Bueno H, Dean V, Deaton C, Erol C, Fagard R, Ferrari R, Hasdai D, Hoes AW, Kirchhof P, Knuuti J, Kolh P, Lancellotti P, Linhart A, Nihoyannopoulos P, Piepoli MF, Ponikowski P, Sirnes PA, Tamargo JL, Tendera M, Torbicki A, Wijns W, Windecker S, Document Reviewers, Knuuti J, Valgimigli M, Bueno H, Claeys MJ, Donner-Banzhoff N, Erol C, Frank H, Funck-Brentano C, Gaemperli O, Gonzalez-Juanatey JR, Hamilos M, Hasdai D, Husted S, James SK, Kervinen K, Kolh P, Kristensen SD, Lancellotti P, Maggioni AP, Piepoli MF, Pries AR, Romeo F, Rydén L, Simoons ML, Sirnes PA, Steg PG, Timmis A, Wijns W, Windecker S, Yildirir A, Zamorano JL (2013) 2013 ESC guidelines on the management of stable coronary artery disease: the Task Force on the management of stable coronary artery disease of the European Society of Cardiology. Eur Heart J 34(38):2949–3003
2. Rybicki FJ, Udelson JE, Peacock WF, Goldhaber SZ, Isselbacher EM, Kazerooni E, Kontos MC, Litt H, Woodard PK (2016) 2015 ACR/ACC/AHA/AATS/ACEP/ASNC/NASCI/SAEM/SCCT/SCMR/SCPC/SNMMI/STR/STS appropriate utilization of Cardiovascular imaging in emergency department Patients with Chest Pain: a joint document of the American College of Radiology Appropriateness Criteria Committee and the American College of Cardiology Appropriate Use Criteria Task Force. JACR 13(2):e1–e29
3. Baptista SB, Raposo L, Santos L, Ramos R, Calé R, Jorge E, Machado C, Costa M, Infante de Oliveira E, Costa J, Pipa J, Fonseca N, Guardado J, Silva B, Sousa MJ, Silva JC, Rodrigues A, Seca L, Fernandes R (2016) Impact of routine fractional flow reserve evaluation during coronary angiography on management strategy and clinical outcome: one-year results of the POST-IT, Circ Cardiovasc Interv 9(7):pii: e003288
4. Götberg M, Christiansen EH, Gudmundsdottir IJ, Sandhall L, Danielewicz M, Jakobsen L, Olsson SE, Öhagen P, Olsson H, Omerovic E, Calais F, Lindroos P, Maeng M, Tödt T, Venetsanos D, James SK, Kåregren A, Nilsson M, Carlsson J, Hauer D, Jensen J, Karlsson AC, Panayi G, Erlinge D, Fröbert O (2017) Instantaneous wave-free ratio versus fractional flow reserve to guide PCI. N Engl J Med 376(19):1813–1823
5. Cury RC,Abbara S, Achenbach S, Agatston A, Berman DS, Budoff MJ, Dill KE, Jacobs JE, Maroules CD, Rubin GD, Rybicki FJ, Schoepf UJ, Shaw LJ, Stillman AE, White CS, Woodard PK, Leipsic JA (2016) CAD-RADS(TM) Coronary Artery Disease—Reporting and Data System. An expert consensus document of the Society of Cardiovascular Computed Tomography (SCCT), the American College of Radiology (ACR) and the North American Society for Cardiovascular Imaging (NASCI). Endorsed by the American College of Cardiology. J Cardiovasc Comput Tomogr 10(4):269–281
6. Wolk MJ, Bailey SR, Doherty JU, Douglas PS, Hendel RC, Kramer CM, Min JK, Patel MR, Rosenbaum L, Shaw LJ, Stainback RF, Allen JM; Technical Panel, Brindis RG, Kramer CM, Shaw LJ, Cerqueira MD, Chen J, Dean LS, Fazel R, Hundley WG, Itchhaporia D, Kligfield P, Lockwood R, Marine JE, McCully RB, Messer JV, O'Gara PT, Shemin RJ, Wann LS, Wong JB; Appropriate Use Criteria Task Force, Patel MR, Kramer CM, Bailey SR, Brown AS, Doherty JU, Douglas PS, Hendel RC, Lindsay BD, Min JK, Shaw LJ, Stainback RF, Wann LS, Wolk MJ, Allen JM (2014) ACCF/AHA/ASE/ASNC/HFSA/HRS/SCAI/SCCT/SCMR/STS 2013 multimodality appropriate use criteria for the detection and risk assessment of stable ischemic heart disease: a report of the American College of Cardiology Foundation Appropriate Use Criteria Task Force, American Heart Association, American Society of Echocardiography, American Society of Nuclear Cardiology, Heart Failure Society of America, Heart Rhythm Society, Society for Cardiovascular Angiography and Interventions, Society of Cardiovascular Computed Tomography, Society for Cardiovascular Magnetic Resonance, and Society of Thoracic

Surgeons. J Card Fail 20(2):65–90 (Multimodality Writing Group for Stable Ischemic Heart Disease)

7. Taylor AJ, Cerqueira M, Hodgson JM, Mark D, Min J, O'Gara P, Rubin GD (2010) ACCF/SCCT/ACR/AHA/ASE/ASNC/NASCI/SCAI/SCMR 2010 appropriate use criteria for cardiac computed tomography. A report of the American College of Cardiology Foundation appropriate use criteria task force, the society of cardiovascular computed tomography, the American College of Radiology, the American Heart Association, the American Society of Echocardiography, the American Society of Nuclear Cardiology, the North American Society for Cardiovascular Imaging, the Society for Cardiovascular Angiography and Interventions, and the Society for Cardiovascular Magnetic Resonance. J Cardiovasc Comput Tomogr 4(6):407.e1-33
8. Halliburton SS, Abbara S, Chen MY, Gentry R, Mahesh M, Raff GL, Shaw LJ, Hausleiter J (2011) SCCT guidelines on radiation dose and dose-optimization strategies in cardiovascular CT. J Cardiovasc Comput Tomogr 5(4):198–224
9. Erbel R, Aboyans V, Boileau C, Bossone E, Bartolomeo RD, Eggebrecht H, Evangelista A, Falk V, Frank H, Gaemperli O, Grabenwöger M, Haverich A, Iung B, Manolis AJ, Meijboom F, Nienaber CA, Roffi M, Rousseau H, Sechtem U, Sirnes PA, Allmen RS, Vrints CJ (2014) ESC Guidelines on the diagnosis and treatment of aortic diseases: document covering acute and chronic aortic diseases of the thoracic and abdominal aorta of the adult. The Task Force for the Diagnosis and Treatment of Aortic Diseases of the European Society of Cardiology (ESC). Eur Heart J 35(41):2873–926
10. Chen MY, Rochitte CE, Arbab-Zadeh A, Dewey M, George RT, Miller JM, Niinuma H, Yoshioka K, Kitagawa K, Sakuma H, Laham R, Vavere AL, Cerci RJ, Mehra VC, Nomura C, Kofoed KF, Jinzaki M, Kuribayashi S, Scholte AJ, Laule M, Tan SY, Hoe J, Paul N, Rybicki FJ, Brinker JA, Arai AE, Matheson MB, Cox C, Clouse ME, Di Carli MF, João AC (2017) Prognostic value of combined CT angiography and myocardial perfusion imaging versus invasive Coronary Angiography and nuclear stress perfusion imaging in the prediction of major adverse cardiovascular events: the CORE320 multicenter Study. Radiology 284(1):55–65
11. Douglas PS, Pontone G, Hlatky MA, Patel MR, Norgaard BL, Byrne RA, Curzen N, Purcell I, Gutberlet M, Rioufol G, Hink U, Schuchlenz HW, Feuchtner G, Gilard M, Andreini D, Jensen JM, Hadamitzky M, Chiswell K, Cyr D, Wilk A, Wang F, Rogers C, De Bruyne B, Clinical outcomes of fractional flow reserve by computed tomographic angiography-guided diagnostic strategies vs. usual Verberne HJ[1], Acampa W[2], Anagnostopoulos C[3], Ballinger J[4], Bengel F[5], De Bondt P[6], Buechel RR[7], Cuocolo A[8], van Eck-Smit BL[9], Flotats A[10], Hacker M[11], Hindorf C[12], Kaufmann PA[7], Lindner O[13], Ljungberg M[14], Lonsdale M[15], Manrique A[16], Minarik D[17], Scholte AJ[18], Slart RH[19], Trägårdh E[20], de Wit TC[9], Hesse B care in patients with suspected coronary artery disease: the prospective longitudinal trial of FFR(CT): outcome and resource impacts study. Eur Heart J 36(47):3359–3367
12. Verberne HJ, Acampa W, Anagnostopoulos C, Ballinger J, Bengel F, De Bondt P, Buechel RR, Cuocolo A, van Eck-Smit BL, Flotats A, Hacker M, Hindorf C, Kaufmann PA, Lindner O, Ljungberg M, Lonsdale M, Manrique A, Minarik D, Scholte AJ, Slart RH, Trägårdh E, de Wit TC, Hesse B (2015) EANM procedural guidelines for radionuclide myocardial perfusion imaging with SPECT and SPECT/CT: 2015 revision. Eur J Nucl Med Mol Imaging 42(12):1929–1940
13. Lang RM, Badano LP, Mor-Avi V, Afilalo J, Armstrong A, Ernande L, Flachskampf FA, Foster E, Goldstein SA, Kuznetsova T, Lancellotti P, Muraru D, Picard MH, Rietzschel ER, Rudski L, Spencer KT, Tsang W, Voigt JU (2015) Recommendations for cardiac chamber quantification by echocardiography in adults: an update from the American Society of Echocardiography and the European Association of Cardiovascular Imaging. Eur Heart J Cardiovasc Imaging 16(3):233–270
14. Lancellotti P, Tribouilloy C, Hagendorff A, Popescu BA, Edvardsen T, Pierard LA, Badano L, Zamorano JL (2013) Recommendations for the echocardiographic assessment of native valvular regurgitation: an executive summary from the European Association of Cardiovascular Imaging. Eur Heart J Cardiovasc Imaging 14(7):611–644

15. Rudski LG, Lai WW, Afilalo J, Hua L, Handschumacher MD, Chandrasekaran K, Solomon SD, Louie EK, Schiller NB (2010) Guidelines for the echocardiographic assessment of the right heart in adults: a report from the American Society of Echocardiography endorsed by the European Association of Echocardiography, a registered branch of the European Society of Cardiology, and the Canadian Society of Echocardiography. J Am Soc Echocardiogr 23(7):685–713, quiz 786–788
16. Habib G, Lancellotti P, Antunes MJ, Bongiorni MG, Casalta JP, Del Zotti F, Dulgheru R, El Khoury G, Erba PA, Iung B, Miro JM, Mulder BJ, Plonska-Gosciniak E, Price S, Roos-Hesselink J, Snygg-Martin U, Thuny F, Tornos Mas P, Vilacosta I, Zamorano JL (2015) 2015 ESC Guidelines for the management of infective endocarditis: The Task Force for the Management of Infective Endocarditis of the European Society of Cardiology (ESC). Endorsed by: European Association for Cardio-Thoracic Surgery (EACTS), the European Association of Nuclear Medicine (EANM). Eur Heart J 36(44):3075–3128
17. Haugaa KH, Basso C, Badano LP, Bucciarelli-Ducci C, Cardim N, Gaemperli O, Galderisi M, Habib G, Knuuti J, Lancellotti P, McKenna W, Neglia D, Popescu BA, Edvardsen T (2017) Comprehensive multi-modality imaging approach in arrhythmogenic cardiomyopathy-an expert consensus document of the European Association of Cardiovascular Imaging. Eur Heart J Cardiovasc Imaging 18(3):237–253
18. Cardim N, Galderisi M, Edvardsen T, Plein S, Popescu BA, D'Andrea A, Bruder O, Cosyns B, Davin L, Donal E, Freitas A, Habib G, Kitsiou A, Petersen SE, Schroeder S, Lancellotti P, Camici P, Dulgheru R, Hagendorff A, Lombardi M, Muraru D, Sicari R (2015) Role of multimodality cardiac imaging in the management of patients with hypertrophic cardiomyopathy: an expert consensus of the European Association of Cardiovascular Imaging Endorsed by the Saudi Heart Association. Eur Heart J Cardiovasc Imaging 16(3):280
19. Galiè N, Humbert M, Vachiery JL, Gibbs S, Lang I, Torbicki A, Simonneau G, Peacock A, Vonk Noordegraaf A, Beghetti M, Ghofrani A, Gomez Sanchez MA, Hansmann G, Klepetko W, Lancellotti P, Matucci M, McDonagh T, Pierard LA, Trindade PT, Zompatori M, Hoeper M (2016) 2015 ESC/ERS Guidelines for the diagnosis and treatment of pulmonary hypertension: the joint task force for the diagnosis and treatment of Pulmonary Hypertension of the European Society of Cardiology (ESC) and the European Respiratory Society (ERS): Endorsed by: Association for European Paediatric and Congenital Cardiology (AEPC), International Society for Heart and Lung Transplantation (ISHLT). Eur Heart J 37(1):67–119
20. Erbel R, Aboyans V, Boileau C, Bossone E, Di Bartolomeo R, Eggebrecht H, Evangelista A, Falk V, Frank H, Gaemperli O, Grabenwoger M, Haverich A, Iung B, John Manolis A, Meijboom F, Nienaber CA, Roffi M, Rousseau H, Sechtem U, Sirnes PA, von Allmen RS, Vrints CJ (2015) Corrigendum to: 2014 ESC Guidelines on the diagnosis and treatment of aortic diseases. Eur Heart J 36(41):2779
21. Lanzer P, Botvinick EH, Schiller NB, Crooks LE, Arakawa M, Kaufman L et al (1984) Cardiac imaging using gated magnetic resonance. Radiology 1(150):121–127
22. Ordidge RJ, Mansfield P, Doyle M, Coupland RE (1982) Real time movie images by NMR. Br J Radiol 55(658)
23. Oppelt A, Graumann R, Barfuss H, Fischer H, Hartl W, Schajor W (1986) FISP—a new fast MRI sequence. Electromedica 54:15–18
24. Moran PR (1982) A flow velocity zeugmatographic interlace for NMR imaging in humans. Magn Reson Imaging 1:197–203
25. Hofman MB, Visser FC, van Rossum AC, Vink GQM, Sprenger M, Westerhof N (1995) In: vivo validation of MRI blood volume flow measurements with limited spatial resolution in small vessels.pdf. Magn Reson Med 33:778–84
26. Kim RJ, Fieno DS, Parrish TB, Harris K, Chen E, Simonetti O et al (1999) Relationship of MRI delayed contrast enhancement to irreversible injury, infarct age, and contractile function. Circulation 100(19):1992–2003
27. Sörensson P, Heiberg E, Saleh N, Bouvier F, Caidahl K, Tornvall P et al (2010) Assessment of myocardium at risk with contrast enhanced steady-state free precession cine cardiovascular

magnetic resonance compared to single-photon emission computed tomography. J Cardiovasc Magn Reson 12(1):25

28. Messroghli DR, Radjenovic A, Kozerke S, Higgins DM, Sivananthan MU, Ridgway JP (2004) Modified look-locker inversion recovery (MOLLI) for high-resolution T1 mapping of the heart. Magn Reson Med 146:141–146
29. Arheden H, Saeed M, Higgins CB, Gao DW, Bremerich J, Wyttenbach R et al (1999) Measurement of the distribution volume of gadopentetate dimeglumine at echo-planar MR imaging to quantify myocardial infarction: comparison with 99mTc-DTPA autoradiography in rats. Radiology 3(211):698–708
30. Kellman P, Aletras AH, Mancini C, McVeigh ER, Arai AE (2007) T2-prepared SSFP improves diagnostic confidence in edema imaging in acute myocardial infarction compared to Turbo Spin Echo. Magn Reson Med 57(5):891–897
31. Anderson LJ, Holden S, Davis B, Prescott E, Charrier CC, Bunce NH et al (2001) Cardiovascular T2-star (T2*) magnetic resonance for the early diagnosis of myocardial iron overload. Eur Heart J 22:2171–2179
32. Pruessmann KP, Weiger M, Scheidegger MB, Boesiger P (1999) SENSE: sensitivity encoding for fast MRI. Magn Reson Med 42(5):952–962
33. Griswold MA, Jakob PM, Heidemann RM, Nittka M, Jellus V, Wang J, Kiefer B, Haase A (2002) Generalized autocalibrating partially parallel acquisitions (GRAPPA). Magn Reson Med 47(6):1202–1210
34. Candes EJ, Romberg J, Tao T (2006) Robust uncertainty principles: exact signal reconstruction from highly incomplete frequency information. IEEE Trans Inf Theory 52(2):489–509
35. Donoho DL (2006) Compressed sensing. IEEE Trans Inf Theory 52(4):1289–1306
36. Lustig M, Donoho D, Pauly JM (2007) Sparse MRI: the application of compressed sensing for rapid MR imaging. Magn Reson Med 58(6):1182–1195
37. Ravishankar S, Bresler Y (2011) MR image reconstruction from highly undersampled k-space data by dictionary learning. IEEE Trans Med Imaging 30(5):1028–1041
38. Wang Y, Ying L (2014) Compressed sensing dynamic cardiac cine MRI using learned spatiotemporal dictionary. IEEE Trans Biomed Eng 61(4):1109–1120
39. Block KT, Uecker M, Frahm J (2007) Undersampled radial MRI with multiple coils. Iterative image reconstruction using a total variation constraint. Magn Reson Med 57(6):1086–1098
40. Tropp JA, Wright SJ (2010) Computational methods for sparse solution of linear inverse problems. Proc IEEE 98(6):948–958
41. Hoang V, Grounds J, Pham D, Virani S, Hamzeh I, Qureshi AM, Lakkis N, Alam M (2016) The role of intracoronary plaque imaging with intravascular ultrasound optical coherence tomography, and near-infrared spectroscopy in patients with coronary artery disease. Curr Atheroscler Rep 18(9):57
42. Schoenhagen P, Nissen S (2002) Understanding coronary artery disease: tomographic imaging with intravascular ultrasound. Heart 88(1):91–96
43. Huang D, Swanson EA, Lin CP, Schuman JS, Stinson WG, Chang W, Hee MR, Flotte T, Gregory K, Puliafito CA et al (1991) Opt Coherence Tomogr. Science 254(5035):1178–1181
44. Gardner CM, Tan H, Hull EL, Lisauskas JB, Sum ST, Meese TM, Jiang C, Madden SP, Caplan JD, Burke AP, Virmani R, Goldstein J, Muller JE (2008) Detection of lipid core coronary plaques in autopsy specimens with a novel catheter-based near-infrared spectroscopy system. JACC Cardiovasc Imaging 1(5):638–648
45. Evertsson M, Cinthio M, Fredriksson S, Olsson F, Persson H, Jansson T (2013) Frequency- and phase-sensitive magnetomotive ultrasound imaging of superparamagnetic iron oxide nanoparticles. IEEE Trans Ultrason Ferroelectr Freq Control 60(3):481–491

Part II
Analysis of Cardiovascular Signals

Cardiac Mechanical Signals

Ramon Casanella, Farzad Khosrow-khavar, Samuel Schmidt, John Zanetti and Kouhyar Tavakolian

Abstract Over the past century, extensive research has been conducted on interpretation of vibration signals created by the heart and their potential use in noninvasive cardiology. Today, new microelectronics and signal processing technologies have provided unprecedented opportunities to reintroduce some of these techniques as useful cardiovascular assessment tools. The purpose of this book chapter is to review these recent efforts and to study these signals in two categories of local pulses and whole-body signals. The present challenges and opportunities in the field are also investigated.

1 Introduction

Every heartbeat creates small vibrations that shake the human body and the mechanically coupled environment around it. These vibrations can be recorded using sensors

John Zanetti passed away on November 30th 2017.

R. Casanella
Universitat Polytecnica Catalunya, Barcelona, Spain
e-mail: ramon.casanella@upc.edu

F. Khosrow-khavar
Simon Fraser University, Burnaby, Canada
e-mail: fkhosrow@sfu.ca

S. Schmidt
Aalborg University, Aalborg, Denmark
e-mail: sschmidt@hst.aau.dk

J. Zanetti
Acceleron Medical, North Andover, USA
e-mail: jmzsenior@gmail.com

K. Tavakolian (✉)
University of North Dakota, North Dakota, USA
e-mail: kouhyar@und.edu

S. Golemati and K. S. Nikita (eds.), *Cardiovascular Computing—Methodologies and Clinical Applications*, Series in BioEngineering,
https://doi.org/10.1007/978-981-10-5092-3_3

placed on the body or on the platforms upon which the body rests. Although what all these signals have in common is the beating of the heart as their main source, these signals have different morphologies and different relationships to cardiovascular dynamics, depending on the placement and type of the sensor.

Over the past century, extensive research has been conducted on interpretation of these signals in terms of their relationship to cardiovascular dynamics and their potential use in diagnostic cardiology. Today, new microelectronics and signal processing technologies have provided unprecedented opportunities to reintroduce some of these relatively old techniques as useful cardiac diagnostic and monitoring tools, creating a new surge of research in this field. The accelerometers and gyroscopes embedded in new cellphones have enough sensitivity to record many of these cardiac signals and the same cell phones have all the processing capability required to extract clinically relevant information from the recorded signals.

The main purpose of this book chapter is to review these recent efforts recording and analysis of mechanical vibration signals and introduce some of the present challenges and opportunities in the field.

2 Different Categories of Cardiac Mechanical Signals

Cardiac mechanical signals are recordings performed by either placing sensors on the body (torso), and recording the *local pulses*, or embedding the sensors in platforms on which the body rests, such as weighing scales, beds and chairs, thus recording *whole-body* movements. The recording of the reaction movement of the centre of gravity of the body caused by the heart action has been traditionally called ballistocardiogram (BCG) [1], whereas the local pulses include several signals with different names depending on the placement and the type of sensor used (See Fig. 1). It should be noticed that in certain situations, where the body and the platform on which it rests, are allowed to freely move in certain axis, such as zero-g in space missions [2], or ultra-low frequency beds [3], the local pulses, measured at the center of gravity of the body, and the and platform signals can be very similar to each other.

2.1 Local Pulses

The pulsatile phenomena of the body's surface with every heart beat have attracted the attention of physicians since the beginning of medicine [4]. Precordial examination or cardiac examination is performed as part of the regular physical examination for the purpose of the detection of cardiovascular pathologies. These tests include palpation and auscultation. With auscultation the audible sounds created by the heart are picked up by a mechanical magnifier in a stethoscope. Signals recorded from the stethoscope are called a phonocardiogram.

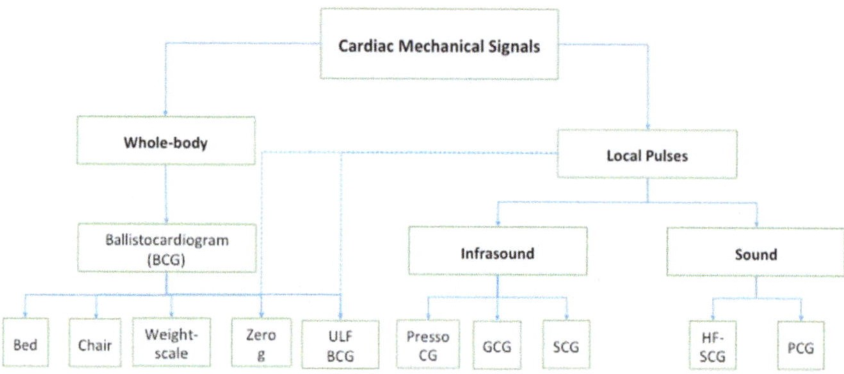

Fig. 1 Different categories of cardiac vibration signals based on the root cause of the signals and also the frequency ranges

With palpation, the sub-audible pulsations of the heart and greater arteries, transmitted to the chest wall, are qualitatively assessed through tactile observations. Different sensors have been used to record the low frequency vibrations (mainly in infrasound range) such as these and have been given different names. This is shown in Fig. 1, where we also separated the pulse signals to those in the audible range and those that are sub-audible. Current advances in transducer technology have provided us with possibilities to record such mechanical signals using small wearable sensors.

2.1.1 Audible Signals: Phonocardiograms

The phonocardiogram (PCG) is quantified heart sounds, which originate from high frequency myocardial vibrations. The PCG has a long history since its discovery in 1908 by Willem Einthoven and auscultation of the heart is still one of the most common medical procedures. Before the introduction of echocardiography, auscultation and PCG were some of the primary tools in cardiology. Today cardiac auscultation is mainly used as an initial screening tool to direct further examination or rule-out cardiac disease. After playing a limited clinical role for several years, PCG is currently being reintroduced by a range of innovative products [5–9]. The PCG signal is often recorded using air-coupled microphones or piezo crystals sensors embedded in digital stethoscopes.

The normal heart sounds comprise the first and second heart sounds (S1 and S2). S1 is caused by the closure of the atrioventricular valves and defines the onset of the mechanical systole, while S2 is caused by closure of the semilunar valves and defines the onset of the diastole period. Common abnormal hearts sounds are Murmurs, the third (S3) and fourth (S4) hearts sounds. Murmurs are noise from turbulent flow often caused from flow constriction as a valve stenosis or by a leaking valve (*regurgitation*).

The S3 sounds occur in early diastolic and the S4 sound occurs in the late diastole, both sounds are pathological in adults above 40 years.

2.1.2 Sub-audible Signals

Different transducers have been placed on different spots on the torso recording low frequency cardiac vibrations. Shape changes and movements of the heart during ejection and filling are believed to cause these low frequency signals. The interest in such precordial recordings dates back to 1885 when Marey studied the movements of the pericardium with the use of a capsule; however, systematic study started after the work of Dressler on pulsations of the chest [10, 11]. As mentioned before, there has always been difficulty in the interpretation of different precordial recordings because of a variety of names and apparatuses used for recording these signals. In the past, precordial recordings were extensively studied in two categories of relative displacement records such as apexcardiography, and absolute displacement records such as kinetocardiography. In the first category, the frame of reference was locally on the chest, and in the second was a point outside the body [12].

Kinetocardiogram and impulse cardiogram were basically the same systems, and the frame of reference for both is outside the body; in apexcardiogam (ACG), and vibrocardiogram (VCG) the reference was on the chest [13]. Pressocardiography is a more recent version of apexcardiography, which has been validated in catheterization lab studies [14].

Another distinct group of precordial recordings were those directly measuring precordial accelerations. Seismocardiogram, which are the best known signals of this category, belongs to this later group of precordial recordings and was first recorded in 60s by Russian researchers including Baevskii [15]. Baevskiy borrowed the technology and concepts from seismology and recorded precordial accelerations calling them seismocardiograms. The initial research was mostly limited to monitoring astronaut's health in space missions. In the late 80 s Salerno and Zanetti used the same technology for clinical purposes [16, 17]. The advent of small and sensitive accelerometers started a new era in this research [18, 19]. Gyrocardiography is a new advent in this field where a gyroscope is placed on the chest instead of an accelerometer as in Seimocardiogram (SCG) [20].

2.2 *Whole Body Signals*

After having observed the pointer of a weighing scale moving in time to his heartbeat, Gordon made the first reported attempt to acquire this movement of his whole body in reaction to his heart action, in 1877 [21], by using a bed suspended from the ceiling. The idea behind the suspended bed was to have a pendulum-like instrument with a resonant frequency below that of the heart rate (about 1 Hz), so that the bed and the body will move together in reaction to heart movement.

The recording of this reaction movement of the centre of gravity of the body caused by the heart action was called ballistocardiogram (BCG) [1] and these kinds of suspended beds, widely used in the past, were called ultra-low-frequency (ULF) ballistocardiographs. That name was given in opposition to a different type of instruments, called high-frequency (HF) ballistocardiographs, in which, once loaded with the body, the natural frequency is much higher than that of the heartbeat. A first example of this second type of instruments, was a chair connected to its base with a very stiff spring developed by Abramson in 1933 [1]. This chair had a resonance frequency, when loaded with 70 kg of iron, of 70 Hz.

The main advantage of the HF systems compared to the ULF ones was that the recording was not interfered with by respiration. It was also not necessary to hold one's breath to use them, which was especially difficult in case of sick patients. With that idea, in 1939 a first HF BCG bed was developed by Starr et al. [22] in which its motion was opposed by using stiff springs. Nevertheless, it was soon noticed that these instruments created some overshoot of part of the waves, which were distorted by after-vibrations especially in the latter systole and diastole parts of the waveform. These limitation motivated, A. Noordergraaf to come up with modelling of different BCG types [23]. This and advances in instrumentation allowed the measurement not only of movement in ULF beds, but also to obtain velocity and acceleration, and therefore to avoid the respiration problem and these instruments were again preferred as the best choice to record BCG's.

Nevertheless, ULF beds required high ceilings and a significant amount of space to be installed and this was one of the reasons the technique was progressively displaced by other newly developed technologies, such as echocardiography. Nevertheless, the field has emerged again in the last few years [24], thanks to the current capability to embed powerful analogue and digital signal processors in a reduced space. This has allowed one to easily acquire BCG's in the most common objects such as chairs [25, 26], beds [27], or weighing scales [28, 29], making that signal very promising for the fast developing field of home health monitoring.

A simultaneous recording of BCG, SCG, PCG together with ECG and impedance cardiogram signal (ICG) is shown in Fig. 2. It should be mentioned that in terms of the frequency range the BCGs are also in the infrasound, sub-audible, signals.

3 Clinical Applications

Many studies during the past century have demonstrated changes in the morphology of mechanical cardiac signals due to different cardiac diseases. For the *local pulse* signals, as mentioned before, auscultation and palpation have been used by physicians for centuries, as part of the cardiac examination, to qualitatively look for signs of cardiac abnormality. Recording of local pulses using accelerometers or gyroscopes could provide quantitative tools for the same assessments. For the *whole body* signals, there was a 20 years longitudinal study by I. Starr, monitoring 211

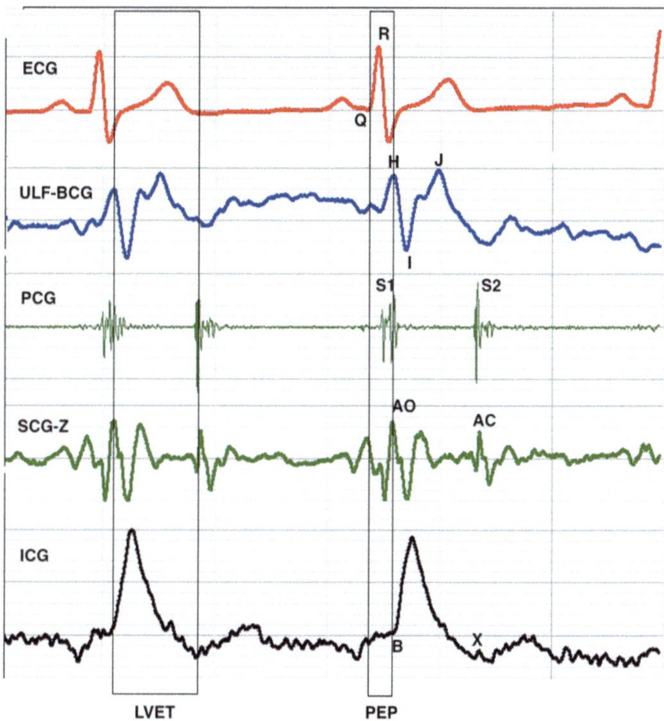

Fig. 2 Simultaneous recording of cardiac mechanical signals (middle three traces) and ECG and impedance cardiogram (ICG) signals as reference from a 36 years old male normal subject. The systolic time intervals of pre-ejection period (PEP) and left ventricular ejection time (LVET) are also shown. BCG was recorded from an ultra-low frequency bed and SCG was recorded in dorso-ventral direction

elderly participants, and showing how the BCG morphology changed by age and different cardiac diseases [30].

For BCG, as there is no need to attach any electrode or sensor when measuring the BCG on a bed and respiration can also be obtained from it, even for babies [31]. This signal has found interesting applications for evaluating the sleep stages [32] and sleep related disorders by using heart rate variability (HRV) related parameters obtained from BCG [33, 34]. This advantage of BCG with respect to other signals for unobtrusive monitoring has been also shown in a very recent application [35] in which heartbeat cycle length was measured during sinus rhythm (SR) and also during atrial fibrillation (AF), showing that this signal is a very promising candidate for prolonged regular heart monitoring to detect silent AF episodes instead of the ECG.

In most recent works in this field a major body of the research is dedicated to measurement of heart rate and in many of them there is a further step to perform heart rate variability analysis using the cardiac time intervals, estimated from mechanical vibration signals. A review of these works is presented in [24] and won't be repeated here. Some of the other research works have focused on extraction of systolic timing intervals from such signals, where these timings could change due to different cardiac abnormalities [36]. In some of the recent works coronary artery disease, myocardial ischemia, heart failure, diastolic dysfunction and hemorrhage detection have been used as example clinical applications for these signals, and they will be reviewed in this section.

3.1 Heart Failure and Cardiac Pacing

S. Wang et al. demonstrated that the presence of the PCG's S3 sound and a systolic dysfunction index was a mortality predictor in patients with severe heart failure [37]. BCGs extracted from modified bathroom scales were also proposed, with preliminary results, to monitor heart failure patients [38].

3.1.1 Cardiac Pacing and Resynchronization Therapy

Pacemakers are being heavily used as a treatment method for heart acute failure patients and cardiac resynchronization therapy (CRT) is one of the more recent advances in cardiac pacemakers. Where on the myocardium to place the electrodes, and how much delay to give between electrode firings, is an important factor how the treatment would work and if the heart failure patient could get back to a normal life. Some of the local pulse signals have been studied in the past for their use in adjusting the CRT procedure and follow ups.

It is demonstrated that biventricular pacing increased the amplitude of PCG's S1 thereby confirming that the amplitude of S1 is related to contraction force [39]. Cardiac timings as measured by SCG were shown to change due to biventricular pacing [40] and feasibility of these signals for CRT was evaluated [41, 42].

3.2 Coronary Artery Disease and Ischemic Heart Disease

Coronary artery diseases (CAD) account for more than 10% of mortalities every year. Diagnostics methods such as coronary tomography angiography and coronary angiography are well established; however, these diagnostics are all expensive image modalities located at specialized hospital units. As such, nonintrusive methods could make a difference in earlier out of hospital diagnosis of CAD or myocardial ischemia, finally leading to CAD.

The accuracy of SCG compared to ECG for detection of coronary artery disease, with exercise test, was studied on 129 patients and it was demonstrated that SCG had more sensitivity in detecting CAD patients [43]. In a separate study the coronary artery was partially obstructed and the effects on SCG were observed [44]. There is a more recent study on the myocardial ischemia and its relation to SCG [45].

Initially PCG based methods for detection of CAD were based on detection of weak murmurs related to post stenotic flow in the coronary arteries, while some of the recent methods combine a range of PCG measures to estimate the risk of CAD [46].

3.3 Hemodynamic Parameters

There has been a long effort to extract or correlate known hemodynamic parameters to indices extracted from cardiac vibration signals [22]. There are recent efforts in this area as briefly reported in this section.

3.3.1 Cardiac Timings

Systolic time intervals have been studied, for the past few decades, as an indirect measure of cardiac contractility [47]. Recent advances in sensor technology have started a new approach to unobtrusive measurement of these signals [36]. Cardiac vibration signals have been proposed to measure these timings.

Seimocardiography was originally proposed in early 90s to be used for estimation of systolic time intervals [48] and many of those findings were further confirmed in more recent studies using MEMS accelerometers [49–51].

The I and J peaks of BCG have also been used to estimated pre-ejection period. R to J timing was introduced as the surrogate of PEP [24, 52, 53]. It is also investigated whether R-I interval was a better surrogate for PEP and also compared the I-J time interval to detect changes in pulse transit time (PTT) [54].

A novel application of the cardiac timing was determining the quiescent periods of cardiac cycle where better image qualities could be achieved using seimocardiography [55].

3.3.2 Cardiac Output

Detection of cardiac output and stroke volume changes could be of important application in different cardiac diseases. Recent studies have been performed on relating the changes on BCG signals and SCG timings to cardiac output and stroke volume [56, 57].

3.3.3 Blood Pressure Estimation Using Pulse Transition Time

The time it takes the blood volume to travel between two points in an artery is inversely proportional to blood pressure and with a proper calibration it could be used to estimate blood pressure for every individual [58]. Mechanical vibration signals have been proposed to be used as the proximal reference for measuring pulse transition time and pulse-plethysmogram signal is normally used as the distal reference for this estimation [50, 54, 59, 60].

4 Analysis Methods

In general, there are three common methodologies for analyzing cardio-mechanical signals:

Whole-signal analysis: The signal is mathematically represented by extracting features that represent its complexity. Examples of such features include Lyapunov exponent, fractional dimensions, power/root mean square and signal entropy. The objective of this type of analysis is to show how the complexity of signal changes with either an external effect or different physiological conditions. For instance, this type of analysis is used to show the effect of the stress exercise test in change of the complexity of the morphology in comparison to the rest conditions for both the healthy and diseased population [61]. The changes of the root mean square of the signal and its relationship with cardiac output in BCG is another example of such methods [52].

Beat-by-beat analysis: The cardio-mechanical signals are divided into periodic cardiac cycles or beats. This is either accomplished by using other bio-signals, such as ECG or PCG, or by using the signal itself [62]. ECG is commonly used for beat extractions since the QRS-complex of the ECG contains the highest energy of the signals and hence it is suitable reference point. The objective of this type of analysis is to extract important events within the cardiac cycle (delineation) or to analyze the variability of specific features in multiple cardiac cycles.

Window-by-window analysis: This type of analysis doesn't model the whole cardiac cycle but only analyzes a portion of the signal. For instance, if only the systolic analysis of the signal is of interest, the algorithm should extract a window where the systolic portion resides. Another example is the delineation algorithm where only specific location or amplitude of fiducial points are only of interest [63].

4.1 Overview of Cardio-Mechanical Delineation Algorithms

Cardio-mechanical delineation algorithms could be either implemented using beat-by-beat or window-by-window methods. In either strategies, the algorithms could either be filter or probabilistic based. The filter based algorithms have been used extensively in analysis of ECG and PPG signals. In the former case, a high-energy narrow-band signal is derived such that its peak is the indication of the QRS-complex [64]. For the latter case, the derivative of the signal is used to delineate the peak and valley of the PPG signal [65]. For cardio-mechanical signals a significant number of algorithms have been developed in the recent years, that can be divided among those that use an auxiliary signal as timing reference, typically ECG, [66, 67], and for the cases in which the use of this auxiliary reference signal is not possible or desirable, those that use the signal by itself. Among this last type, there are also several approaches, such as those based on template matching [68], envelope detection, like the Bseg++ [69] and its very recent improved version, JDet [70], those based on continuous or discrete wavelet transforms [71–74], those based on classification or clustering procedures [75–78] and also some based on the Hilbert transform [79].

Nevertheless, due to the aforementioned limitations regarding the sensitivity of the cardio-mechanical signals, filter based algorithms could not be the recommended approach in some cases. This is due to the fact that the fiducial points of cardio-mechanical signals have similar time and frequency features compared to their adjacent peaks. As a result, misprediction will lead to significant high-prediction error. If beat-by-beat analysis is not required, the median of the results would discard such cases. However, for the individuals that have significantly high beat to beat variation in their morphology, the final prediction could be unreliable [67].

Probabilistic based algorithms overcome the lack of robustness of filter-based algorithms, by assigning a probability or equivalently a signal quality index (SQI) to each cardiac beat. Consequently, decision-making process based on SQI would make the algorithm robust to tackle different heart conditions and abnormalities. This is accomplished by discarding the cardiac cycles that have low SQI's. This is very important since in cases with heart abnormalities, the algorithm would only select high reliable cycles for parameter extraction.

In the beat-by-beat model, each beat is modeled with prior knowledge representing the morphology of the signals. The most prominent methodology is to use "dynamical systems" to represent each cardiac beat. Different models could be used based on different heart conditions. Each model is applied to the signal with the parameters uniquely representing desired fiducial points. The set of parameters that maximizes the posterior probability of the signal is used as the selected model. The extracted parameters are used for further analysis or other classifications.

4.2 Case Study—Seismocardiography Delineation to Extract Systolic Time Intervals

Systolic time intervals are important timing parameters based on events within the cardiac cycle. These parameters are used for the purpose of assessing the performance of the heart [36]. The combination of electrocardiogram and seimocardiogram has been used to extract systolic time intervals, in particular, pre-ejection period

(PEP), and left ventricular ejection time (LVET). The former is extracted from ECG Q-wave to aortic-valve opening (AO) of SCG, whereas, the latter is extracted from SCG aortic-valve opening to SCG aortic valve closing. The ratio of PEP/LVET is one of the most important cardiac time intervals for diagnosis of heart failure [36].

Khosrow-khavar et al., proposed a probabilistic window-by-window based algorithm [63]. The algorithm selected the systolic and diastolic window with respect to ECG R-wave or a SCG-derived envelope depending whether ECG signal was present. Within each systolic and diastolic window, time and frequency features were used to extract SQI. A fixed and automatic SQI threshold mechanism was used for discarding the low-quality cardiac cycles. This algorithm was robust in discarding low-quality beats while maintaining accurate estimation of systolic time intervals for different heart conditions such as patients with prior heart disease.

5 Limitations and Future Prospective

Lack of standardization and common terminologies has encouraged the researchers in the field to get together every year at IEEE Engineering in Medicine and Biology conference in mini-symposiums presenting their latest results. On the other hand, there have been two workshops in Vancouver, Canada (2012 and 2016), where researchers recorded signals together. These efforts also showed itself in a common paper back in 2014 to review the fields of ballistocardiography and seismocardiography [24]. This book chapter is also co-authored by some of the participants of these workshops.

There have been two major limitations for designing algorithms for annotation of cardiomechanical signals are (1) Lack of a manually annotated public database: The "Physionet" database contains multiple ECG datasets with thousands of manually annotated cardiac cycles by the experts in the field. Such a database does not exist for the cardio-mechanical signals in general and an effort was made to annotate about 40,000 cycles of SCG in 2011 [57], which will be publically available on Physionet in a near future. (2) Lack of accepted standard for the cardio-mechanical fiducial points and morphologies: The cardio-mechanical signals have complex morphologies. In particular, the signal morphology consists of many extrema's occurring nearby of each other. Furthermore, the signal morphology changes significantly between different individuals and it is affected by factors such as heart conditions, age, and sex.

5.1 Local Pulses

For local pulse signals such as SCG, subjects can often suffer from a significant degree of motion artifacts caused by postural changes, tremble, or respiration. In depth, studies haven't been conducted to quantify changes on both the morphology and fiducial points. As a result, it is very difficult to pursue the beat analysis method unless only normal morphologies are extracted. Despite the current effort in collaborating with multiple research groups, still a global standard for the SCG morphology and associated fiducial points does not exist [17].

Regarding phonocardiogram signal analysis, a large focus area of recent research in digital PCG has focused on automated and robust identification of abnormal murmurs related to defect heart valves. The aim of this research is to develop intelligent acoustic analyses to support doctor's auscultation of patients. Recently this research was boosted due a Physionet challenge in 2016 aiming at differentiating abnormal from normal heart sounds. The challenge managed to build a database consisting of more than 4000 heart recordings where of many of them are obtained in real-life scenarios.

5.2 *Whole-Body Signals*

There are currently two main limitations to be mentioned regarding BCG analysis. The first is related to the mechanism for the genesis of BCG waves, which is still not fully understood and it is still under investigation. In the old BCG era, A. Noordergraaf proposed a model based on evaluating the changes in the movement of the center of gravity of the body as the pressure waves propagate along the arterial tree in each cardiac cycle [1]. That model explained the BCG signals obtained with different beds, and their relationships with each other, and this was fully accepted by the scientific community then, despite the existing differences in the signals obtained with ULF and HF systems previously mentioned in this chapter.

Nevertheless, as the most common systems used nowadays to obtain the BCG, such as weighing scales, chairs or beds, with the exception of zero g methods [80], are not ULF systems, the understanding of these differences has become a very relevant unsolved problem that needs to be addressed. To this respect, a new simple model has been very recently proposed [81], which attributes the genesis of the BCG waves mainly to blood pressure gradients in the ascending and descending aorta. Although this model has not been validated with real BCG measurements yet, it has shown a potential, as it predicted the relationship between the IJ interval and the aortic PTT, that has been experimentally observed independently in the most recent times [54] and that remained unexplained by the old models.

The second main current limitation in the field is the lack of standardization and characterization of the different mechanical and electronic interfaces used to obtain the BCG signal. Regarding the electronic interfaces, although the possible effects of J peak timing of some of the most common analog and digital conditioning blocks employed has been already determined [53], clear standards regarding the shape and the timing of the rest of BCG waves the necessary frequency bandwidth for them has still to be established and accepted by the BCG scientific community.

Regarding the mechanical interfaces, it has been recently observed that weighing scales with too low natural resonant frequency can distort BCG waves [82]. Although this effect could also be present in BCG signals acquired in beds or chairs, most of these interfaces have still not been properly characterized and this is a very relevant work that needs to be done in the near future to avoid a similar degree of confusion to that introduced by the un-calibrated but very popular Dock shin-bar BCG systems in the old BCG era [1].

Finally, in some of the recent research developed in the field, local pulse measurements have been performed by placing accelerometers on several points of the body surface, which has been termed wearable ballistocardiography [83]. Although some of these works have contributed to determine the effect of posture-dependent distortions in BCG waves [84] and the relationship between local measurements and whole body measurements [85, 86], the use of a BCG terminology for these local measurements, especially those performed far from the center of gravity of the body, can also be an additional cause of confusion that shows that the efforts towards a higher standardization in the field are, with no doubt, one of the most relevant tasks to be undertaken in the promising field of cardiac mechanical signals, in the near future.

References

1. Starr A, Noordergraaf I (1967) Ballistocardiography in cardiovascular research. Lippincott Company, Philadelphia
2. Lejeune L, Caiani EG, Prisk GK, Migeotte P (2014) Evaluation of ensemble averaging methods in 3D ballistocardiography. In: IEEE EMBC, pp 5176–5179
3. Ngai B, Tavakolian K, Akhbardeh A, Blaber AP, Kaminska B, Noordergraaf A (2009) Comparative analysis of seismocardiogram waves with the ultra-low frequency ballistocardiogram. In: IEEE EMBC, vol 2009, pp 2851–2854
4. Weissler AM, Harris WS, Schoenfeld CD (1968) Systolic time intervals in heart failure in man. Circulation 37(2):149–159
5. Rijuven (2017). http://www.rijuven.com/ (Online)
6. 3M (2017). http://www.littmann.ca/ (Online)
7. Inovise. http://www.inovise.com/ (Online)
8. Eko (2017). https://ekodevices.com/ (Online)
9. Acarix. http://www.acarix.com/ (Online)
10. Dressler W (1937) Pulsations of the wall of the chest. Arch Intern Med 225–239
11. Droitcour A (2006) Non-contact measurment of heart and respiration rates with a single-chip microwave doppler radar. Stanford University
12. Schweizer W, Bertrab RV, Reist P (1965) Kinetocardiography in coronary artery disease. Br Heart J 27(2):263–268
13. Eddleman E (1974) Kinetocardiography. In: Noninvasive cardiology. Gtune & Stratton, New York, pp 227–273
14. Manolas J (2016) Assessment of diastolic behavior of patients with hypertension vs. other myocardial diseases using an external pressure transducer and short handgrip exercise. J. Hypertens. Manag. 2(1):1–3
15. Baevskii RM, Egorov AD, Kazarian LA (1964) The method of seismocardiography. Kardiologiia 18:87–89
16. Salerno D, Zanetti J (1991) Seismocardiography for monitoring changes in left ventricular function during ischemia. Chest 100(4):991–993

17. Zanetti JM, Tavakolian K (2013) Seismocardiography : past, present and future. In: IEEE engineering in medicine and biology society conference, pp 7004–7007
18. Castiglioni P, Faini A, Parati G, Di Rienzo M (2007) Wearable seismocardiography. In: IEEE EMBC conference, pp 3954–3957
19. Tavakolian K (2010) Characterization and analysis of seismocardiogram for estimation of hemodynamic parameters. PhD diss
20. Tadi MJ, Lehtonen E, Saraste A, Vasankari T, Koivisto T (2016) Gyrocardiography : a new non-invasive approach in the study of mechanical motions of the heart. Concept, method and initial observations. In: IEEE EMBC conference, pp 2034–2037
21. Gordon JW (1877) Certain molar movements of the human body produced by the circulation of the blood. J Anat Physiol 11:533–536
22. Starr I, Rawson AJ, Schroeder HA, Joseph NR (1939) Studies on the estimation of cardiac ouptut in man, and of abnormalities in cardiac function, from the heart's recoil and the blood's impacts; the ballistocardiogram. Am J Physiol 127(1):1–28
23. Noordergraaf A (1956) Physical basis of ballistocardiography. Utrech University
24. Inan O et al (2015) Ballistocardiography and seismocardiography: a review of recent advances. IEEE J Biomed Heal Inform 19(4):1414–1427
25. Junnila S, Akhbardeh A, Värri A, Koivistoinen T (2005) An EMFi-film sensor based ballistocardiographic chair: performance and cycle extraction method. In: IEEE workshop on signal processing systems (SiPS) design and implementation, vol 2005, pp 373–377
26. Luna-Lozano PS, Alvarado-Serrano C (2012) Time and amplitude relationships of the ballistocardiogram in vertical and horizontal direction. In: CCE 2012—2012 9th international conference on electrical engineering, computer science automatic control, no September
27. Chee Y, Han J, Youn J, Park K (2005) Air mattress sensor system with balancing tube for unconstrained measurement of respiration and heart beat movements. Physiol Meas 26(4):413–422
28. González-Landaeta R, Casas O, Pallàs-Areny R (2008) Heart rate detection from an electronic weighing scale. Physiol Meas 29(8):979–988
29. Inan OT, Etemadi M, Wiard RM, Giovangrandi L, Kovacs GT (2009) Robust ballistocardiogram acquisition for home monitoring. Physiol Meas 30(2): 169–185
30. Starr I, Wood FC (1961) Twenty-year studies with the ballistocardiograph the relation between the amplitude of the first record of 'healthy'. Circulation 23:714–732
31. Lee WK, Yoon H, Jung DW, Hwang SH, Park KS (2015) Ballistocardiogram of baby during sleep. In: Proceedings of annual international conference IEEE engineering in medicine and biology society (EMBS), vol 2015–Novem, pp 7167–7170
32. Watanabe K, Watanabe T, Watanabe H, Ando H, Ishikawa T, Kobayashi K (2005) Noninvasive measurement of heartbeat, respiration, snoring and body movements of a subject in bed via a pneumatic method. IEEE Trans Biomed Eng 52(12):2100–2107
33. Jung DW, Hwang SH, Yoon HN, Lee Y-JG, Jeong D-U, Park KS (2014) Nocturnal awakening and sleep efficiency estimation using unobtrusively measured ballistocardiogram. IEEE Trans Biomed Eng 61(1): 131–138
34. Zhao W, Ni H, Zhou X, Song Y, Wang T (2015) Identifying sleep apnea syndrome using heart rate and breathing effort variation analysis based on ballistocardiography. In: 2015 37th Annual International Conference on IEEE Engineering Medicine and Biology Society, vol 2015, pp 4536–4539
35. Zink MD et al (2015) Heartbeat cycle length detection by a ballistocardiographic sensor in atrial fibrillation and sinus rhythm. Biomed Res Int 2015:840356
36. Tavakolian K (2016) Systolic time intervals and new measurement methods. Cardiovasc Eng Technol 7(2):118–125
37. Eleuteri E et al (2016) Prognostic value of angiopoietin-2 in patients with chronic heart failure. Int J Cardiol 212:364–368
38. Etemadi M et al (2014) Tracking clinical status for heart failure patients using ballistocardiography and electrocardiography signal features. In: 2014 36th Annual International Conference on IEEE Engineering Medicine and Biology Society, EMBC 2014, vol 94143, pp 5188–5191

39. Jensen AS et al (2014) Effects of cardiac resynchronization therapy on the first heart sound energy. Comput Cardiol 2014(41):29–32
40. Marcus FI et al (2007) Accelerometer-derived time intervals during various pacing modes in patients with biventricular pacemakers: comparison with normals. PACE 30(12):1476–1481
41. Giorgis L et al (2008) Analysis of cardiac micro-acceleration signals for the estimation of systolic and diastolic time intervals in cardiac resynchronization therapy. In: Computing in cardiology, pp 393–396
42. Donal E et al (2011) Endocardial acceleration (sonR) vs. ultrasound-derived time intervals in recipients of cardiac resynchronization therapy systems. Europace 13(3):402–408
43. Wilson R, Bamrah V, Lindsay J Diagnostic accuracy of seismocardiography compared with electrocardiography for the anatomic and physiologic diagnosis of coronary artery disease during exercise. Am J 71(August 1989, 1993)
44. Salerno DM, Zanetti JM, Green LA, Mooney MR, Madison JD, Van Tassel RA (1991) Seismocardiographic changes associated with obstruction of coronary blood flow during balloon angioplasty. Am J Cardiol 68(2): 201–207
45. Becker M et al (2013) Simplified detection of myocardial ischemia by seismocardiography: differentiation between causes of altered myocardial function. Herz (April): 1–7
46. Winther S et al (2016) Diagnosing coronary artery disease by sound analysis from coronary stenosis induced turbulent blood flow: diagnostic performance in patients with stable angina pectoris. Int J Cardiovasc Imaging 32(2):235–245
47. Lewis RP, Leighton RF, Forester WF, Weissler AM (1974) Systolic time intervals. In: Noninvasive cardiology. Grune & Stratton, New York, p 300:400
48. Crow R, Hannan P, Jacobs D, Hedquist L, Salerno D (1994) Relationship between seismocardiogram and echocardiogram for events in the cardiac cycle. Am J Noninvasive Cardiol 8(39):39–46
49. Tavakolian K, Blaber AP, Ngai B, Kaminska B (2010) Estimation of hemodynamic parameters from seismocardiogram. In: Computing in cardiology, pp 1055–1058
50. Di Rienzo M, Vaini E, Lombardi P (2015) Use of seismocardiogram for the beat-to-beat assessment of the pulse transit time: a pilot study. In: Proceedings of annual international conference IEEE engineering in medicine and biology society (EMBS), vol 2015–November, pp 7184–7187
51. Javaid AQ, Fesmire NF, Weitnauer MA, Inan OT (2015) Towards robust estimation of systolic time intervals using head-to-foot and dorso-ventral components of sternal acceleration signals. In: 2015 IEEE 12th international conference on wearable and implantable body sensor networks, BSN 2015
52. Inan OT, Etemadi M, Paloma A, Giovangrandi L, Kovacs GTA (2009) Non-invasive cardiac output trending during exercise recovery on a bathroom-scale-based ballistocardiograph. Physiol Meas 30(3): 261–274
53. Gomez-Clapers J, Serra-Rocamora A, Casanella R, Pallas-Areny R (2014) Towards the standardization of ballistocardiography systems for J-peak timing measurement. Meas J Int Meas Confed 58:310–316
54. Gomez-clapers J, Casanella R, Pallas-areny R (2016) Direct pulse transit time measurement from an electronic weighing scale. In: Computing in cardiology, pp 773–776
55. Wick CA, McClellan JH, Inan OT, Tridandapani S (2015) Seismocardiography-based detection of cardiac quiescence. IEEE Trans Biomed Eng 62(8): 2025–2032
56. Ashouri H, Orlandic L, Inan OT (2016) Unobtrusive estimation of cardiac contractility and stroke volume changes using ballistocardiogram measurements on a high bandwidth force plate. Sensors (Switzerland), 16(6)
57. Tavakolian K, Dumont GA, Houlton G, Blaber AP (2014) Precordial vibrations provide noninvasive detection of early-stage hemorrhage. Shock 41(2): 91–96
58. Mukkamala R et al (2015) Toward ubiquitous blood pressure monitoring via pulse transit time: theory and practice. IEEE Trans Biomed Eng 62(8):1879–1901
59. Kim CS, Carek AM, Mukkamala R, Inan OT, Hahn JO (2015) Ballistocardiogram as proximal timing reference for pulse transit time measurement: potential for cuffless blood pressure monitoring. IEEE Trans Biomed Eng 62(11):2657–2664

60. Verma AK, Fazel-rezai R, Blaber A, Tavakolian K (2015) Pulse transit time extraction from seismocardiogram and its relationship with pulse pressure. In: Computing in cardiology, pp 2–5
61. Ahlström C (2008) Nonlinear phonocardiographic signal processing. Linkoping University
62. Khosrow-Khavar F, Tavakolian K, Blaber A, Zanetti J, Fazel-Rezai R, Menon C (2014) Automatic annotation of seismocardiogram with high frequency precordial accelerations. IEEE J Biomed Heal Inform. (in Press)
63. Khosrow-Khavar F, Tavakolin K, Blaber A, Menon C (2016) Automatic and robust delineation of the fiducial points of the seismocardiogram signal for non-invasive estimation of cardiac time intervals. IEEE Trans Biomed Eng
64. Pan J, Tompkins WJ (1985) A real-time QRS detection algorithm. IEEE Trans Biomed Eng 32(3):230–236
65. Jang DG, Park SH, Hahn M (2014) Framework for automatic delineation of second derivative of photoplethysmogram: a knowledge-based approach. J Med Biol Eng 34(6):547–553
66. Pandia K, Inan OT, Kovacs GTA, Giovangrandi L (2012) Extracting respiratory information from seismocardiogram signals acquired on the chest using a miniature accelerometer. Physiol Meas 33(10): 1643–1660
67. Khosrow-khavar F et al (2015) Automatic annotation of seismocardiogram with high frequency precordial accelerations. IEEE J Biomed Heal Inform 19(4):1428–1434
68. Shin JH, Choi BH, Lim YG, Jeong DU, Park KS (2008) Automatic ballistocardiogram (BCG) beat detection using a template matching approach. In: Conference proceedings of IEEE engineering medicine and biology society, vol 2008, no c, pp 1144–1146
69. Akhbardeh A, Kaminska B, Tavakolian K (2007) BSeg++: a modified blind segmentation method for ballistocardiogram cycle extraction. In: IEEE EMBC, vol 2007, pp 1896–1899
70. Gomez-clapers J, Casanella R, Pallas-areny R (2016) A novel algorithm for fast BCG cycle extraction in ambulatory scenarios. In: Computing in cardiology, pp 357–360
71. Xu W, Sandham WA, Fisherm AC, Conway M (1996) Wavelet transform analysis of the seismocardiogram. In: Proceedings of IEEE-SP international symposium on time-frequency time-scale analysis, pp 481–484
72. Postolache O, Girao PS, Postolache G, Pereira M (2007) Vital signs monitoring system based on EMFi sensors and wavelet analysis. In: 2007 IEEE instrumentation & measurement technology conference IMTC 2007, pp 1–4
73. Gilaberte S, Gómez-Clapers J, Casanella R, Pallas-Areny R (2010) Heart and respiratory rate detection on a bathroom scale based on the ballistocardiogram and the continuous wavelet transform. In: 2010 Annual international conference on IEEE engineering and medicine biology society EMBC'10, pp 2557–2560
74. Alvarado-Serrano C, Luna-Lozano PS, Pallàs-Areny R (2016) An algorithm for beat-to-beat heart rate detection from the BCG based on the continuous spline wavelet transform. Biomed Signal Process Control 27(May):96–102
75. Bruser C, Stadlthanner K, Brauers A, Leonhardt S (2010) Applying machine learning to detect individual heart beats in ballistocardiograms. In: Conference proceedings of IEEE engineering and medicine biology society, vol 2010, pp 1926–1929
76. Bruser C, Stadlthanner K, de Waele S, Leonhardt S (2011) Adaptive beat-to-beat heart rate estimation in ballistocardiograms. IEEE Trans Inf Technol Biomed 15(5):778–786
77. Brueser C, Winter S, Leonhardt S (2013) Robust inter-beat interval estimation in cardiac vibration signals. Physiol Meas 34(2):123–138
78. Paalasmaa J, Toivonen H, Partinen M (2015) Adaptive heartbeat modeling for beat-to-beat heart rate measurement in ballistocardiograms. IEEE J Biomed Heal Inform 19(6):1945–1952
79. Jafari Tadi M et al (2016) A real-time approach for heart rate monitoring using a Hilbert transform in seismocardiograms. Physiol Meas 37(11): 1885–1909
80. De Ridder S, Migeotte PF, Neyt X, Pattyn N, Prisk GK (2011) Three-dimensional ballistocardiography in microgravity: a review of past research. In: Proceedings of annual international conference IEEE engineering in medicine and biology society (EMBS), pp 4267–4270

81. Kim C-S et al (2016) Ballistocardiogram: mechanism and potential for unobtrusive cardiovascular health monitoring. Sci Rep 6:1–6
82. Casanella R, Gomez-clapers J, Hernandez-urrea M, Pallas-areny R (2016) Impact of the mechanical interface on BCG signals obtained from electronic weighing scales. In: Computing in cardiology, pp 285–288
83. Da He D, Winokur ES, Sodini CG (2011) A continuous, wearable, and wireless heart monitor using head ballistocardiogram (BCG) and head electrocardiogram (ECG). In: Proceedings of annual international conference IEEE engineering in medicine and biology society (EMBS), pp 4729–4732
84. Javaid AQ, Wiens AD, Fesmire NF, Weitnauer MA, Inan OT (2015) Quantifying and reducing posture-dependent distortion in ballistocardiogram measurements. IEEE J Biomed Heal Inform 19(5):1549–1556
85. Wiens A, Etemadi M, Klein L, Roy S, Inan OT (2014) Wearable ballistocardiography: preliminary methods for mapping surface vibration measurements to whole body forces. In: 2014 36th Annual international conference IEEE engineering in medicine and biology society EMBS, 2014, vol 94143, pp 5172–5175
86. Wiens A, Etemadi M, Roy S, Klein L, Inan O (2014) Towards continuous, non-invasive assessment of ventricular function and hemodynamics: wearable ballistocardiography. IEEE J Biomed Heal Inform. PP(99): 1

Time-Domain Analysis of the Electrocardiogram

Ioanna Chouvarda, Dimitris Filos and Nicos Maglaveras

Abstract The electrocardiogram (ECG) is an affordable and well-studied biosignal, which has a wide presence in clinical research and practice, especially as a frontline diagnostic tool that measures the evolution of the electrical activity of the heart, with characteristic morphologies for atrial and ventricular activity, depending also on the position of recording. Time domain analysis of ECG includes: (a) preprocessing for quality characterization and improvement, (b) recognition of ECG waves, (c) analysis of ECG waves morphology, durations, amplitudes, as well as distances among waves, (d) variability analysis, as regards evolution in time. Numerous application areas are based on these analysis building blocks, with arrhythmia detection, and risk analysis among them. Analysis of the ECG signals in the time domain has been a continuous research field, although later complemented by frequency and time-frequency analysis This chapter aims to provide an overview of ECG analysis methods along with the main clinical application areas. A description of the general characteristics and challenges of ECG in the time domain, is followed by summarizing the basic types of ECG analysis and reviewing analytics methods in the context of their clinical use. Finally, the current methods and future directions are discussed.

Keywords ECG · Time domain analysis

1 Introduction

A century of research and clinical practice [1] constitutes electrocardiography a clinically mature technique and a first line diagnostic tool in clinical practice, applied as part of the initial evaluation for any patient with cardiac complaints. The Electrocardiogram (ECG) is a biosignal that reflects cardiac electrophysiology and can

I. Chouvarda (✉) · D. Filos · N. Maglaveras
Laboratory of Computing, Medical Informatics and Biomedical-Imaging Technologies, Medical School, Faculty of Health Sciences, Aristotle University of Thessaloniki, Thessaloniki, Greece
e-mail: ioannach@auth.gr

S. Golemati and K. S. Nikita (eds.), *Cardiovascular Computing—Methodologies and Clinical Applications*, Series in BioEngineering,
https://doi.org/10.1007/978-981-10-5092-3_4

be acquired in a non-invasive and safe manner, which is nowadays easily monitored also in home and ambulatory settings.

ECG analysis has attracted numerous scientists in the quest of achieving diagnostic information from ECG. Over the years, numerous digital signal processing and machine learning techniques have been tested with ECGs. Factors contributing to the continuous scientific activity in ECG analysis can be divided in three categories:

- **Clinical**, including the availability in healthcare environments of ECGs in legacy clinical databases of specific research purpose (e.g. response to treatment), and a series of clinical problems and challenges that have been well defined with clear clinical benefit, such detection of alerting events, or patient prognosis.
- **Academic**, as concerns the wide availability of ECG signals in public and research oriented databases (e.g. Physionet[1] and THEW [2]), which provided the testbed for proving the virtue of biomedical analysis techniques (e.g. arrhythmia detection), as well as a scientifically nurturing environment supporting new challenges, such as the Computing in Cardiology Conference.[2]
- **Industrial**, with respect to industrial policies towards affordable devices, easily accessible and standardized recordings and formats [3] and embodiment of analytics with increasingly accurate diagnostic capabilities, such as the implantable defibrillators.

Analysis of the ECG signals in the time domain has been a continuous research field, although later complemented by frequency and time-frequency analysis. The main areas of time-domain analysis (TDA) of ECG in the clinical routine are: (a) recognition of ECG waves and their durations, amplitudes and specific morphologies, (b) distances among waves, (c) generation of average signals, and (d) heart rate statistics. These methods are characterized by simplicity and low computation burden, as well as straightforward clinical interpretation. Other time domain methods applied in research include sophisticated denoising methods, complexity analysis features, and various machine learning techniques.

This chapter aims to provide an overview of ECG analysis methods along with the main clinical application areas. Section 2 presents the general characteristics and challenges of ECG in the time domain. Section 3 describes the basic types of ECG analysis and Sect. 4 reviews analytics methods in the context of their clinical use. Finally, Sect. 5 discusses the main issues arising in current TDA and links them with the future directions and opportunities that are offered by the advancements in information and communication technology, as well as electronics, coupled with the new health services expanding beyond the clinical settings.

---

[1] http://www.physionet.org.

[2] https://physionet.org/challenge/.

2 The ECG Signal and its Nature

2.1 ECG Recordings

Many decades ago, Gezelowitz stated that over 90% of the heart's electric activity can be explained with a dipole source model [4]. To evaluate this dipole, it is sufficient to measure its three independent components. The purpose of the vectorcardiographic (VCG) systems is to detect the equivalent dipole of the heart, in leads X, Y and Z, and the trajectory of VCG vector, which can then be visually inspected and computationally analyzed [5]. Several lead systems have been proposed for capturing the three-dimensional extent of the heart dipole, such as Frank lead system [6]. In common clinical practice, a more redundant system is usually adopted, i.e. the 12 lead consisting of the leads I, II, III, aVR, aVL, aVF, V1, V2, V3, V4, V5, V6, and as each lead reflects the projection of the electrical activity of the heart from different angles, it enhances pattern recognition and facilitates diagnosis. Recent studies suggest also the use of 80-lead body surface map electrocardiogram system in emergency care, as it promises greater sensitivity for detecting MI events [7]. On the other hand, long term ambulatory electrocardiography or 24 h ECG Holter setups typically include 1–3 leads and are widely used for detection and monitoring of arrhythmias. Recent devices, including wearables, for recordings in daily life do not follow strictly the clinically specified recording positions. With respect to temporal resolution, it spans from high resolution (1000 Hz), usually for short recordings, to regular clinical measurements at 250 Hz, also applicable in Holter long term recordings.

2.2 ECG Fiducial Points

ECG, as recorded at the body surface, reflects the conduction of electrical activity through the different chambers of the heart, from the atria to the ventricles. It is composed of distinct waves: the P-wave that corresponds to atrial depolarization and has a unipolar or bipolar morphology, the QRS wave, being the most prominent wave and corresponding to ventricular depolarization, and the T-wave representing the ventricular repolarization (Fig. 1). The morphology of these waves depends heavily on the recording lead, and on the potential pathology. In some cases, the U-wave, a positive flat deflection after the T-wave, is visible, and its origin has been attributed to the repolarization of the Purkinje fibers, or papillary muscle, or mid myocardium. Usually its presence or absence is not considered to have clinical significance, although some morphologies are of diagnostic value (acute ischemia, hypokalemia, or severe aortic valve incompetence). The fusion of the T-wave with the U-wave, leading to a TU wave, is possible, in which cases, the U-wave creates an ambiguity in detecting the end of T-wave. In most normal ECGs the junction (J) point can be seen as the point that defines the end of the QRS complex and the beginning of the ST segment, and is a point close to the isoelectric line.

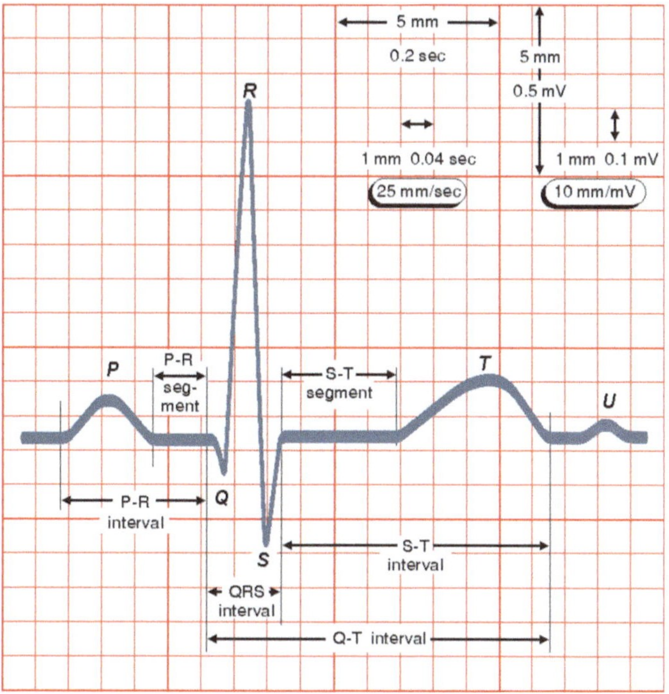

Fig. 1 ECG fiducial points [8]

ECG wave delineation is the determination of the Fiducial Points (FPs) in an ECG signal, i.e. the locations of peak, onset and offset of the aforementioned waves, on a beat by beat basis. These waves' amplitudes and durations contain clinically useful information. Thus, accurate "Fiducial Point Extraction" or "ECG wave delineation" is a first step in many ECG analysis tasks. Besides a potential temporal and spatial dispersion of these morphologies, and the challenges posed by noisy recordings, it is important to note that specific changes in the morphological properties of ECG reflect altered cardiac cell properties, i.e. membrane ionic currents and action potential properties [9].

2.3 The Challenges of ECG Analysis in the Time-Domain

As ECG is recorded in diverse conditions, spanning from controlled clinical recordings at rest, to exercise stress test, Intensive Care Unit (ICU) recordings, ambulatory and Holter recordings, or even telehealth related ECG from wearable sensors during daily life, data quality is an important challenge, in order to ensure the recognition of ECG waves, and especially their start and end. ECG is recorded in different standard positions, and this multilead information is not only useful as the necessary redundancy to increase signal reliability, but also towards increasing the information content. Thus, the development of multichannel timeseries approaches is a challenge in this field. Furthermore, non-stationarity and morphological variation, both intraperson and interperson, need to be addressed in order to achieve reproducible results, and 'Normative' values of clinical relevance. Further processing steps, including machine learning methods, heavily depend on the preprocessing steps and the assumptions made, thus pipelines have to be end-to-end optimized, taking into account all steps, and the propagating consequences, and the need for standardization of methods at large.

Considering that different leads of the ECG represent the propagation of the electrical activity on the myocardium from different projections, the major challenge of the TDA consists the association of potential underline pathology for the observation of the time domain characteristics of the ECG. In this respect the conduction properties of the myocardium could be associated with the morphological characteristics of the ECG.

3 Types of Time-Domain Analysis

ECG signal is a quasiperiodic signal whose components reflect physiological activity of the heart. Thus, it is always important to follow a certain series of steps to extract the main characteristics of ECG, either in the form of time intervals, or waveform morphology, as described in the following subsections.

3.1 ECG Preprocessing and Denoising Fiducial Point Extraction

3.1.1 Denoising

Noise is typically embedded in an ECG signal during acquisition and transmission. This includes muscle artifacts, baseline drift with respiration (0.15–3 Hz), powerline interference (50/60 Hz and harmonics) and electrode motion. ECG denoising and wave delineation constitute the typical preprocessing steps, and are implemented either in a sequential or in a combined manner.

Adaptive filtering has been typically used for baseline wandering and powerline interference. An interesting two step approach is proposed by Der Lin [10], where the presence of powerline interference is first detected by linear discriminant analysis, and upon detection the noise suppressed by a recursive least-squares (RLS) adaptive notch filter. Efficient implementations of adaptive filtering, such as Fast Block MS (FBLMS) algorithm, have been proposed for removing artifacts while preserving the low frequency components [11]. Band-pass digital filters have been used for the removal of interference (either high or low frequency, or even in narrow zones), and the need for their careful design in order to avoid signal distortion has been identified [12]. Blind source separation techniques, focusing on independent component analysis based techniques, such as constrained Independent Component Analysis (ICA), have been applied to motion artifact removal [13]. For ECG denoising, Kuzilek et al. [14] propose an ICA-based method that relies on supervised algorithms for training the detection of noise and the separation of the noise components from signal ones. It has to be noted that most methods have been tested in MIT-Arrhythmia database, which makes them comparable in terms of performance. Yet their applicability in a wider range of acquisition conditions needs to be addressed, as well as the efficiency of these preprocessing steps with respect to the application and main processing demands.

As regards the detection and rejection of artifactual segments in recordings, especially in non-resting clinical settings, a well-accepted semi-automatic method is template based, i.e. based on the definition of a high quality segment, and the rejection of candidate beats that are not adequately correlated.

3.1.2 Wave Delineation—Fiducial Point Extraction

Fiducial point extraction follows the ECG signal improvement and denoising [15]. A popular algorithm for QRS detection is the algorithm based on low pass, high pass filtering and on differentiation as well as on the application of adaptive thresholding proposed by Pan and Tompkins [16], widely used due to its simplicity. Another robust and simple single-lead ECG delineator was proposed by Martínez et al. [17]. Based on phasor transform and the derivative of the signal produced the algorithm achieves QRS detection with an average sensitivity of 99.81% and positive predictivity of 99.89% while it also presents high sensitivity on the detection of P and T waves. Kalman filtering has been recently used for denoising and fiducial point extraction [18]. This approach is based on a dynamic model with (a) modelling of ECG waveforms with Gaussian functions, (b) representing parameters of Gaussian functions and of ECG waveforms (P-wave, QRS complex and T-wave) as state variables. A Kalman filter is used for estimating the model parameters. A multilead approach for ECG wave delineation was proposed by Almeida [19] towards accurate QT interval estimation.

3.1.3 Cancellation of ECG Waves

Cancellation of ECG waves has been attempted for more focused and accurate study of specific waves' dynamics. Characteristically, due to the much higher amplitude of the electrical ventricular activity (VA) on the surface ECG, cancellation of the ventricular wave is important in the study of atrial activity in Atrial Fibrillation on ECGs.

Two approaches are generally used to perform this task. Template based approaches are based on the subtraction of a template calculated as an average beat [20], under the assumption of QRS stability over time, an assumption sensitive to noise and other reasons for subtle changes. Source separation approaches have employed Principal Component Analysis (PCA) or ICA, under the assumption of uncorrelated or independent components respectively [21]. Machine learning techniques have also been employed [22].

3.2 Signal Averaged ECG Versus Beat to Beat Analysis

The ECG is a quasi-stationary signal, having a morphology that is loosely repeated in every beat. This fact has led to signal averaging approaches, which meant to result in a mean ECG waveform playing the role of a template ECG that preserves the main characteristics under investigation. Signal Averaged ECG (SAECG) not only has decreased Gaussian noise, but also facilitates analysis, features extraction and comparison from the template morphology [23, 24], under the assumption that ECG beats were well synchronized before averaging. It has to be highlighted that synchronization has to take place with respect to the wave that needs to be averaged and processed, be it QRS or P-wave [25].

SAECG is heavily based on the assumption of stationarity and the need for noise reduction. In long term recordings, stationarity assumption could not be universally assumed, not only due to potential arrhythmias, but also due to the change of ECG in higher heart rate (exercise) or circadian variations. This issue has been approached by segmenting the total (e.g. 24 h) recording in smaller sections with presumably similar conditions and signal characteristics. More recent approaches do not heavily rely on this assumption, and furthermore can capitalize on technological advancements for quality signal measurements and signal enhancements. Thus, there is an emerging trend for morphological analysis on a beat by beat basis, which explores the morphological variability of ECG waves.

T-wave alternans [26] was the first characteristic example of beat to beat fluctuation analysis with diagnostic value, while later fluctuation of QRS-T waves was analyzed for myocardial ischemia and infarction [27] and P-wave variability with respect to atrial fibrillation [28]. Figure 2 depicts consecutive and synchronized P-waves from a normal subject. While an average P-wave can be subsequently calculated, their morphological analysis on a beat by beat basis can reveal how consistent this morphology is over time.

3.3 Heart Rate and Its Variability

Among the most valuable measurements that are derived from an ECG is the Heart Rate (HR), i.e. the rate of consecutive beats. While the average HR value at resting

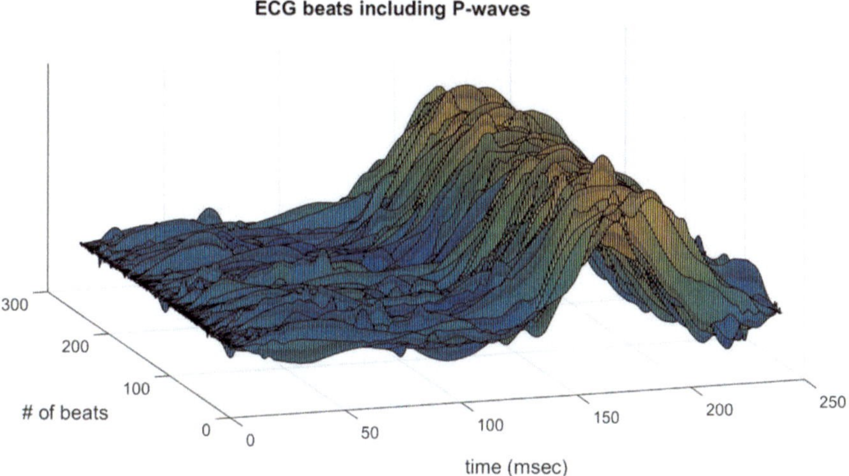

Fig. 2 Aligned P-waves from consecutive beats

conditions (in beats per minute) is a standard measure, available also by other types of measurements (e.g. blood pressure devices produce pulse), the dynamics of HR have also drawn attention during the last decades. In aerobic exercise and stress test, the HR increase is related to the oxygen consumption, used to measure cardiovascular fitness. HR during recovery from exercise stress test has been proposed as predictor of mortality [29].

HR variability (HRV), the beat-to-beat variation in either HR or in R-R intervals, has become an established clinical research tool. In [30] a series of HRV measures were studied, including statistical (SDNN, SDANN, RMSSD, SDNN index, SDSD, pNN50), geometric (HRV triangular index, TINN), and frequency (ULF, VLF, LF, HF, LF/HF) measures, (see Table 1) and their suitability in short term and long term recordings was examined. The HRV is modulated by the interplay between the two branches of the Autonomic Nervous System (ANS); the sympathetic ANS branch increases HR and has a slow response, while the parasympathetic branch decreases HR and the response is faster. In Fig. 3, the decrease of HRV with increasing involvement of sympathetic nervous system (higher exercise intensity and higher HR) is depicted. HRV is also affected by numerous factors, including long term conditions such as age and cardiovascular status, or short term ones, such as stress, exercise, medication, and therefore stationarity with respect to long-term recordings has to be taken into account.

Numerous studies have suggested the value of HRV as a predictor of cardiovascular deterioration or mortality [32]. HR dynamics were modelled as stochastic point process methods in [33], and the proposed descriptors were employed in different dynamic conditions. Non-linear and complexity features have been proposed for the characterization of HR dynamics [34], including Poincare indices, Sample entropy, Detrended fluctuation analysis, which provide new insights into the HRV changes

Table 1 Time-domain measures of HRV [30]

Variable	Description	Equation
Standard deviation of the NN interval	SDNN	$SDSD = \sqrt{\frac{1}{N-1}\sum_{j=1}^{N}\left(RR_j - \overline{RR}\right)^2}$
Standard deviation of the average of NN intervals calculated over short periods (usually 5 min)	SDANN	
Root mean square of successive differences	RMSSD	$SDSD = \sqrt{\frac{1}{N-1}\sum_{j=1}^{N}\left(\Delta RR_j\right)^2}$
Mean of the standard deviation of all NN intervals calculated over the windowed RR intervals, (usually 5 min)	SDNN index	
Standard deviation of successive differences	SDSD	$SDSD = \sqrt{\frac{1}{N-1}\sum_{j=1}^{N}\left(\Delta RR_j - \overline{\Delta RR}\right)^2}$
Percentage of differences between adjacent RR intervals that are greater than 50 ms to the total number of RR intervals	pNN50	$pNN50 = \left(\sum NN50/\sum NN\right)$
Integral of the density distribution (that is, the number of all RR intervals) divided by the maximum of the density distribution	HRV triangular index	HRV triangular index $= \sum_{j=1}^{N} RR/Y$
The baseline width of the RR distribution measured as the base of a triangle	TINN	$TINN = M - N$

$NN50$ is the number of interval differences of successive RR intervals greater than 50 ms

The most frequent NN interval length X is established, that is $Y = D(X)$ the maximum of the sample density distribution D. N and M are calculated as the time so that $g(t) = 0$ for $t \leq N$ and $t \geq M$ and $q(t) = Y$ and $\int_0^\infty (D(t) - q(t))^2 dt$ is the minimum among all selections of the values N and M

under various physiological and pathophysiological conditions, linking decreased HRV complexity decrease with aging and disease. The parameters and settings (e.g. window length) for calculation of HR complexity need careful consideration rather than default use. In addition, as a single feature may not be enough, these methods need to be considered in a multivariate approach in order to describe the complex

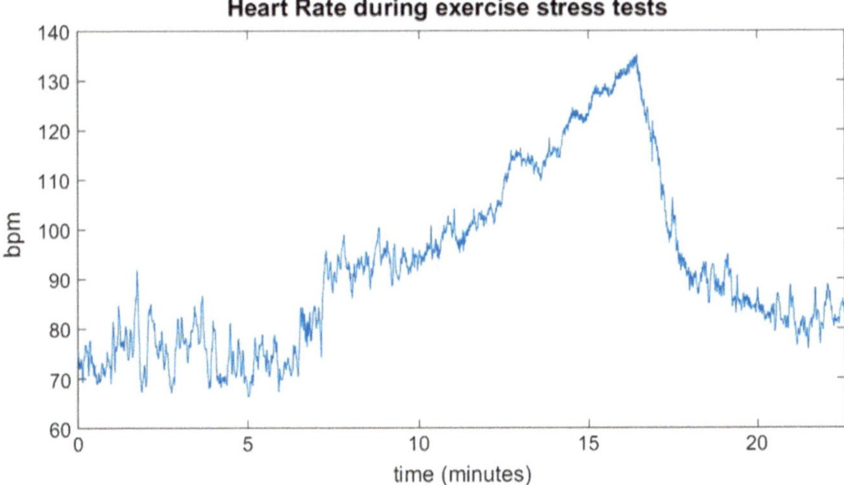

Fig. 3 The HR of an individual underwent exercise stress test from the physionet's MIT-BIH ST change database [31]. As expected, the HRV is higher when the HR is low while it decreases when the HR is high

HR control system. In [35], a machine learning approach including feature selection and classification, showed that a combination of nonlinear features and linear HRV features best predicted cardiovascular and cerebrovascular events.

4 Methods and Clinical Use

4.1 Analysis of ECG Waves: Features and Use

For reader facilitation, the methods that have been proposed are divided according to the specific ECG wave that they are focused to.

4.1.1 P-Wave Analysis

The atrial depolarization is represented on the surface ECG as the P-wave. The first part of this wave corresponds mainly to right atrial depolarization, while the second part to the left atrial depolarization [8, 36]. Surface ECG closely correlates with the conduction in specific parts of the atria [37, 38] and thus any deflection of the P-wave characteristics implies regional changes in atrial activation time and conduction route.

There are different approaches dealing with the analysis of the P-wave. The first approach is based on the extraction of an average P-wave which is supposed to represent all the P-waves of the signal. Several methods describe the methods for the extraction of the averaged P-wave and those methods can be categorized as those referred as QRS complex triggered and P-wave triggered. Both methods have advantages and disadvantages mainly based on the PQ and PR interval variability [39]. Some of the time domain characteristics include P-wave duration [40], P-wave dispersion [41], defined as the difference between the longest and the shortest P-wave duration in a 10 s ECG as they are recorded from multiple ECG leads, the duration of the high frequency (40–250 Hz) P-wave and the root mean square amplitude [42]. Additional time domain characteristics were also proposed including P-wave variance which is defined as the square of the standard deviation of the P-waves duration and it is considered less independent on P-wave morphology and more reproducible [43], or PR interval [44].

An alternative approach that gets increasingly popular relies on the analysis of the time domain characteristics of the P-waves in a beat-to-beat basis [45] and the results demonstrate the increased variability of specific features as Paroxysmal AF onset approximates suggesting a distributed conduction in the atrial substrate. The parameters inspected are the distance between the P-wave peak and its onset and offset as well as the intervals from the onset, the peak and the offset of the P-wave up to the R peak.

The last approach focuses on the analysis of the morphological characteristics of the P-waves. This approach gained the attention of research community in order to detect any local conduction disturbances as it reflects the three-dimensional course of atrial depolarization, as a projection of the depolarization vector on the ECG lead axes. These techniques are based on the extraction of an average P-wave morphology [46] or the consideration of predefined types of morphologies [47]. Later, each P-wave is characterized as following specific types of P-wave morphologies denoting the existence of pathological substrate in the atrial myocardium.

4.1.2 QRS Analysis

The amplitude and the duration of the QRS complex reflects the ventricular depolarization [39]. According to [48] a total of four parameters were proposed to characterize QRS complexes:

1. The duration or width of the QRS complex
2. The maximum amplitude minus the minimum amplitude of the QRS complex
3. The positive or negative vertical distance from the midpoint of the baseline to the center of the QRS complex. The baseline is defined as the straight line connecting the temporal boundary points of the QRS complex. The center is defined as the midpoint between the highest and lowest bounds in amplitude of the QRS complex

4. The area under the QRS waveform rectified with respect to a straight line through the midpoint of the baseline.

The usefulness of measuring the QRS width during exercise for identifying myocardial ischemia has been reported [49] and its prolongation can be considered as a marker of percutaneous transluminal coronary angioplasty success [50]. In [51], the relation between the different types of QRS morphologies, in terms of left bundle-branch block (LBBB), right bundle-branch block (RBBB) and nonspecific intraventricular conduction delay (NIVCD), and the QRS duration was studied in order to verify the benefit from cardiac resynchronization therapy (CRT). QRS fragmentation [52] has been proposed as a marker with prognostic value after Acute Myocardial Infarction (AMI) [53] or a predictor of response to CRT [54]. The latter work employs time-scale QRS morphology to characterize fragmentation.

4.1.3 ST Morphology

ST segment represents the interval between ventricular depolarisation and repolarization. The segment from J-point to the start of T-wave is expected to be close to the baseline, and deviations are related to abnormal conduction of various origins [55]. In [56] two types of ST segment morphology were considered (concave or non-concave). This classification was based on the drawing of a line between the J-point and the peak of the T-wave. Concave was considered a morphology in case an area is noted below the line and above ST segment while non-concave in case an area is noted above the line and be—low the ST segment or the line falls directly on the ST segment. According to the results, non-concave STE morphology is more frequent in acute myocardial infraction patients.

4.1.4 T-Wave Alternans

T-wave alternans (TWA) are defined as a beat-to-beat fluctuation in the morphology and the amplitude of the ST segment of T-wave. This marker reflects the special heterogeneities of repolarization of myocardial regions leading to lethal arrhythmogenesis such as ventricular tachycardia or ventricular fibrillation [26]. The most commonly used time domain method for the analysis of the ST-segment and T-wave is the modified moving average (MMA) method [57]. According to this method, the odd and even beats are separated into different clusters and are averaged. The average complexes are then superimposed and the maximum difference between the odd and even complexes at any point within the JT-segment is averaged for every 10 or 15 s and reported as the TWA value. This method can be used either during 24 h ECG monitoring or during standard exercise test while in contrary to other methods, no HR target is required while no special electrode is needed.

Table 2 Commonly used QT interval variations measures [58]

Variable	Description	Equation
Standard deviation of QT	SDQT	$SDQT = \sqrt{\frac{\sum(QT_n - QT_{mean})^2}{N}}$
Variance of QT interval normalized to the squared mean QT interval	QTVN	$QTVN = \frac{SDQT^2}{QT_{mean}^2}$
Short-term variability of QT	STVQT	$STVQT = \sum \frac{\lvert QT_{n+1} - QT_n \rvert}{N\sqrt{2}}$
Long-term variability of QT	LTVQT	$LTVQT = \sum \frac{\lvert QT_{n+1} - QT_n - 2QT_{mean} \rvert}{N\sqrt{2}}$
QT interval variability-to-HRV ratio	QTVi	$QTVi = log \frac{QTVN}{HRVN}$
Short-term variability of QT to Short-term variability of RR	Variability ratio; VR	$VR = \frac{STVQT}{STVRR}$

$STVRR = \sum \frac{\lvert RR_{n+1} - RR_n \rvert}{N\sqrt{2}}$ and $HRVN = \frac{HR_{var}}{HR_{mean}^2}$, where HR_{var} is the variance of the HR time series and N is the total number of beats

4.1.5 QT Interval Variability

QT interval variability (QTV) is defined as the fluctuation of the distance between Q and the end of the T-wave (Tend) in a beat-to-beat basis. It reflects the variations in ventricular depolarization and repolarization [58]. QTV analysis presents a series of challenges, including the accurate delineation of the T-wave end, and needs careful consideration of the best lead for single lead analysis, stationarity, and recording duration. The T-wave amplitude is inversely related to the QT interval variability and temporal QT interval variations may differ among recording locations, due to lead-specific interference and local repolarization heterogeneity. Table 2 summarizes the most commonly used QTV measures. QTV is widely used for screening patients with CAD, Left Ventricular (LV) hypertrophy and/or LV systolic dysfunction [59].

4.2 Characteristic Clinical Application Areas

The main goal of the analysis of a biosignal, including ECG, consists the extraction of useful information that could assist the clinical expert in the decision making, tailoring the intervention strategy for a patient. In this section the application of the TDA of the ECG, into several clinical areas are described.

4.2.1 Prediction of Pathological Atrial Electrical Activity

The main factors which influence the P-wave morphology include: [18] the origin of the sinus rhythm, [1] the left atrial breakthrough and [19] both the shape and the size of the atrial chambers which affect the time required for the depolarization process completion. Apart from the aforementioned factors, any structural abnormalities contributing to the slowing and propagation of the electrical activation may influence the P-wave morphology [60].

Based on the time domain analysis, specific thresholds were set on the P-wave duration in order to discriminate Atrial Fibrillation (AF) patients from healthy subjects and its prolongation (>120 ms) has been associated with a history of AF [61]. P-wave dispersion [41] and it is widely used for predicting the subjects prone to AF (>58 ms). Additionally, the duration of the high frequency (40–250 Hz) P-wave and the root mean square amplitude was also studied [42] and it was shown that these parameters may be helpful for the identification of patients underwent direct-current cardioversion and who are prone to recurrences. All these studies denoted statistical significant differences between AF patients and healthy subjects.

However, patients without structural heart disease may not have any impressive P-wave prolongation [62] and thus time characteristics may not reveal the development of AF. The analysis of the time domain characteristics in a beat to beat basis was studied in [45] and the results demonstrate the increased variability of specific features as Paroxysmal AF onset approximates suggesting a distributed conduction in the atrial substrate. The parameters inspected was the distance between the P-wave peak and its onset and offset as well as the intervals from the onset, the peak and the offset of the P-wave up to the R peak.

Regarding the analysis of the morphological characteristics of the P-waves, most of the studies combine beat-to-beat analysis of the P-wave with correlation techniques in order to extract the average P-wave [47, 63]. The idea behind the beat-to-beat analysis is that mild to moderate remodeling may not change the P-wave morphology constantly. In [47], the outcome of the circumferential pulmonary vein isolation (CPVI) was studied in terms of P-wave morphology. According to this study, each beat was classified, according to its morphology, into one of five predefined classes. The most common P-wave morphology observed was defined as the dominant morphology. Additionally, the percentage of the P-waves with non-dominant morphology (PMV) is extracted and it is reported that an increased PMV can be associated with CPVI success. In [63], the P-wave morphology of the average P-wave is modelled by fitting a combination of Gaussian functions. The results demonstrate that the P-wave morphology can be effectively modeled. The results denote that the morphological parameters extracted can effectively identify patients of different risks for AF development.

The results can be further improved in case time-domain and morphological parameters are combined. In [46] a semi-automated algorithm is proposed and applied to healthy subjects in order to explore the changes in P-wave morphology. Via k-means clustering, each beat is classified, under the strong assumption that two clusters exist in the P-wave morphology in each signal. The need for standardization of time domain analysis for assessing atrial fibrillation has been highlighted in [64].

4.2.2 Heart Rhythm and Arrhythmic Beat Detection

An "arrhythmia" refers generally to a problem of the HR (too fast or too slow) or the rhythm (irregular pattern of the heartbeat). The HR provides the necessary information for tachycardia/bradycardia characterization, but ECG morphology is required in detection of other types.

In [65] an attempt was made towards the classification of the heart beats, based on the morphological characteristics of the QRS complexes in the time domain, including QRS complex width, maximal point of positive and negative peak, area of QRS complex, onset to maximum negative/positive peak, VCG vector maximum, QRS slope velocity. The study focused on the arrhythmias which have effect on the QRS waveforms like Premature Ventricular Contractions (PVC), Left Bundle Branch Blocks (LBBB), Right Bundle Branch Blocks (RBBB) and Paced Beats (PB).

Typically, arrhythmia beat classification follows the five types of arrhythmia recommended by the Association for Advancement of Medical Instrumentation: non-ectopic beats (N), supra-ventricular ectopic beats (S), ventricular ectopic beats (V), fusion beats (F) and unclassifiable and paced beats (U), while some methods also distinguished RBBB and LBBB. Machine learning techniques have been extensively used for arrhythmic beat detection [66], Including Higher Order Statistics (HOS) and PCA [67], time-frequency features (wavelet or S-transform) [68] in combination with RR-based features and sophisticated classifiers, such as Support Vector Machine (SVM) classifiers. The database principally used was the MIT-BIH Arrhythmia database, and high accuracy (over 90%) was reached. The ability for generalization beyond this reference database is sparsely examined.

4.2.3 Detection of Acute Myocardial Infarction (AMI) and Ischemia

There exist two types of AMI. The first type, so-called ST-elevation myocardial infraction (STEMI), occurs when a complete vascular occlusion exists resulting transmural ischemia. In the ECG a ST-elevation is observed. The patient in this category are in higher risk for adverse events [69]. On the other hand, the non ST-elevation myocardial infraction (NSTEMI) is most common and it results in ST-depression, T-wave inversion or no ECG change at all. It is mentioned [70], that 25% of patient with AMI have no detectable ECG abnormalities. This is the reason why the most important challenge in current research is on the early detection of Coronary Artery Disease (CAD) and of exercise induced myocardial ischemia before the occurrence of the first AMI. In this respect, ST-segment depression criterion have been used for years however the clinical usefulness has been limited by poor sensitivity.

Apart from observation of the ST-segment and T-wave changes representing the ventricular repolarization, the analysis of the T-waves and T-loops morphology from a vectorcardiography can be used as a marker of myocardial infraction [71]. However, myocardial infraction also affects the depolarization of the ventricles, which occurs during the QRS complex, the analysis of which is more challenging because of its subtle changes, non-detectable by a clinical expert's eye. The amplitude of the R and S waves [72, 73] and the changes of the QRS slope and morphological QRS angles changes [74] and vectors have been used for the detection of ischemia.

More sophisticated methods include the observation of the amplitude and morphology of the high frequency components of the QRS (HF-QRS) [75] while those signals decrease in the existence of ischemia. Finally, a promising QRS score has been proposed [76] for the detection of myocardial ischemia. For this score, the amplitude of the Q, R and S wave were subtracted from the values prior to an exercise test. In [77], prediction of thrombolysis success after AMI was based on morphological features of QRS and ST, which however were calculated via time-frequency areas and amplitudes.

4.2.4 Risk Stratification of Sudden Cardiac Death

The stratification of patient for Sudden Cardiac Death (SCD) is of high importance in order to select the optimal treatment. The existence of ventricular arrhythmias, such as ventricular tachycardia and fibrillation is responsible for the half of SCD events. Several ECG markers have been proposed in order to assess either the ventricular depolarization or repolarization.

QRS duration (QRSd) was found to correlate with mortality in patients with structural heart disease [78]. A QRS score, based on 54 criteria form 10 leads has been also used for assessing the viability after myocardial infraction [79] and a value greater than 5 has been associated with increased mortality [80]. Apart from QRS score, fragmentation of the QRS (fQRS) complexes can also been used for the assessment of myocardial scar and fibrosis [52]. Fragmented QRS are defined as presence of one of more additional R wave (R′) or notching in the nadir of the S wave and can be also been associated with increased mortality. The existence of ventricular late potentials (VLP) has been suggested with [24]. Existence of VLP is typically quantified by time domain features of the high resolution signal averaged ECG, root mean square amplitude of the last 40 ms (RMS40), high frequency low amplitude signals less than 40 mV (HFLAS40), in addition to frequency domain methods (power spectral density of the last 40 ms) and time-frequency methods.

In addition to the ventricular depolarization, the repolarization heterogeneities of the ventricles can be assessed either by the use of the QRS-T angle [81], as measured between the QRS and T-wave vectors, or corrected QT interval (QTc) which is an estimation of the distance between Q and T at a HR of 60 bpm, while prolongation of this marker is predictive of SCD [82]. In addition the dispersion of the QT-interval, measured as the difference between the shortest and the longest QT in 12 leads ECG, can also quantify the heterogeneities during the repolarization of the ventricles [83]. Finally, T-wave peak to T-wave end interval (Tpe) is a marker which also shown to reveal the ventricular heterogeneities [84].

5 Discussion

A series of time domain methods for ECG analysis were presented, linked with their clinical application. The signal improvement, delineation of ECG waves, and the heart beat characterisation have been investigated in numerous studies with a wide range of time-domain biosignal processing and machine learning methods, although usually not in a multilead manner. Testing and comparison against available benchmark databases has been a positive widely adopted step so far, which would need to be complemented by further evaluation in data derived from different contexts.

The most characteristic group of clinically adopted methods focuses on ECG wave intervals or amplitudes, as measured in the average signals. As these methods have been evaluated specific clinical setups, their robustness in beat to beat ECG analysis and ECGs recorded in different unsupervised setups and physiological factors needs further elaboration, including normative values.

A second group of methods revolves around the temporal variability of wave intervals or of morphologies (RR, QT, T-wave alternans, P-wave clusters). While these approaches are dynamic and promising, also in terms of systemic approach, and have incorporated a series of sophisticated measures, the main factors that affect these dynamics have to be modelled and incorporated in such analysis. In addition, taking into account findings of spatial dispersion of morphologies, and elaboration of methods investigating spatiotemporal dynamics [85], and meticulously linking them with smaller scale phenomena (e.g. electrograms and action potentials) would leverage the computational electrocardiology within a systems medicine and 'in silico cardiology' framework.

The typical clinical electrocardiology approaches have been focusing on univariate analysis towards validating simple practical markers of a disease. Investing on multiparametric models, although more resource demanding, is expected to lead to more accurate and personalized approaches. Such approaches could combine morphological information (e.g. from wavelet analysis) and temporal information (e.g. wave durations), along with rhythm/rate information. Overall, while more sophisticated timescale measures and machine learning methods have been proposed and tested, either in benchmark or legacy databases, they have not been widely adopted. The two main barriers are (a) the reproducibility and validation of various methods in a wide range of clinical datasets, including a clear specification of the setups and parameters in each dataset, and (b) the availability of published methods in for testing by clinicians in user friendly analytics frameworks that can be accessible in clinical practice. The generation of big ECG databases with recordings at different conditions could help towards offering new challenging benchmarking frameworks for the evaluation and further leverage of computational electrocardiology.

Moving beyond the current landscape, the progress of electronics, information and communication technologies is gradually leading to the adoption of cost-effective strategies for ambulatory ECG monitoring and remote patient monitoring services. Holter smartphone applications [86] coupled with non-invasive sensors and wearable sensors, are suggested for the detection of arrhythmia and other events of clinical importance in the home environment and during activities of daily life. Therefore, relevant methods need to be extended and validated with noisy data [87], non-standard leads, different contextual parameters in uncontrolled environments, in order to ensure robustness of medical (not just consumer) quality and decrease false alarms. Smart techniques, data fusion, information redundancy can contribute in this direction.

The remote patient monitoring employing ECG and relevant biosignals is expected to lead to an unprecedented amount of ECG data that would require real time analysis embedded in the monitoring and response technology, both for robust real time alarming and even intervention (e.g. defibrillators), and for storing to be reused. These developments are constituting the electrocardiology as a big data domain [88], in terms of data management and analytics. As the necessary data is gradually getting available, big data approaches for predictive modelling in electrocardiology, such as deep learning [89], are emerging and expected to offer new knowledge and open new perspectives.

References

1. AlGhatrif M, Lindsay J (2012) A brief review: history to understand fundamentals of electrocardiography. J Community Hosp Intern Med Perspect 2(1):1–5
2. Couderc JP (2012) The telemetric and holter ECG warehouse (THEW): the first three years of development and research. J Electrocardiol 45(6):677–683
3. Badilini F (1998) The ISHNE holter standard output file format. Ann. Noninvasive Electrocardiol 3(3 I): 263–266
4. Geselowitz DB (1964) Dipole theory in electrocardiography. Am J Cardiol 14(3):301–306
5. Yang H, Bukkapatnam STS, Komanduri R (2012) Spatiotemporal representation of cardiac vectorcardiogram (VCG) signals. Biomed Eng (Online) 11(1):16
6. Frank E (1956) An accurate, clinically practical system for spatial vectorcardiography. Circulation 13(5):737–749
7. Ornato JP et al (2009) Body surface mapping vs 12-lead electrocardiography to detect ST-elevation myocardial infarction. Am J Emerg Med 27(7):779–784
8. Malmivuo J, Plonsey R (2012) Bioelectromagnetism: principles and applications of bioelectric and biomagnetic fields. Oxford University Press, USA
9. Gima K, Rudy Y (2002) Ionic current basis of electrocardiographic waveforms: a model study. Circ Res 90(8):889–896
10. Lin YD, Hu YH (2008) Power-line interference detection and suppression in ECG signal processing. IEEE Trans Biomed Eng 55(1):354–357
11. Rahman MZU, Shaik RA, Reddy DVRK (2011) Cancellation of artifacts in ECG signals using block adaptive filtering techniques. In: Arabnia HR, Tran Q-N (eds) Software tools and algorithms for biological systems. Springer New York, New York, NY, pp 505–513
12. Luo S, Johnston P (2010) A review of electrocardiogram filtering. J Electrocardiol 486–496
13. Milanesi M et al (2008) Independent component analysis applied to the removal of motion artifacts from electrocardiographic signals. Med Biol Eng Compu 46(3):251–261
14. Kuzilek J et al (2014) Independent component analysis and decision trees for ECG holter recording de-noising. PLoS ONE, 9(6)
15. Martis RJ, Acharya UR, Adeli H (2014) Current methods in electrocardiogram characterization. Comput Biol Med 48(1):133–149

16. Pan J, Tompkins WJ (1985) A real-time QRS detection algorithm. IEEE transactions on biomedical engineering 32(3):230–236
17. Martínez A, Alcaraz R, Rieta JJ (2010) Application of the phasor transform for automatic delineation of single-lead ECG fiducial points. Physiol Meas 31(11):1467–1485
18. Akhbari M et al (2016) ECG denoising and fiducial point extraction using an extended Kalman filtering framework with linear and nonlinear phase observations. Physiol Meas 37(2):203–226
19. Almeida R et al (2009) Multilead ECG delineation using spatially projected leads from wavelet transform loops. IEEE Trans Biomed Eng 56(8):1996–2005
20. Slocum J, Sahakian A, Swiryn S (1992) Diagnosis of atrial fibrillation from surface electrocardiograms based on computer-detected atrial activity. J Electrocardiol 25(1):1–8
21. Vaya C et al (2007) Convolutive blind source separation algorithms applied to the electrocardiogram of atrial fibrillation: Study of performance. IEEE Trans Biomed Eng 54(8):1530–1533
22. Mateo J, Joaquín Rieta J (2013) Radial basis function neural networks applied to efficient QRST cancellation in atrial fibrillation. Comput Biol Med 43(2):154–163
23. Brembilla-Perrot B et al (2002) Absence of change of signal-averaged electrocardiogram identifies patients with ventricular arrhythmias who are non-responders to amiodarone. Int J Cardiol 83(1):47–55
24. Kamath GS et al (2011) Value of the signal-averaged electrocardiogram in arrhythmogenic right ventricular cardiomyopathy/dysplasia. Heart Rhythm 8(2):256–262
25. Tuzcu V et al (2000) P wave signal-averaged electrocardiogram as a new marker foratrial tachyarrhythmias in postoperative Fontan patients. J Am Coll Cardiol 36(2):602–607
26. Verrier R et al (2010) T-wave alternans as a therapeutic marker for antiarrhythmic agents. J Cardiovasc Pharmacol 55(6):544–554
27. Demidova MM et al (2014) Transient and rapid QRS-widening associated with a J-wave pattern predicts impending ventricular fibrillation in experimental myocardial infarction. Heart Rhythm 11(7):1195–1201
28. Censi F et al (2016) P-wave variability and atrial fibrillation. Sci Rep 6:26799
29. Cole CR et al (1999) Heart-rate recovery immediately after exercise as a predictor of mortality. N Engl J Med 341(18):1351–1357
30. Task-force (1996) Heart rate variability. Standards of measurement, physiological interpretation, and clinical use. Task Force of the European Society of Cardiology and the North American Society of Pacing and Electrophysiology. Eur Heart J 17(3): 354–381
31. Goldberger AL et al (2000) PhysioBank, PhysioToolkit, and PhysioNet: components of a new research resource for complex physiologic signals. Circulation 101(23):e215–e220
32. Brateanu A (2015) Heart rate variability after myocardial infarction: what we know and what we still need to find out. Curr Med Res Opin 31(10):1855–1860
33. Barbieri R et al (2005) A point-process model of human heartbeat intervals: new definitions of heart rate and heart rate variability. Am J Physiol Heart Circ Physiol 288(1):H424–H435
34. Voss A et al (2009) Methods derived from nonlinear dynamics for analysing heart rate variability. Philos Trans Ser A Math Phys Eng Sci 367(1887):277–296
35. Melillo P et al (2015) Automatic prediction of cardiovascular and cerebrovascular events using heart rate variability analysis. PLoS One 10(3)
36. Michelucci A et al (2002) P wave assessment: state of the art update. Cardiac Electrophysiol Rev 6(3):215–220
37. Dilaveris PE, Gialafos JE (2002) Future concepts in P wave morphological analyses. Card Electrophysiol Rev 6(3):221–224
38. Ndrepepa G et al (2000) Relationship between surface electrocardiogram characteristics and endocardial activation sequence in patients with typical atrial flutter. Z Kardiol 89(6):527–537
39. Poli S et al (2003) Prediction of atrial fibrillation from surface ECG: review of methods and algorithms. Annali dell'Istituto Superiore di Sanita 39(2):195–203
40. Hofmann M et al (1996) Analysis of the p wave in the signal-averaged electrocardiogram: normal values and reproducibility. Pacing Clin Electrophysiol 19(11):1928–1932
41. Dilaveris PE, Gialafos JE (2001) P-wave dispersion: a novel predictor of paroxysmal atrial fibrillation. Ann Noninvasive Electrocardiol Off J Int Soc Holter Noninvasive Electrocardiology, Inc 6(2): 159–165

42. Opolski G et al (1997) Detection of patients at risk for recurrence of atrial fibrillation after successful electrical cardioversion by signal-averaged p-wave ECG. Int J Cardiol 60(2):181–185
43. Andrikopoulos GK et al (2000) Increased variance of P wave duration on the electrocardiogram distinguishes patients with idiopathic paroxysmal atrial fihrillation 23(July)
44. Passman R et al (2001) Predicting post—coronary bypass surgery atrial arrhythmias from the preoperative electrocardiogram. Am Heart J 142(5):806–810
45. Martínez A, Alcaraz R, Rieta JJ (2012) Study on the P-wave feature time course as early predictors of paroxysmal atrial fibrillation. Physiol Meas 33(12):1959–1974
46. Herreros A et al (2009) Analysis of changes in the beat-to-beat P-wave morphology using clustering techniques. Biomed Signal Process Control 4(4):309–316
47. Huo Y et al (2015) Variability of P-wave morphology predicts the outcome of circumferential pulmonary vein isolation in patients with recurrent atrial fibrillation. J Electrocardiol 48(2):218–225
48. Rangayyan RM (2002) Biomedical signal analysis: a case-study approach. Signals 552
49. Michaelides A et al (1993) Exercise-induced QRS prolongation in patients with coronary artery disease: a marker of myocardial ischemia. Am Heart J 126(6):1320–1325
50. Takaki H et al (1999) Exercise-induced QRS prolongation in patients with mild coronary artery disease: computer analysis of the digitized multilead ECGs. J Electrocardiol 32 Suppl(0022–0736 (Print)): 206–211
51. Birnie DH et al (2013) Impact of QRS morphology and duration on outcomes after cardiac resynchronization therapy results from the resynchronization defibrillation for ambulatory heart failure trial (RAFT). Circ Heart Fail 6(6):1190–1198
52. Pietrasik G, Zareba W (2012) QRS fragmentation: diagnostic and prognostic significance. Cardiol J 19(2):114–121
53. Lorgis L et al (2013) Prognostic value of fragmented QRS on a 12-lead ECG in patients with acute myocardial infarction. Heart Lung J Acute Crit Care 42(5):326–331
54. Vassilikos VP et al (2014) QRS analysis using wavelet transformation for the prediction of response to cardiac resynchronization therapy: a prospective pilot study. J Electrocardiol 47(1):59–65
55. Dodd KW, Elm KD, Smith SW (2016) Comparison of the QRS complex, ST-segment, and T-wave among patients with left bundle branch block with and without acute myocardial infarction. J Emerg Med 51(1):1–8
56. Brady WJ et al (2001) Electrocardiographic ST-segment elevation: the diagnosis of acute myocardial infarction by morphologic analysis of the ST segment. Acad Emerg Med Off J Soc Acad Emerg Med 8(10):961–967
57. Verrier RL, Nearing BD (2002) Modified moving average analysis of T-wave alternans to predict ventricular fibrillation with high accuracy. J Appl Physiol 92(2):541–549
58. Baumert M et al (2016) QT interval variability in body surface ECG: measurement, physiological basis, and clinical value: position statement and consensus guidance endorsed by the European Heart Rhythm Association jointly with the ESC Working Group on Cardiac Cellular Electroph. Europace : European pacing, arrhythmias, and cardiac electrophysiology : journal of the working groups on cardiac pacing, arrhythmias, and cardiac cellular electrophysiology of the European Society of Cardiology, p euv405
59. Schlegel TT et al (2010) Accuracy of advanced versus strictly conventional 12-lead ECG for detection and screening of coronary artery disease, left ventricular hypertrophy and left ventricular systolic dysfunction. BMC Cardiovasc Disord 10:28
60. Platonov PG (2012) P-wave morphology: Underlying mechanisms and clinical implications. Ann Noninvasive Electrocardiol 17(3):161–169
61. Stafford PJ, Turner I, Vincent R (1991) Quantitative analysis of signal averaged p wave in idiopathic paroxysmal atrial fibrillation. Am J Cardiol 751–755
62. Jurkko R et al (2008) High-resolution signal-averaged analysis of atrial paroxysmal lone atrial fibrillation. Ann Noninvasive Electrocardiol 13(4):378–385
63. Censi F et al (2007) P-wave morphology assessment by a Gaussian functions-based model in atrial fibrillation patients. IEEE Trans Biomed Eng 54(4):663–672

64. Schotten U, Maesen B, Zeemering S (2012) The need for standardization of time-and frequency-domain analysis of body surface electrocardiograms for assessment of the atrial fibrillation substrate. Europace 14(8):1072–1075
65. Christov I et al (2006) Comparative study of morphological and time-frequency ECG descriptors for heartbeat classification. Med Eng Phys 28(9):876–887
66. Luz EJS et al (2016) ECG-based heartbeat classification for arrhythmia detection: a survey. Comput Methods Programs Biomed 127: 144–164
67. Elhaj FA et al (2016) Arrhythmia recognition and classification using combined linear and nonlinear features of ECG signals. Comput Methods Programs Biomed 127:52–63
68. Raj S, Ray KC, Shankar O (2016) Cardiac arrhythmia beat classification using DOST and PSO tuned SVM. Comput Methods Programs Biomed 136:163–177
69. Steg PG et al (2012) ESC guidelines for the management of acute myocardial infarction in patients presenting with ST-segment elevation. Eur Heart J 33(20):2569–2619
70. Reichlin T et al (2009) Early diagnosis of myocardial infarction with sensitive cardiac troponin assays. N Engl J Med 361:858–867
71. Rubulis A et al (2004) T vector and loop characteristics in coronary artery disease and during acute ischemia. Heart Rhythm 1(3):317–325
72. Barnhill JE et al (1989) Depolarization changes early in the course of myocardial infarction: significance of changes in the terminal portion of the QRS complex. J Am Coll Cardiol 14(1):143–149
73. Surawicz B et al (1997) QRS changes during percutaneous transluminal coronary angioplasty and their possible mechanisms. J Am Coll Cardiol 30(2):452–458
74. Romero D et al (2016) Ischemia detection from morphological QRS angle changes. Physiol Meas 37(7):1004–1023
75. Pettersson J et al (2000) Changes in high-frequency QRS components are more sensitive than ST-segment deviation for detecting acute coronary artery occlusion. J Am Coll Cardiol 36(6):1827–1834
76. van Campen CM, Visser FC, Visser CA (1996) The QRS score: a promising new exercise score for detecting coronary artery disease based on exercise-induced changes of Q-, R- and S-waves: a relationship with myocardial ischaemia. Eur Heart J 17(5):699–708
77. Chouvarda J et al (2003) Wigner-Ville analysis and classification of electrocardiograms during thrombolysis. Med Biol Eng Comput 41(6):609–617
78. Kalahasti V et al (2003) QRS duration and prediction of mortality in patients undergoing risk stratification for ventricular arrhythmias. Am J Cardiol 92(7)(United States PT-Journal Article LG-English): 798–803
79. Strauss DG et al (2008) ECG quantification of myocardial scar in cardiomyopathy patients with or without conduction defects: correlation with cardiac magnetic resonance and arrhythmogenesis. Circ Arrhythm Electrophysiol 1(5):327–336
80. Strauss DG et al (2013) Screening entire health system ECG databases to identify patients at increased risk of death. Circ Arrhythm Electrophysiol 6(6): 1156–1162
81. Gotsman I et al (2013) Usefulness of electrocardiographic frontal qrs-t angle to predict increased morbidity and mortality in patients with chronic heart failure. Am J Cardiol 111(10):1452–1459
82. Chugh SS et al (2009) Determinants of prolonged QT interval and their contribution to sudden death risk in coronary artery disease: the Oregon sudden unexpected death study. Circulation 119(5):663–670
83. Glancy JM et al (1995) QT dispersion and mortality after myocardial infarction. Lancet 345(0140–6736):945–948
84. Patel C et al (2009) Is there a significant transmural gradient in repolarization time in the intact heart?: cellular basis of the T wave: a century of controversy. Circ Arrhythm Electrophysiol 2(1): 80–88
85. Erem B et al (2016) Extensions to a manifold learning framework for time-series analysis on dynamic manifolds in bioelectric signals. Phys Rev E Stat Nonlinear Soft Matter Phys 93(4)
86. Kennedy HL (2013) The evolution of ambulatory ECG monitoring. Prog Cardiovasc Dis 56(2):127–132

87. Clifford GD et al (2011) Signal quality indices and data fusion for determining acceptability of electrocardiograms collected in noisy ambulatory environments. In: 2011 Computing in cardiology (CinC), vol 1419, pp 285–288
88. Deserno TM, Marx N (2016) Computational electrocardiography: revisiting holter ECG monitoring. Methods Inf Med 55(4):305–311
89. Choi E et al (2016) Using recurrent neural network models for early detection of heart failure onset. J Am Med Inform Assoc JAMIA 292(3):344–350

Estimation of Cardiovascular Variability

George Manis

Abstract The heart is a complex system. Its activity is affected by and affects most of the vital organs of the human body. The large number of factors influencing it results into a complicated functionality, characterized by physiological variability, difficult to be predicted and modeled. This variability hides valuable information expressing the ability of the heart to respond to normal autonomic functions of the body and to react to external events. It is used in clinical practice for both diagnosis and prognosis. It can be described with many indices, like the heart rate variability, the QT variability, the ST variability, the deceleration capacity, etc. A large number of methods have been proposed for estimating these indices, including statistical methods, frequency domain methods and non-linear ones. The research in the field is very active. A large number of papers has been published during the last two decades in the field and this number increases day by day with a continuously increasing rate.

1 Introduction

With the term *Cardiovascular Variability* we refer to any kind of variability related to the functionality of the heart and/or the vascular system. The most popular one is *Heart Rate Variability*, but other kinds of variability, like *QT variability*, *T-wave alternans* or indexes like *Deceleration Capacity* are also in the center of the attention of the research community.

The cardiovascular system consists of the heart and the blood vessels, which transfer the oxygen and other useful or waste materials through the blood to the rest of the body. The heart coordinates the cardiovascular system, a difficult and

G. Manis (✉)
Department of Computer Science & Engineering, University of Ioannina,
Ioannina, Greece
e-mail: manis@cs.uoi.gr

S. Golemati and K. S. Nikita (eds.), *Cardiovascular Computing—Methodologies and Clinical Applications*, Series in BioEngineering,
https://doi.org/10.1007/978-981-10-5092-3_5

complicated task, affected by several factors and affecting almost every organ in our body. It is not difficult to realize that the heart is a complex system and the large number of factors affecting it results in a complicated, non-linear and difficult to be predicted functionality. Increased variability indicates an increased capability to respond to those factors, thus revealing a healthy situation. Decreased variability shows a decreased capability to react, a definitely unwanted behavior.

Cardiovascular variability is affected by (i) physiological parameters, like age and gender, (ii) lifestyle factors, like sporting activity, increased body weight, smoking and alcohol abuse, (iii) diseases including heart diseases, lung diseases and diabetes and (iv) external factors, like harmful substances and medication [31]. The heart is accelerated by the *sympathetic nervous system (SNS)* which is related to responses for external events. Those events can be considered as threads, or generally, need rapid reactions or extra body effort. On the other hand, the *parasympathetic nervous system (PSNS)* functions as decelerator of the heart rhythm and is connected to vital body activities like rest and digest.

2 Heart Rate Variability

Heart Rate Variability (*HRV*) expresses the variation of time intervals between successive heart beats. HRV is a physiological phenomenon and high variability is an indication of healthy heart functionality.

In Fig. 1, a part of an electrocardiogram is depicted, where *R* (peak) points and the time intervals between them are marked. The series of these intervals constitutes the HRV time series, which is what we study.

In 1996, guidelines for measurements, physiological interpretation and clinical use for HRV were published [36] from the European Society of Cardiology and the North American Society of Pacing and Electrophysiology. This article is the most cited one and commonly accepted as a standard in the field. The most common methods for HRV analysis are described there. Several other methods can be found in the literature, perhaps more than one hundred, the most important of which are described in the following. They can be divided into linear and non linear methods.

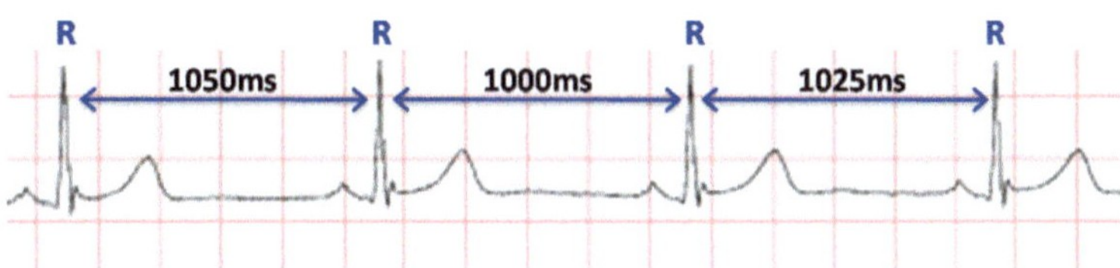

Fig. 1 Variability of heart rate

2.1 Linear Methods

Linear methods can be further divided into time domain, frequency domain and time-frequency domain methods. Time and frequency domain methods are described in [36]. In the same paper, geometrical methods are also discussed, but since they are not often used in practice, we selected not to present them here.

Linear methods in the time domain express the amount of the existing variability. Methods in frequency domain quantify the underlying rhythms and the amount of power in these rhythms. Time-frequency domain methods are somewhere in the middle. Non-linear methods investigate the complexity of the system.

2.1.1 Time Domain Methods

Time domain methods include the statistical ones. We mention here the:

- standard deviation of NN intervals ($SDNN$)
- root mean square of successive differences of adjacent intervals ($RMSSD$)
- standard deviation of the averages in 5 min segments of the entire recording ($SDANN$)
- mean of the standard deviations in 5 min segments of the entire recording ($SDNNindex$)
- standard deviation of successive differences of adjacent intervals ($SDSD$)
- probability adjacent NN intervals to differ more than 50 ms ($pNN50$)

Please note that we refer to NN and not to RR intervals, i.e. *Normal to Normal* beats. R points not considered as *normal*, e.g. ectopic beats, should be excluded from computations. Normal values reported in [36] for time-domain methods are: $SDNN = 141 \pm 39$ ms, $SDANN = 127 \pm 35$ ms, $RMSSD = 27 \pm 12$ ms.

In Fig. 2 we can see the discrimination achieved with time-domain methods, when applied on a dataset with two different groups of subjects (*fantasia* dataset [19]). The database is available on the internet [14]. Fantasia consists of 40 recordings, 20 from young subjects (21–34 years old) and 20 from elderly (68–85 years old), all healthy. All subjects remained in a resting state in sinus rhythm during recording while watching the movie Fantasia (Disney, 1940) to help maintain wakefulness. The continuous ECG signals were 120 min long. From the box plots in Fig. 2 it is not difficult to conclude that all metrics presented a statistically significant discrimination, and that the box plots do not overlap in any case. The most clear discrimination in this dataset is exhibited by $pNN50$.

2.1.2 Frequency Domain Methods

Frequency domain methods are based on spectral analysis. They use different metrics when considering short and long recordings. For short (5 min) recordings we compute the:

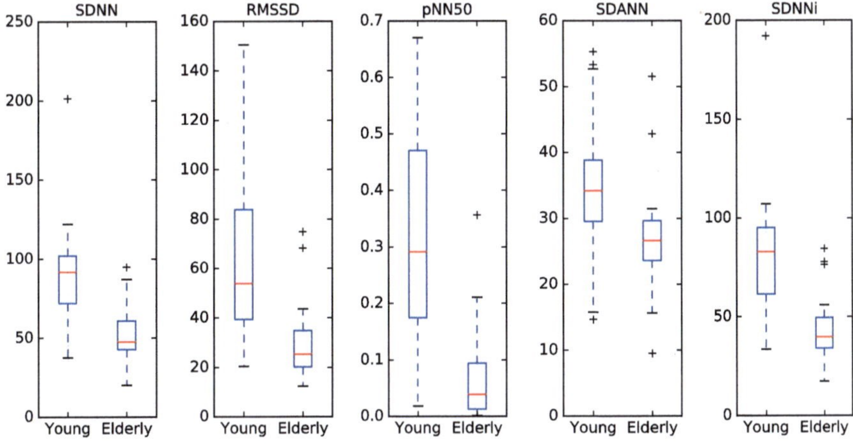

Fig. 2 Discrimination of young end elderly subject with time-domain methods

- total power TP ($f < 0.4$ Hz)
- power in very low frequencies VLF ($f < 0.04$)
- power in low frequencies LF ($0.04\,\text{Hz} < f < 0.15$ Hz)
- power in high frequencies HF ($0.15\,\text{Hz} < f < 0.4$ Hz).

The power in low and high frequencies can also be expressed in normalized units, with the amount $100 \times (TP - VLF)$ being the normalization factor:

- $LF_n = {}^{LF}/_{100 \times (TP - VLF)}$
- $HF_n = {}^{HF}/_{100 \times (TP - VLF)}$

The ratio LF/HF is also considered a useful index. Normal values for stationary 5 min recordings, as given in [36], are: $TP = 3466 \pm 1018\,\text{ms}^2$, $LF = 1170 \pm 416\,\text{ms}^2$, $HF = 975 \pm 203\,\text{ms}^2$, $LF_n = 54 \pm 4$, $HF_n = 29 \pm 3$, $LF/HF = 1.5$–2.0.

For long (24 h) recordings we compute again the:

- total power (TP)
- power in ultra low frequencies ULF ($f < 0.003$ Hz)
- power in low frequencies LF ($0.003\,\text{Hz} < f < 0.15$ Hz)
- power in high frequencies HF ($0.15\,\text{Hz} < f < 0.4$ Hz)

In Fig. 3 we can see the power spectral density of a short recording. There are two distinct frequency areas (one for low and one for high frequencies) in which the energy is increased. In this figure, the power at low frequencies seems to be higher than higher frequencies, indicating increased parasympathetic activity. Figure 4 presents the power spectrum of a long recording. The shape of the expected curve and the frequency areas in which we compute the indexes are shown.

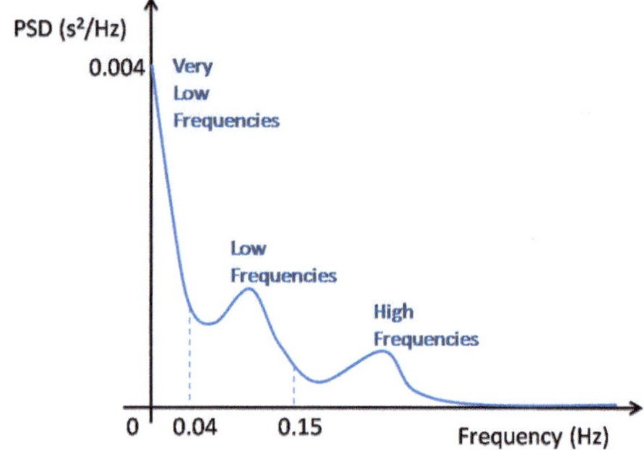

Fig. 3 Spectral analysis for short recordings

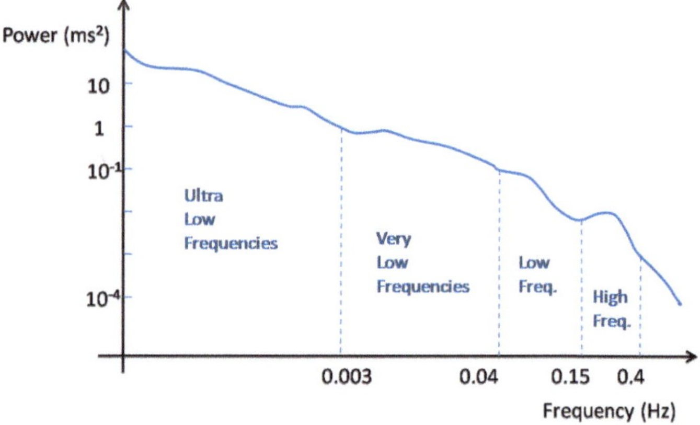

Fig. 4 Spectral analysis for long recordings

2.1.3 Time-Frequency Domain Methods

Time-frequency domain methods include the multiresolution wavelet analysis as described in [37]. *RR* time series are decomposed into wavelet coefficients in different scales of analysis with smaller scales corresponding to more rapid changes. Various wavelet families have been tested and can be used, but the *Haar* wavelet seems to be the most popular. In each scale, approximation and detail coefficients are produced. The approximation coefficients are used as input for the analysis of the next scale, while the standard deviation of the detailed coefficients serves as a measure of variability.

In [37], the authors report discrimination of healthy subjects from those with cardiac pathology in scales 4 and 5. In [23] the authors investigates different measures of variability for different scales of analysis, showing that a measure detecting

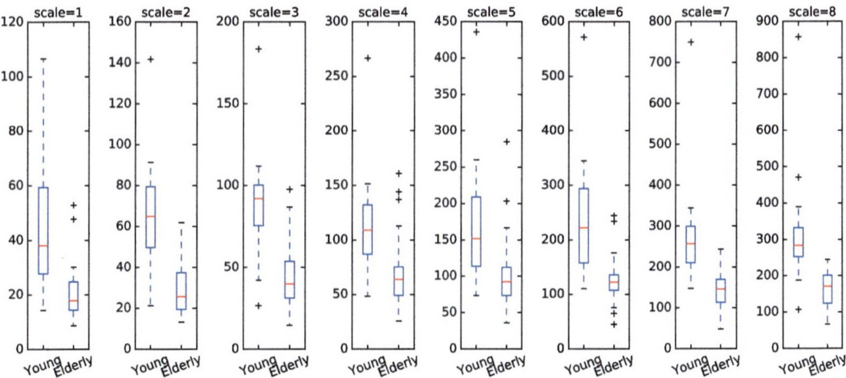

Fig. 5 Discrimination of young end elderly subject with wavelet analysis

adjacent point variations is more descriptive in smaller scales than the standard deviation which works better in larger scales.

Box plots for the fantasia dataset and for several scales of analysis are presented in Fig. 5. All scales exhibit a remarkable discrimination, with scales 2 and 3 presenting the clearest one for this dataset.

2.2 Non-linear Methods

In HRV guidelines [36], non-linear methods were also referred as means to analyze *RR* signals, but they were not given the same attention with the linear ones. This might was due to the limited use of non-linear methods in the analysis of HRV until then. Non-linear methods play today an important role in HRV, have gained the attention of the research community and are also used in clinical practice. Non linear methods attempt to extract deeper or more irregular correlations, which cannot be captured by the more traditional linear methods. They act complementary and do not replace the linear methods.

Twenty years after the publication of the guidelines in 1996, the e-Cardiology ESC Working Group and the European Heart Rhythm Association co-endorsed by the Asia Pacific Heart Rhythm Society published a new article [32]. In this article, methods not reported in 1996 guidelines were investigated. Well defined criteria for the selection of these methods were set, based on the number of publications, the quality of the journals and the size of the databases on which the methods were applied. Approximation Entropy (*ApEn*), Detrended Fluctuation Analysis (*DFA*) and the Poincaré plot satisfied best these criteria. In the following we will investigate each of them.

2.2.1 Approximate and Sample Entropy

Entropy is a measure of irregularity. It expresses the disorder in a system. It is also connected to the capability of a system to produce energy. In Information Technology, entropy describes the possible states of a system.

Approximate entropy is a definition of entropy based on self similarity of time series. It is also a *conditional entropy*, meaning that it compares entropy of a system described in a given dimension with the entropy of the same system described in a higher dimension. The method has been suggested by Pincus [28] and a detailed description follows.

Given the time series: $x = x_1, x_2, ..., x_N$, we select the value of m and create a new series of vectors:

$$\mathbf{x} = \mathbf{x}_1, \mathbf{x}_2, ..., \mathbf{x}_{N-m+1}, \quad \mathbf{x}_i = (x_i, x_{i+1}, x_{i+2}, ..., x_{i+m-1}).$$

We also select a value for the threshold r. The distance between the vectors $\mathbf{x}_i$ and $\mathbf{x}_j$ (of size m) is smaller than r when:

$$\left|x_{i+k} - x_{j+k}\right| < r, \quad \forall k, \quad 0 \leq k \leq m-1.$$

In this case we consider the two vectors as *similar* i.e. $\left\|\mathbf{x}_i - \mathbf{x}_j\right\|_m < r$.

Given the distance r, the probability a vector $\mathbf{x}_i$ of size m to be similar with the vector $\mathbf{x}_j$ of the same size is:

$$C_i^m(r) = \frac{\sum_{j=1}^{N-m+1} \Theta(i,j,m,r)}{N-m+1}, \quad \Theta(i,j,m,r) = \begin{cases} 1, \ \left\|\mathbf{x}_i - \mathbf{x}_j\right\|_m < r \\ 0, \ otherwise \end{cases}. \quad (1)$$

We define:

$$\Phi^m(r) = \frac{\sum_{i=1}^{N-m+1} \ln C_i^m(r)}{N-m+1}.$$

Approximate entropy is given by the difference:

$$ApEn(m,r) = \Phi^m(r) - \Phi^{m+1}(r).$$

The method has been extensively used in biomedical signal analysis, and other research fields as well, with very good results. Soon after it was proposed, it became a standard in non-linear analysis. At the same time, the method became subject to criticism and was accused as biased, mainly due to *self-matching*, i.e. checking if a vector is similar to itself (see Eq. 1 when $i = j$). Of course, every vector is similar to itself, something that makes the computed value dependent on the length of the time series. On the other hand, self-matching increases the stability and reduces the effect of outliers.

Taking into account the above concerns, a new method was suggested: *Sample Entropy* (*SampEn*) [29]. The last years *SampEn* increased its impact, became popular, is an evolution or at least modification of *ApEn*, and therefore, we included it in this section.

The description of *SampEn* is exactly the same with the description of *ApEn* up to the definition of similar points. After that, Eq. (1) is replaced by the definitions of $n_m(r)$ and $n_{m+1}(r)$, the probabilities a point to be similar with another point for embedding dimensions m and m+1 respectively:

$$n_m(r) = \sum_{j=1}^{N-m} \Theta(i, j, m, r), i \neq j \quad \text{and} \quad n_{m+1}(r) = \sum_{j=1}^{N-m} \Theta(i, j, m+1, r), i \neq j,$$

where $\Theta(i, j, m, r) = \begin{cases} 1, \ \left\|\mathbf{x}_i - \mathbf{x}_j\right\|_m < r \quad \text{and} \quad j > i \\ 0, \ otherwise \end{cases}.$

The quantities $B_i^m(r)$ and $A_i^m(r)$ are measures of similarity:

$$B_i^m(r) = \frac{1}{N-m-1} n_m, \quad i = 1 \ldots N-m, \quad \text{and}$$

$$A_i^m(r) = \frac{1}{N-m-1} n_{m+1}, \quad i = 1 \ldots N-m.$$

We compute the mean values:

$$B^m(r) = \frac{1}{N-m} \sum_{i=1}^{N-m} B_i^m(r) \quad \text{and} \quad A^m(r) = \frac{1}{N-m} \sum_{i=1}^{N-m} A_i^m(r).$$

Sample Entropy is given by the ratio:

$$SampEn(m, r) = \ln \frac{B^m(r)}{A^m(r)}.$$

Approximate and Sample entropy have found application in many studies. They are the most popular metrics of non-linear analysis. The main drawback of both methods is the existence of the two parameters, r and m. The results and their descriptive capability heavily rely on the estimation of those parameters. After extensive use, the researchers have concluded and agreed that the values $m = 2$ and $r = 0.2std(x)$, where $std(x)$ is the standard deviation of the signal, are the most typical values and should be preferred.

2.2.2 Detrended Fluctuation Analysis

Detrended Fluctuation Analysis (*DFA*) has been suggested by Peng [27]. Given the heartbeat time series $x = x_1, x_2, ..., x_N.$, we compute the integrated series:

$$y(k) = \sum_{i=1}^{k} (x_i - x_{avg}),$$

where x_{avg} is the average value of x. Next, we split $y(k)$ into non-overlapping windows of equal length n. We approximate the points in each window with a least squares line, which represents the *trend* in each window. The y coordinate of the line is denoted with $y_n(k)$. Then, we remove the trend, by subtracting the local trend in each window. The fluctuation of the detrended time series is given by the formula:

$$F(n) = \sqrt{\frac{1}{N} \sum_{k=1}^{N} [y(k) - y_n(k)]^2}$$

The computation is repeated for all values of n. $F(n)$ is plotted in a log to log plot. The slop a_1 of the curve in small scales ($4 \leq n \leq 16$) and the slop a_2 in large scales ($16 \leq n \leq 64$), as well as the ration a_1/a_2 are reported as the three indexes expressing the time series variability.

2.2.3 Poincaré Plot

Poincaré plot is generally used to examine self-similarities in time series. Given the time series: $x = x_1, x_2, ..., x_N$, we create all possible pairs (x_i, x_{i+1}) and plot them on a graph, so that x_i is the abscissa and x_{i+1} the ordinate. Using a curve fitting technique, we fit an ellipse to the resulting plot. Figure 6 shows the plotted pairs (x_i, x_{i+1}) and the fitted ellipse for a time series of *RR* intervals. SD_1 and SD_2 represent the dispersion along minor and major axis of the fitted ellipse and quantify the variability. Increased similarity between successive beats results in gathering of points close to the line of identity, i.e. smaller SD_1. Wide range of *RR* values increases the value of SD_2.

2.3 Clinical Use and Significance

Reduced heart rate variability is related to several specific pathologies, especially cardiovascular ones. Many researchers have shown that HRV is affected by myocardial infarction and low HRV is an indicator of mortality after myocardial infarction. We must mention here the landmark paper [22] and two review papers [9, 18] which

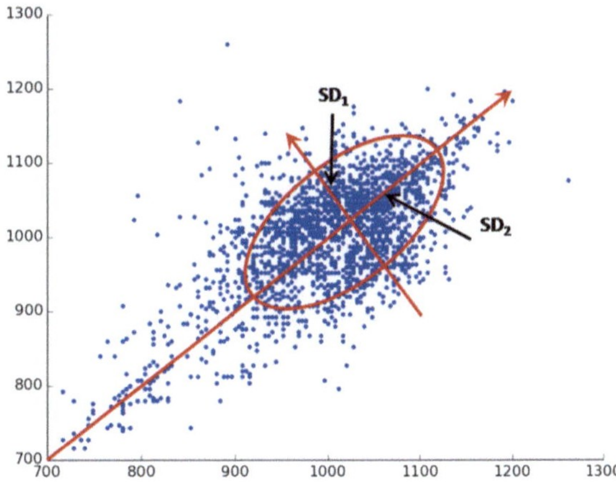

Fig. 6 Poincare plot of an *RR* time series

summarizes research work related to HRV and myocardial infarction. There is also a number of publications connecting findings from Holter recordings after HRV analysis and congestive heart failure [15, 39], as well as sudden cardiac death or heart arrest [2]. Dysfunction of the autonomous nervous system also results in hypertension [33].

We have already shown earlier in this section that HRV is affected by age when we showed a clear discrimination of young and elderly subjects using statistical time domain methods, as well as methods from the time-frequency domain. Publications with similar subject and results are [19, 20].

HRV is also decreased by several other pathologies which are not characterized as cardiovascular. We mention the reduction of HRV in patients with Diabetes Mellitus [10]. HRV is also connected to stress [34], smoking [17, 21], emotional situations [8] as well as several other factors.

3 Other Indexes Expressing Cardiovascular Variability

HRV methods are the most common means to study cardiovascular variability. It is not the only one way to do it, though. Other methods, based on the heart rate or not, are also be used expressing other types of variability. We will study here the deceleration capacity of heart rate, the QT variability and the T-wave alternans.

3.1 Deceleration Capacity

Deceleration Capacity of heart rate (DC) [4] is a measure of variability aiming to express the capability of the heart to decelerate its rhythm. It is based on the *PRSA*

(*Phase Rectified Signal Averaging*) method [5], according to which the whole signal is split into equal sized line segments and, after aligning, the average of these segments is computed. Let's see in detail, how DC is defined.

The first step is to detect the *anchor* points. An RR_i interval is considered as *anchor*, if it is longer than its preceding interval: $RR_i > RR_{i-1}$. At this point the heart decelerates its rhythm. From the anchor points we exclude as artifacts those which differ more than 5% from their preceding interval. Then, for each anchor RR_i we consider the four-interval segment: $RR_{i-2}, RR_{i-1}, RR_i, RR_{i+1}$. All segments are aligned and the averaged segment $\bar{RR}_{i-2}, \bar{RR}_{i-1}, \bar{RR}_i, \bar{RR}_{i+1}$ is computed. DC is given by the following formula:

$$DC = \frac{\bar{RR}_{i+1} + \bar{RR}_i - \bar{RR}_{i-1} - \bar{RR}_{i-2}}{4}.$$

Acceleration Capacity (AC) is defined in a similar way.

A modified version of Deceleration Capacity (DC_{sgn}) has been proposed in [3]. Two main modifications have been proposed there:

- all three points RR_{i+1}, RR_i and RR_{i-1} in a four-interval segment are checked if they differ more than 5% from their preceding interval. If at least one of them differs more than 5% from its preceding interval then the four-beat segment is excluded from computations. The original method allows beats that have been considered as artifacts during the anchor points detection to participate in the averaging process when they are not anchors.
- deceleration segments are considered those segments for which:

$$RR_{i+1} + RR_i - RR_{i-1} - RR_{i-2} > 0,$$

  eliminating the possibility to compute negative values for DC. A negative value in the computation of DC_{sign} is considered as acceleration. The original methods considers as deceleration segments those segments for which: $RR_i - RR_{i-1} > 0$.

In the same paper, *Beat to Beat Deceleration Capacity* ($BBDC$) is also proposed. In the computation of $BBDC$ two-beat segments are examined, i.e. only anchor points and their preceding intervals participate in the computations. $BBDC$ is a reduction of the original method and a reduction of DC_{sgn} to two-interval segments.

Deceleration capacity of heart rate was proposed as a predictor of mortality after myocardial infarction [4]. It has been shown that DC is also an independent predictor for mortality in patients with non-ischemic dilated cardiomyopathy [11]. In [35] the authors use a modification of the method to discriminate between healthy and IUGR fetuses, according to the gestational week. Recently, the index has increased its popularity and new applications of the method in diverse problems are expected to appear in the near future.

3.2 QT Variability

The segment QT is defined from the start of the QRS complex (point Q) and the end of the T wave (Fig. 7). It represents the depolarization and repolarization phases of the heart cycle.

Since the duration of QT depends on the duration of the heart cycle (RR), the normalization of QT was suggested. The new index (QT_c, stands for *QT corrected*) makes the QT segment comparable with other QT segments in the same or different recordings. Various normalization factors have been proposed by several researchers, we list the most significant ones here:

- $QT_cB = QT/\sqrt{RR}$, Bazett [6]
- $QT_cF = QT/\sqrt[3]{RR}$, Fridericia [13]
- $QTl_c = QT + 0.154(1 - RR)$, Sagie et al. [30]

Berger et al., in order to express the variability of QT using a more stable metric, proposed $QTVI$ (*QT Variability Index*) [7]. This metric is based on pattern matching and not on point detection. In a semi-automatic way and using a visualizing tool, a template segment with representative shape is selected. The user marks the start of the depolarization phase (Q point), the start of repolarization phase (S point) and the end of it (end of T wave). This template segment is then compared with all succeeding beats, compressing or stretching it until the best fit is achieved. From the resulting QT intervals we compute the *QT Variability Index* index:

$$QTVI = \log \frac{QT_V/QT_m{}^2}{RR_V/RR_m{}^2},$$

where QT_V is the variance of QT, QT_m the mean of QT, RR_V is the variance and RR_m the mean of RR intervals. The index:

$$QTVN = QT_V/QT_m{}^2,$$

i.e. the nominator of the fraction gives the variability of QT without the adjustment for the heart rate.

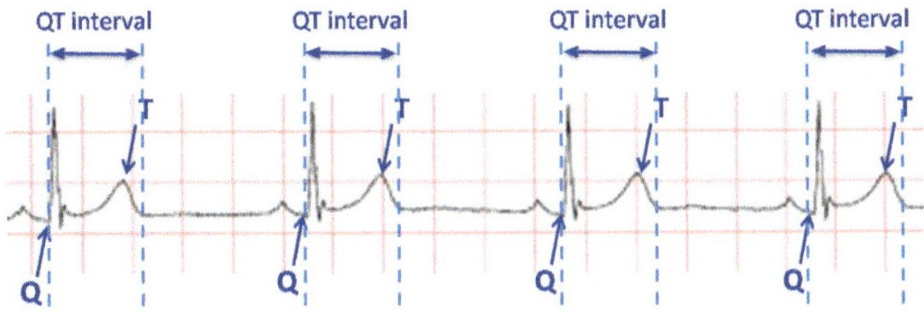

Fig. 7 *QT* variability

A extensive review on the clinical applications of $QTVI$ can be found in [12]. We mention here the fundamental work [7] which investigated $QTVI$ for ischemic and non-ischemic dilated cardiomyopathy, the study [26] which showed that $QTVI$ can predict sudden cardiac death and [16] which showed that $QTVI$ increases for patients with ventricular tachycardia or fibrillation.

3.3 T-Wave Alternans

With the term *T-Wave Variability* (*TWV*) we refer to the beat to beat variations of the duration, the height and generally the shape of the T wave. In Fig. 8 we have aligned T waves from the same recording. It is easy to see that T waves differ, not only in the duration and height, but also in the shape.

T-Wave Alternans (*TWA*) is a repeated fluctuation in the morphology and amplitude of T-waves with two distinct forms of T-waves appearing in alteration. In other words, we expect the morphology and amplitude of T-wave to follow a pattern of the form: *ABABAB*.

Microvolt T-Wave Alternans (*MTWA*) [1] exploit the recent technology to detect T-wave Alternans at the level of microvolts, very small in amplitude to be detected visually. An interesting review in the Microvolt TWA can be found in [38], while methods for computing TWA are examined in [24]. From all available methods we

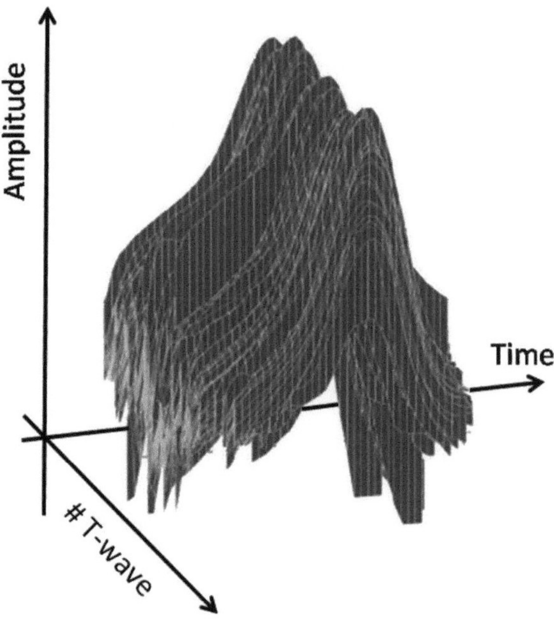

Fig. 8 Aligned T waves from the same recording

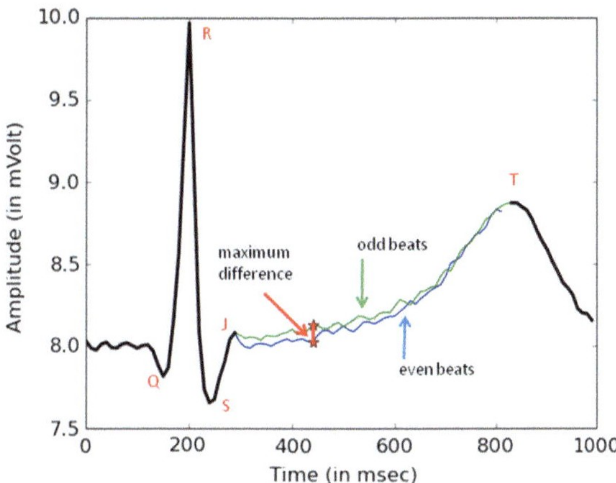

Fig. 9 Maximum difference between averaged odd and even waves

selected to present here the *Modified Moving Average Method* (*MMA*), a time domain method included in both [24, 38], while initially appeared in [25].

The methods separates the *QRS* patterns in odd and even beats. Then, odd and even patterns are aligned, averaged and superimposed. The maximum difference between superimposed patterns at any point within the *JT* segment is averaged for every 10–15 s. This averaged value is reported as the result of the method. Figure 9 shows the superimposed odd and even patterns and the segment on which the the maximum difference is averaged.

In [38], there is an extensive review of literature related to TWA. The clinical significance is also discussed. We mention here the connection of TWA to heart failure, myocardial ischemia, ventricular tachycardia and fibrillation, and sudden cardiac death.

4 Challenges

Even though the research in the field of cardiovascular variability is active many many years, starting even before computers facilitated fast and accurate computations, there is still much research to be done. Until now, we can only observe a complex behavior, only part of which we can explain, or even worse, predict.

A large number of methods have been suggested and, many of them, are used today in clinical practice. Some of them are more popular, not because they produce more reliable results, but due to their support by medical devices and, thus, medical doctors are used to use them. The exploitation of a larger number of methods in clinical practice is a challenge, which requires knowhow and expertise.

On the other hand, even though the large number of available methods is a versatile approach with many advantages, it is also of increased complexity and difficult to be exploited. The selection, or suggestion of a single method describing cardiovascular variability is far away from reality, even if we focus on a specific pathology. And this is the greatest chance of all.

Machine learning technology seems to offer an attractive solution. Training in multidimensional space can combine information from diverse methods, selecting the useful information of each of them. Medical doctors could use the expert system as a black box. Huge amount of data is necessary to train the system and produce reliable results. The good news is that, in the near future, data will not be a problem any more.

References

1. Adam D, Akselrod S, Cohen R (1981) Estimation of ventricular vulnerability to fibrillation through T-wave time series analysis. Comput Cardiol 8:307–310
2. Algra A, Tijssen J, Roelandt J, Pool J, Lubsen J (1993) Heart rate variability from 24-hour electrocardiography and the 2-year risk for sudden death. Circulation 88(1):180–185
3. Arsenos P, Manis G (2014) Deceleration capacity of heart rate: two new methods of computation. Biomed Signal Process Control 14:158–163
4. Bauer A, Kantelhardt JW, Barthel P, Schneider R, Mkikallio T, Ulm K, Hnatkova K, Schmig A, Huikuri H, Bunde A, Malik M, Schmidt G (2006) Deceleration capacity of heart rate as a predictor of mortality after myocardial infarction: cohort study. Lancet 367(9523):1674–1681
5. Bauer A, Kantelhardt JW, Bunde A, Barthel P, Schneider R, Malik M, Schmidt G (2006) Phase-rectified signal averaging detects quasi-periodicities in non-stationary data. Phys A Stat Mech Appl 364:423–434
6. Bazett HC (1920) An analysis of the time-relations of electrocardiograms. Heart 7:353–370
7. Berger RD, Kasper EK, Baughman KL, Marban E, Calkins H, Tomaselli GF (1997) Beat-to-beat QT interval variability: novel evidence for repolarization lability in ischemic and nonischemic dilated cardiomyopathy. Circulation 96(5):1557–1565
8. Brosschot JF, Dijk EV, Thayer JF (2007) Daily worry is related to low heart rate variability during waking and the subsequent nocturnal sleep period. Int J Psychophysiol 63(1):39–47
9. Buccelletti E, Gilardi E, Scaini E, Galiuto L, Persiani R, Biondi A, Basile F, Silveri N (2009) Heart rate variability and myocardial infarction: systematic literature review and metanalysis. Eur Rev Med Pharmacol Sci 13(4):299–307
10. De Souza NM, Vanderlei LCM, Garner DM (2015) Risk evaluation of diabetes mellitus by relation of chaotic globals to HRV. Complexity 20(3):84–92
11. Demming T, Sandrock S, Kuhn C, Kotzott L, Tahmaz N, Bonnemeier H (2016) Deceleration capacity: a novel predictor for total mortality in patients with non-ischemic dilated cardiomyopathy. Int J Cardiol 221:289–293
12. Dobson C, Kim A, Haigney M (2013) QT variability index. Prog Cardiovasc Dis 56(2):186–194
13. Fridericia LS (1920) The duration of systole in the electrocardiogram of normal subjects and of patients with heart disease. Acta Medica Scand 53:469–486
14. Goldberger AL, Amaral LAN, Glass L, Hausdorff JM, Ivanov PC, Mark RG, Mietus JE, Moody GB, Peng CK, Stanley HE (2000) PhysioBank, PhysioToolkit, and PhysioNet: components of a new research resource for complex physiologic signals. Circulation 101(23):e215–e220
15. Guzzetti S, La Rovere M, Pinna G, Maestri R, Borroni E, Porta A, Mortara A, Malliani A (2005) Different spectral components of 24 h heart rate variability are related to different modes of death in chronic heart failure. Eur Heart J 36(4):357–362
16. Haigney MC, Zareba W, Gentlesk PJ, Goldstein RE, Illovsky M, McNitt S, Andrews ML, Moss AJ (2004) QT interval variability and spontaneous ventricular tachycardia or fibrillation in the multicenter automatic defibrillator implantation trial (MADIT) II patients. J Am Coll Cardiol 44(7):1481–1487

17. Harte C, Meston CM (2014) Effects of smoking cessation on heart rate variability among long-term male smokers. Int J Behav Med 21(2):302–309
18. Huikuri H, Stein P (2012) Clinical application of heart rate variability after acute myocardial infarction. Front Physiol 3:41
19. Iyengar N, Peng CK, Morin R, Goldberger AL, Lipsitz LA (1996) Age-related alterations in the fractal scaling of cardiac interbeat interval dynamics. Am J Physiol 271(4 Pt 2):R1078–84
20. Kampouraki A, Manis G, Nikou C (2009) Heartbeat time series classification with support vector machines. Trans Inf Tech Biomed 13:512–518
21. Karakaya O, Barutcu I, Kaya D, Esen A, Saglam M, Melek M, Onrat E, Turkmen M, Esen O, Kaymaz C (2007) Acute effect of cigarette smoking on heart rate variability. Angiology 58(5):620–624
22. Kleiger RE, Miller JP, Bigger JT, Moss AJ (1987) Decreased heart rate variability and its association with increased mortality after acute myocardial infarction. Am J Cardiol 59(4):256–262
23. Manis G, Arsenos P, Nikolopoulos S, Gatzoulis K, Stefanadis C (2013) Details on the application of multiresolution wavelet analysis on heartbeat timeseries. Int J Bioelectromagn 15(1):60–64
24. Martinez J, Olmos S (2005) Methodological principles of T wave alternans analysis: a unified framework. IEEE Trans Biomed Eng 52(4):599–613
25. Nearing B, Verrier R (1985) Modified moving average analysis of T-wave alternans to predict ventricular fibrillation with high accuracy. J Appl Physiol 92(2):541–549
26. Oosterhoff P, Tereshchenko LG, van der Heyden MA, Ghanem RN, Fetics BJ, Berger RD, Vos MA (2011) Short-term variability of repolarization predicts ventricular tachycardia and sudden cardiac death in patients with structural heart disease: a comparison with QT variability index. Heart Rhythm 8(10):1584–1590
27. Peng CK, Havlin S, Stanley HE, Goldberger AL (1995) Quantification of scaling exponents and crossover phenomena in nonstationary heartbeat time series. Chaos Interdiscip J Nonlinear Sci 1:82
28. Pincus S (1995) Approximate entropy (ApEn) as a complexity measure. Chaos 5(1):110–117
29. Richman JS, Moorman JR (2000) Physiological time-series analysis using approximate entropy and sample entropy. Am J Physiol Heart Circ Physiol 278(6):H2039–H2049
30. Sagie A, Larson MG, Goldberg RJ, Bengston JR, Levy D (1992) An improved method for adjusting the QT interval for heart rate (the Framingham heart study). Am J Cardiol 70(7):797–801
31. Sammito S, Bckelmann I (2016) Factors influencing heart rate variability. Int Cardiovasc Forum J 6:18–22
32. Sassi R, Cerutti S, Lombardi F, Malik M, Huikuri HV, Peng CK, Schmidt G, Yamamoto Y, Document Reviewers, Gorenek B, Lip GY, Grassi G, Kudaiberdieva G, Fisher JP, Zabel M, Macfadyen R (2015) Advances in heart rate variability signal analysis: joint position statement by the e-Cardiology ESC Working Group and the European Heart Rhythm Association co-endorsed by the Asia Pacific Heart Rhythm Society. Europace 17(9):1341–1353
33. Schroeder EB, Liao D, Chambless LE, Prineas RJ, Evans GW, Heiss G (2003) Hypertension, blood pressure, and heart rate variability. Hypertension 42(6):1106–1111
34. Schubert C, Lambertz M, Nelesen RA, Bardwell W, Choi J, Dimsdale JE (2009) Effects of stress on heart rate complexity—a comparison between short-term and chronic stress. Biol Psychol 80(3):325–332
35. Tagliaferri S, Fanelli A, Esposito G, Esposito FG, Magenes G, Signorini MG, Campanile M, Martinelli P (2015) Evaluation of the acceleration and deceleration phase-rectified slope to detect and improve IUGR clinical management. Comput Math Methods Med 2015:236896
36. Task Force of the European Society of Cardiology, the North American Society of Pacing and Electrophysiology (1996) Heart rate variability: standards of measurement, physiological interpretation and clinical use. Circulation **93**(5):1043–1065
37. Thurner S, Feurstein MC, Teich MC (1998) Multiresolution wavelet analysis of heartbeat intervals discriminates healthy patients from those with cardiac pathology. Phys Rev Lett 80(7):1544–1547

38. Verrier RL, Klingenheben T, Malik M, El-Sherif N, Exner DV, Hohnloser SH, Ikeda T, Martnez JP, Narayan SM, Nieminen T, Rosenbaum DS (2011) Microvolt T-wave alternans: physiological basis, methods of measurement, and clinical utility—consensus guideline by International Society for Holter and Noninvasive Electrocardiology. J Am Coll Cardiol 58(13):1309–1324
39. Wijbenga J, Balk A, Meij S, Simoons M, Malik M (1998) Heart rate variability index in congestive heart failure: relation to clinical variables and prognosis. Eur Heart J 19(11):1719–1724

Part III
Analysis of Cardiovascular Images

Segmentation of Cardiac Structures

Claudio Fabbri, Maddalena Valinoti, Cristiana Corsi and Martino Alessandrini

Abstract Medical image-based 3D cardiac models have grown rapidly in the last fifteen years due to the advance and consolidation of imaging systems such as magnetic resonance, computed tomography and real-time 3D echocardiography. One of the most challenging task in the development of a 3D cardiac model from in vivo imaging is the segmentation of cardiac structures. This task is the first step towards the analysis of heart anatomy and function. Whole heart segmentation focuses on the localization and detection of the following regions: the left ventricle (LV), which starts at the mitral valve and is composed of the main LV chamber up to the apex and stops at the aortic valve; the right ventricle (RV), which begins at the tricuspid valve, comprises the RV chamber and ends at the pulmonary valves; the left atrium (LA), which start at the pulmonary veins and ends at the mitral valve; the right atrium (RA), which start at the superior and inferior vena cava and ends at the tricuspid valve. In recent years, a variety of methods have been developed for cardiac structure segmentation paving the way for "personalized" medicine in the clinical setting. In this chapter we will briefly review the most recent and advanced approaches for cardiac image segmentation. The chapter is organized in three main sections dealing with the imaging modalities used in clinical practice for cardiac structure and function assessment. A fourth section is focused on the open access validation tools for cardiac structure segmentation nowadays available. Each section is divided in paragraphs in which we will describe the different techniques developed for the specific cardiac structures.

C. Fabbri · M. Valinoti · C. Corsi (✉) · M. Alessandrini
BIOMedical Imaging Group, Dipartimento di Ingegneria dell'Energia Elettrica e dell'Informazione (DEI), Università di Bologna, Bologna, Italy
e-mail: cristiana.corsi3@unibo.it

S. Golemati and K. S. Nikita (eds.), *Cardiovascular Computing—Methodologies and Clinical Applications*, Series in BioEngineering,
https://doi.org/10.1007/978-981-10-5092-3_6

1 Magnetic Resonance Imaging

Cardiac magnetic resonance (CMR) imaging is a non-invasive unique technique that provides a comprehensive evaluation of the heart. Due to its broad applicability including cardiac morphology and function, infarcts and viability assessment, it has gained the definition of "one-stop shop". It is accepted as the gold-standard for cardiac applications.

In order to compute quantitative indices of cardiac structure and function, the delineation of relevant heart boundaries is required. Hereto, manual tracing of chamber boundaries from CMR on multiple slices and frames is a time-consuming and subjective procedure, suffering from intra- and inter-observer variability. Consequently, a lot of research has been dedicated to CMR image segmentation to provide objective assessment of chamber boundaries from which global and regional quantitative indices can be derived. Although CMR is considered to provide the best image quality as compared to the other imaging techniques, accurate and automatic cardiac segmentation remains a challenge due the geometric and dynamic complexity of the heart and to its high anatomical variability between subjects and pathologies.

Segmentation applied to CMR images is a quite complex scenario including a variety of approaches. Existing and most advanced segmentation techniques include patient-specific as well as population-based approaches. Data-driven with or without prior models or model-driven based on a strong a priori knowledge represents the two main segmentation categories. Data-driven approaches operate directly on the image pixels and segmentation is performed by considering the statistical features obtained from the pixels in the specific image. Model driven-approaches rely in a prior knowledge about the objects to detect that is incorporated in the segmentation algorithm. Both approaches include edge-based and region-based techniques.

In the following paragraphs we will provide information about the most effective approaches proposed in literature for the segmentation of left and right ventricles and of the atria from CMR images.

1.1 Left Ventricle Segmentation

The most extensively studied among cardiac chambers is the left ventricle. In the last years, active contours or deformable models were the most widely techniques applied for LV segmentation. Deformable models were introduced by Terzopoulos in the eighties [1–3]. They are curves or surfaces, defined within an image domain, that move under the influence of internal and external forces: internal forces are defined within the curve or surface itself and are designed to keep model smooth during the evolution whilst external forces are computed from the image data and move the model towards image boundaries. Prior information about the object's shape can be incorporated in the model. The first application to CMR image segmentation dates back to Paragios [4]. Their approach is based on the coupled propagation of two

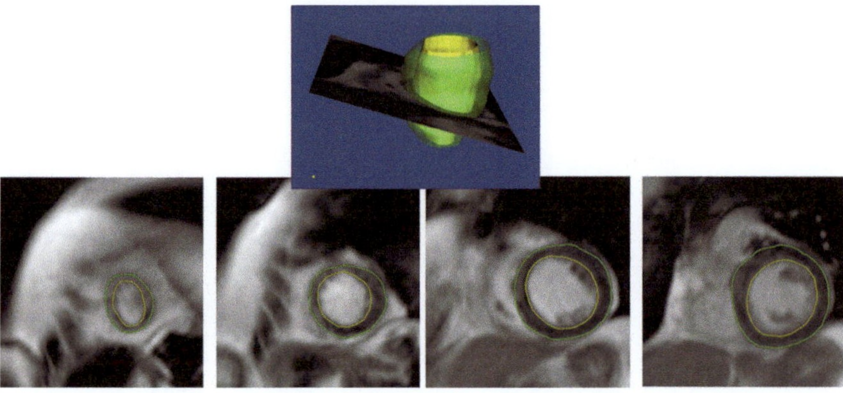

Fig. 1 Example of the endocardial and epicardial contours (bottom panels) at different levels of the left ventricle from apex (left) to base (right) in multiple short-axis slices. Navigation of the surfaces using any arbitrary plane allows verification of the correctness of the detection in any arbitrary cross-sectional plane (top panel) (image modified from [5])

cardiac contours for endocardium and epicardium segmentation through a gradient vector flow snake and an anatomical constraint based on the contour relative distance. The motion equations are implemented using a level set approach. Deformable models and level set approach were also proposed in [5–7] for dynamic endo and epi segmentation of short-axis CMR images, also encoding prior knowledge about cardiac temporal evolution [6, 7]. A typical result is of endocardium and epicardium segmentation in shown in Fig. 1.

Other approaches, semi-automatic or automatic [8, 9] are based on GVF snake and do not require any a priori information. Wu et al. [10] proposed a gradient vector convolution external force for the snake model with the adoption of the circle-shape energy for endocardium segmentation and of a shape similarity energy for epicardium segmentation. It is also worth mentioning other two approaches proposed by Cordero-Grande et al. [11] and Khalifa et al. [12]. The former presents an automated and unsupervised segmentation method for the myocardium in short axis cine images. The segmentation task is modeled as an optimization problem and integrates smoothness, image intensity and gradient related features in an optimal way under a Markov random field framework by maximum likelihood parameter estimation. In the latter, segmentation is performed applying a geometric deformable model guided by a special stochastic speed relationship and wall thickness and thickening function are then assessed. Recently, the B-spline explicit active surface (BEAS), originally proposed for 3D ultrasound and briefly reviewed in the next session, was successfully adapted to the real time 3D segmentation of endo and epicardium from CMR image sequences [13, 14].

More recently, model-based techniques gained a lot of popularity. They rely on a strong prior knowledge mainly based on specific shape variability of the left ventricle. The first study refers to Mitchell et al. [15] and is based on 3D active appearance

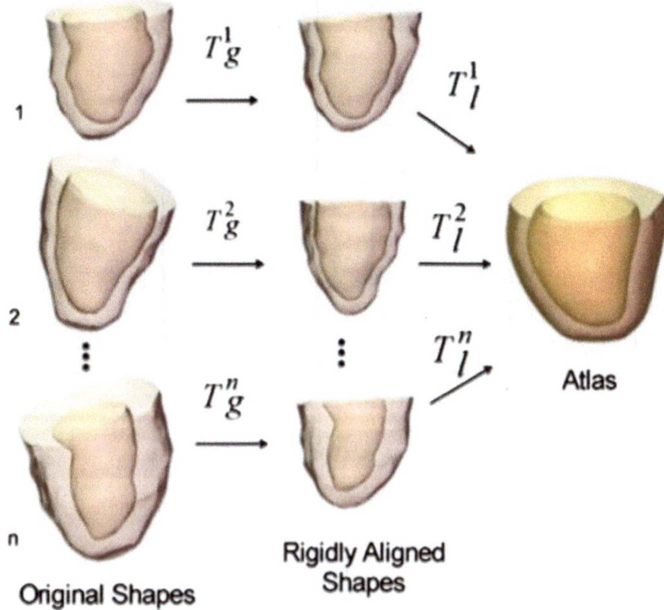

Fig. 2 Schematic layout for atlas construction in which original shapes of a training set are aligned to a mean atlas (modified from [16])

model. Other model-based approaches include active shape models [16, 17] applied to images acquired in arbitrary positions, also with large under-sampled regions [16]. This technique rely on the construction of an atlas from which global and local transformation are obtained (Fig. 2). Lekadir et al. [17] improved this approach by integrating additional shape prior invariant to translation, rotation and scaling, leading to more robust results. Nambakhsh et al. [18] proposed a fast training based left ventricle segmentation via convex relaxation and distribution matching considering shape and intensity constraints; Alba et al. [19] applied a graph cut approach including intensity information, shape and interslice smoothness constraints. Later on, Caiani et al. [20] proposed a nearly automated left ventricular surface segmentation procedure, based on active shape modelling and built on a database of 3D echocardiographic LV surfaces, for CMR images. This is the first study considering the inter-modality application of the active shape models, providing a realistic definition of LV apex and base that may be problematic in CMR images.

Qin et al. [21], in their study, built a shape dictionary dynamically updated to generate patient-specific model by classifying the features and applying a sparse shape model.

1.2 Right Ventricle Segmentation

Accurate automated segmentation of the right ventricle is difficult due to its complex shape and to shape variation between patients. Only few studies on small groups of subjects are proposed in literature and apply image-driven or model-based approaches. Image-driven techniques were developed using graph cut framework [22], also including shape prior based on contours from manually traced CMR images [23]. To improve generalization to complex and pathological cases limited by the use of prior knowledge, some interesting approaches were based on reinforcement learning from user interaction [24]. Simple deformable models and level set approach were also proposed for 3D right ventricular segmentation [25]. This technique requires a rough initialization and it is totally free of geometric assumptions and lead to a 3D patient-specific right ventricular model (Fig. 3). Very recently, a technique based on regularized two level sets was proposed to dynamically segment right and left ventricles [26].

Model-drive approaches for right ventricle segmentation have received considerable attention. Due to the right ventricle variability such models require high adaptability in terms of shape. They are based on active shape models and active appearance model or on a combination of both, thus improving segmentation results overcoming the drawbacks characterizing the two approaches separately. The most recent approaches are based on PCA-based statistical shape model and registration [27, 28], and deformable models guided by a PCA on distance function derived by training contours [29].

For an interesting overview of several state-of-the art techniques for RV segmentation, representing image-driven, model based as well as atlas-based approaches, we refer the reader to the recent [30].

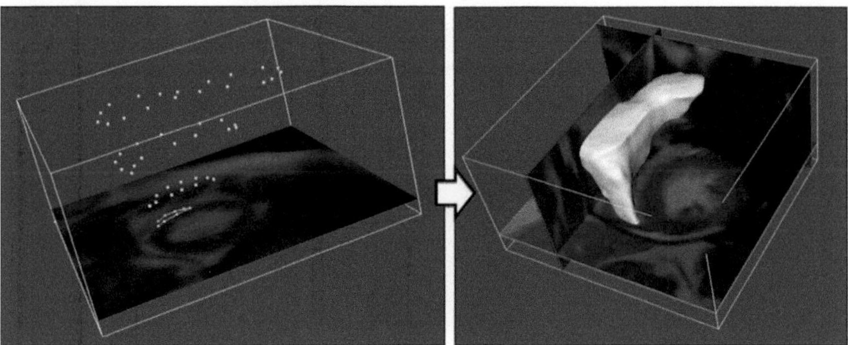

Fig. 3 Endocardial surface assessment with the method proposed in [25] by manual selection of some endocardial points on few planes (left panel) and final detected 3D right ventricular surface (right panel)

1.3 Atria Segmentation

Atria segmentation is the most challenging task compared to ventricle segmentation. In specific clinical scenarios including atrial fibrillation ablation guidance and fibrosis quantification, atria segmentation is crucial. In addition, cardiac computational modeling requires patient specific anatomies of the cardiac chambers, including atria. Magnetic resonance angiography or late-gadolinium enhanced magnetic resonance images are the data usually processed for atrium segmentation. A review of the algorithms submitted for the open challenge that was put to the medical imaging community through the IEEE International Symposium on Biomedical Imaging workshop in 2013 was published by Karim et al. [31] and a benchmark on this topic was recently presented in [32]. The majority of proposed approaches are model-based but were designed to handle significant variational anatomies without user interaction [33–36]. Global fully automatic segmentation of the left atrium based on multi-atlas registration followed by a local refinement by level set was proposed by Tao et al. [33]. Similarly, Wachinger et al. [34] developed an automatic segmentation approach based on an atlas of manually labeled images. Kutra et al. [35] applied a multi-component left atrium segmentation including different patterns which are selected by a trained support vector machine. Very few image-driven approaches are reported in literature including region growing with shape prior represented by Zernike moments [37], and level set approach guided by a phase–based edge detector to obtain the 3D left atrium model with and without pulmonary veins [38] (Fig. 4).

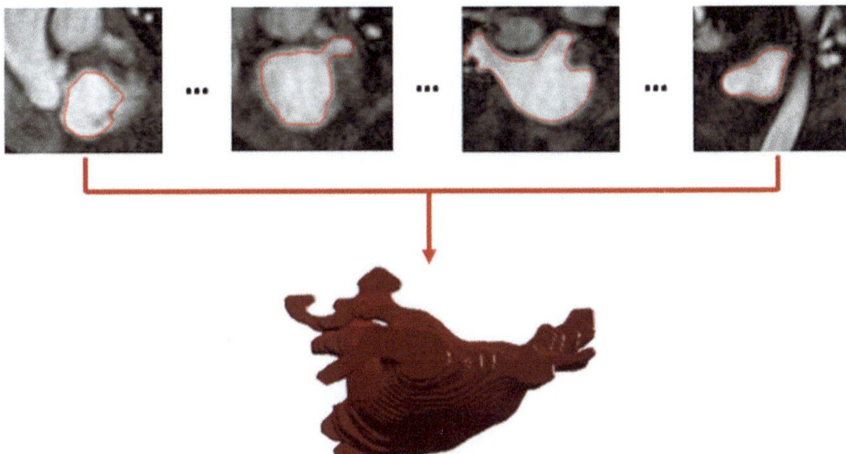

Fig. 4 An example of 3D patient specific LA model derived from the segmentation step. Top panel: 2D detected LA contours including the PVs. Bottom panel: 3D patient specific LA surface derived from the segmented MRA images (modified from [38])

2 Echocardiography

Echocardiography, or cardiac ultrasound (US), offers relevant advantages against other images modalities such as computed tomography (CT) and CMR being cheap, portable (hence, can be employed bedside) and safe for the patient (since it does not make use of ionizing radiations). Moreover, it allows imaging the moving heart with the highest temporal resolution (Fig. 5).

For these reasons, echocardiography has become the modality of choice in clinical diagnostics for the assessment of the heart. Although still mainly a 2D modality, 3D ultrasound, supported by strong research investments, is also gradually entering the clinical practice. 3D ultrasound overcomes some of the limitations of the 2D alternative: it eliminates the need of geometrical assumptions and mitigates foreshortening issues.

Yet, the clinical assessment of ultrasound recordings still mainly relies on visual reading, which is intrinsically dependent on the operator's expertise. Visual reading is particularly problematic in echocardiography due to the low image quality. Moreover, the 3D modality offers additional challenges related to the navigation through the 3D volumes. Therefore, a number of tools have been proposed by academia and industry for the automated quantification of cardiac function from echocardiographic recordings.

In this context, the main attention has been and is still focused on the volumetric and functional assessment of the left ventricle. Yet, there is a recent noticeable shift of interest, although still limited to research feasibility studies, towards the other cardiac chambers. This section provides therefore an overview of the available techniques for the volumetric assessment of the heart chambers with 3D ultrasound. Of note, we will consider applications for the adult heart. Yet, we register a relevant gain of interest towards pediatric and fetal applications [39]. For reasons of space, our overview will be limited to the most representative works. For more extensive reviews, we address the reader to [40, 41] and the very recent [42].

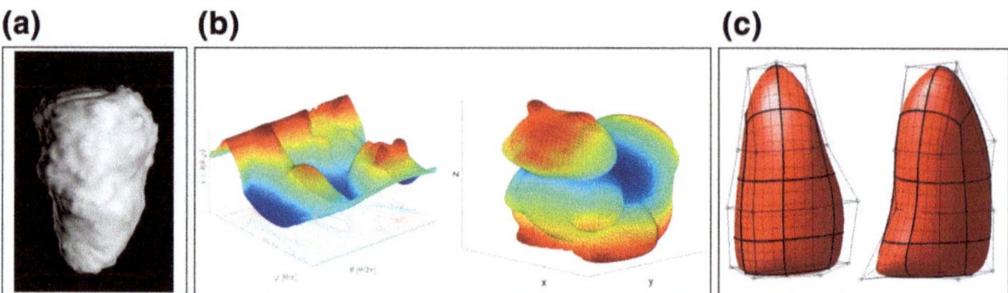

Fig. 5 Comparison between different surface representations. **a** Level sets, modified from [43]; **b** spline explicit active surfaces, modified from [45]; **c** Doo-Sabin subdivision surfaces, modified from [46]

2.1 Left Ventricle Segmentation

Several commercial products are available clinically for the automated analysis of LV shape and function by 3D US [42]. The technology employed is often not known inasmuch covered by trade secret. TomTec Imaging Systems (Unterschleissheim, Germany) distributes the TomTec 4D LV-Analysis tool, in which the 3D endocardial surface is contoured by the software in end of systole and then propagated using speckle tracking. Philips Healthcare (Best, Netherlands) commercializes the QLAB—3DQ Advance (3DQA) software suit, in which five anatomical landmarks must be marked to initialize a deformable shell model. The model is afterwards deformed towards the left ventricular boundaries. More recently, General Electric (GE Vingmed, Horten, Norway) introduced a package, 4D Auto LVQ, for fully or semi-automated segmentation and volume quantification. Toshiba Medical Systems (Tokyo, Japan) distributes the Artida TM system, which was complemented with a software tool for chamber quantification: 3D Wall Motion Tracking (3D-WMT). In it, the user is required to place six markers, used to automatically segment the endocardium. The epicardial contour is propagated over time with a 3D block matching algorithm. Siemens Medical Solutions (Mountain View, California) distributes the tool eSie LVATM. This tool is based on a database of manually annotated RT3DE exams (over 4000). The annotated database is used to train the final classifier which, given an input volume, detects the LV endocardium automatically, with the possibility of manual correction.

Among solutions available in research, early attempts, such as by Corsi et al. [43] and Angelini et al. [44], employed the level-set formalism. One drawback of level set algorithms is the heavy computation time coming from the fact that the 3D contour is handled as the zero level of a large 4D matrix. This conflicts with the intrinsic real time capability of ultrasound and partly explains the loss of interest towards these methods in the last years.

Therefore, more recent techniques exploited lighter parametric expressions of the evolving 3D surface. In [45], Barbosa et al. made use of B-spline explicit active surfaces (BEAS), in which the 3D surface is expressed as a B-spline parametrization on a 2D polar grid. This allowed accomplishing the fully automated 3D LV segmentation in few milliseconds. In [46], Orderud and Rabben exploited instead Doo-Sabin subdivision surfaces, in which the 3D surface is represented by few 3D control points on its convex hull. This technique is now at the core of the Real Time Contour Tracking Library (RCTL) by GE. Different kinds of surface representations are illustrated in Fig. 1.

Given the low image quality, it is essential to constraint a segmentation algorithm towards realistic shapes. Hereto, the use of active shape models (ASM), as by Hansegard et al. [47], and active appearance models (AAM), as by Mitchell et al. [15], in a smaller measure, has become a well-established tool in this sense. Both approaches evolve from the seminal work by Cootes et al. [48]. In ASM's, a database of segmented geometries is used to build a statistical model of LV shapes, e.g. by principal component analysis (PCA). In AAM, the statistical model is built instead on the voxel intensities directly (i.e. not on the shapes).

Most recently, with huge gain in popularity of machine learning, we are witnessing multiple attempts to apply these concepts to the volumetric assessment of cardiac chambers. The technique by Yang et al. [49] exploited marginal space learning and is now part of the Siemens system for LV quantification. In [50] Milletari et al. applied Hough regression forests, a generalization of Hough transform. In [51] Oktay et al. applied the multi atlas propagation principle, which consists in registering a set of labelled images (i.e. the atlas) on the image to be segmented and then combining the labels to produce the final segmentation. Hereto, probabilistic edge maps (PEMs) are used to guide the registration step. PEMs are computed by using structured random forests. In [52] Lempitsky et al. solve LV segmentation by using random forest classification.

For an overview of the most recent advances in the field of ultrasound LV segmentation, we point the reader to the proceedings of the recent Challenge on Endocardial Three-dimensional Ultrasound Segmentation (CETUS) hosted at MICCAI 2014 [53], which shows an interesting head-to-head comparison between more traditional image-based and recent learning based techniques.

2.2 *Right Ventricle Segmentation*

To our knowledge, the only technique available clinically was developed by Tomtec Imaging Systems (Unterschleissheim, Germany), who has made available an offline tool for semi-automatic RV function assessment, called 4D RV-Function [4]. Firstly, the correct anatomical axis must be defined by the user and landmarks placed in both the tricuspid and mitral valves and the apex. The software then automatically delineates the RV endocardial border along the heart cycle.

In general, the literature on RV segmentation with 3D echocardiography is extremely limited. As recognized in [39], one reason is the difficulty in acquiring good images due to the peculiar RV morphology and shape. Another reason is the perceived greater importance of the left heart as compared to the right one.

For the same reason, the research attempts to tackle the problem have also been scarce. In [44], Angelini et al. used level sets to segment left and right ventricles jointly. Following the general trend, more recent techniques shifted towards parametric surface representations, as in [51, 52] where subdivision surfaces are used, or statistical shape models, as in [54].

2.3 *Left Atrium Segmentation*

Given the lower priority, the commercial solutions expressively designed for LA assessment limited. The first the 4D LA Analysis package by TomTec. In it, the user is asked to manually contour the LA endocardium in three different views

(2-, 3- and 4-chamber). A polyhedral mesh is then generated for each of those frames by volumetric interpolation of the 2D contours. Philips' fully automatic Heart Model AI tool was released in August 2015 and performs fully automatic 4 chamber segmentation. Therefore, it also provides LA volumes besides LV [42]. Besides that, the application of software packages for LV analysis has also been documented [42]. Yet, LV analysis tools might not be well suited for LA analysis given the very specific atrial function and morphology.

Solutions available in research are also scarce. Existing techniques are mostly a revisiting of what originally proposed for the LV. Among the image-based techniques, we refer to the very recent works by Almeida et al. [55, 56]. In [55] the BEAS framework was adapted to account for the most complex atrial morphology. In [56] the RCTL library was used to build joint model of LV and LA based on Doo-Sabin subdivision surfaces. Using joint models of LA and LV offers a way to prevent leaking of the contours trough the mitral valve. Moreover, it allows studying the mechanical interactions between the two chambers.

Machine learning solutions include the work by Voigt et al. [57], where marginal space learning by Siemens is used to segment LA, LV and mitral valve with 3D trans esophageal echocardiography (TEE). Another dual chamber model was proposed and evaluated in [58].

3 Computed Tomography

Computed Tomography is also used clinically for the acquisition of cardiac images. The underlying principle of this technology is the emission of ionizing radiation over a spatial region to investigate the permeated tissues. Because of the risk related with exposure to X-rays [59], if possible, other imaging modalities are preferred, such as CMR and echocardiography.

CT images acquisition may be performed with or without a contrast-agent, which, specifically, is a radiopaque substance injected, as a bolus or continuously, that absorbs the travelling radiation and leads to a hyper-intensification of the signal.

Non-contrast CT is a low-exposure method used to detect the presence of coronary artery calcium [60], whereas contrast-enhanced CT is used for the imaging of coronary arteries, the detection of coronary stenosis, the visualization of vessel and heart chamber walls and the quantification and localization of coronary plaques. Besides, CT allows morphological and functional assessment of the heart: it is used to evaluate wall thickness (WT), chamber volume and regional wall motion. Moreover, it is also used to detect diseases of the pericardium, chamber volume and function in patients who are unable to undergo CMR procedures [61].

As for the other imaging modalities reviewed in this chapter, the need for an objective diagnosis and a faster and reproducible image analysis pipeline have motivated the development of techniques for the automatic quantification of cardiac function from CT image sequences. In this section, we will give therefore an overall description of the most successful techniques available in research for the segmentation of heart chambers, walls (i.e. joint segmentation of endo- and epicardium), and coronary arteries.

3.1 Heart Chambers

Since the introduction in the 90th of spiral scanning techniques and, subsequently, of multi-slice CT, the increasing amount of data posed a big burden on the processing workflow and so robust automatic segmentation of the cardiac anatomy remains an open subject [62, 63].

As for MR and echo, most recent approaches make use of atlases of labelled images to constraint the segmentation result to meaningful shapes. As already mentioned, the atlas can be used to build a statistical model of shape or appearance; within a machine learning context, the atlas can be used to train an architecture for regression or classification (neural networks and random forests are gaining popularity in this sense); finally, it can be used in a multi-atlas propagation framework. For a review, we address the reader to [64].

In this regard, an efficient and a fast technique used for full heart (i.e. 4 chamber) segmentation from 3D-CT is based on the concepts of marginal space learning and steerable features [65]. Hereto, a shape model is built from a large set of already segmented CT volumes. The algorithm proceeds in two steps: a preliminary automatic heart localization in 3D, obtained by aligning the learned heart models with the image, followed by a non-rigid point-guided deformation constrained by the shape model to adjust the model features onto the subject anatomy.

A different effective approach is based on the multi-atlas segmentation [66]. In this case, the segmentation is obtained by means of image registration between the image to be segmented (fixed image) and each image of the atlas (moving images). The method requires a cost function used for the registration: most commonly, mutual information (MI) is used, defined as follows [66]:

$$MI(X, Y) = \int_Y \int_X p(x, y) \log(\frac{p(x, y)}{p(x)p(y)})\, dxdy$$

In information and probability theory, mutual information defines the measurement of dependence between two variables. As such, the aim is to find a global maximum of MI to obtain the best fit between the atlas and the subject data. The found transformation, applied to the labels, produces a set of candidate segmentations, which are then fused together (in the simplest case, with majority voting) to produce the final output.

3.2 *Cardiac Walls*

Detecting and tracking the movement of cardiac walls is an important task for the assessment of cardiac function and diagnosis of cardiac diseases. This task poses particular challenge since a wide variability of shape and dimension exist between different patients, and also because of the presence of fat or soft tissues near the right wall, which could hinder the accurate segmentation of thin walls [67].

The same concepts used for heart chamber segmentation have been applied for wall segmentation. Hereto, a sophisticated approach is based on shape segmentation and variational region growing [68].

This particular approach tackles the challenge of subject variability. The algorithm starts by locating the LV, which is the most easily detectable chamber given its mostly cylindrical shape. Then, given subject orientation and position, it searches for the RV. Starting from the apex and analyzing the shape of the boundaries, the ventricular models are cut at the height of the respective valve planes, identified as the turning point of a distance field applied on the isocontour at the difference levels. After this step, where RV and LV were localized as deep concave boundaries, an active contour model using localization constraints is applied to refine the results.

Other methods proposed for the task, like region-based methods [69], still require post processing and manual interaction. Statistical based approaches give good results but problems arise in differentiating the fat from the cardiac wall since the intensities are similar. Active contour models require the definition of initial condition to ensure that the segmentation is accurate. Neural network, atlases and classifiers require big datasets for learning or building and it is difficult for them to account for the anatomical variability between patients. In fact, the current direction of research is by using coarser techniques in the beginning, which can be based on prior knowledge or statistical information, and then refine and consolidate the segmentation results with finer techniques once the solution is near.

3.3 *Coronary Arteries*

Precise vessel volume and diameter assessment is also an invaluable tool for the detection of cardiovascular diseases such as Coronary Artery Disease (CAD). The degree of stenosis is an important clinical index, and early detection is critical to determine a therapy. Also other features play a role such as branching. To obtain this kind of information, the segmentation of the coronary tree is highly desirable [70].

As described by Dehkordi et al. [71], techniques used in clinical practice for assessment of CAD are divided in *vessel enhancement* and *vessel segmentation*. In this particular paragraph the focus will be on vessel segmentation.

Tian et al. [72] proposed the following approach, which is composed by four different steps: in the first, a registration method, which aligns the atlas reference set on the patient images by minimizing the least square distance between image intensities, is applied to obtain and extract the heart region. The second step enhances the vessel tree via image filtering in the vicinity of the heart surfaces. Thresholding and morphological operators are then used to obtain the seed points for the initialization of the last step of the algorithm. Finally, a statistical model region growing is run on every seed. Hereto, all the resulting segmentations are merged and then statistical information is recalculated on all the voxels belonging to it. At last, region growing is applied on the previous segmentation merge until there are no more voxel changes between iterations.

The majority of algorithms for coronary artery segmentation employ a set of different techniques at different steps. An example of this kind of workflow is presented in Zhou et al. [73]. Here, early localization of the heart is completed through thresholding and expectation maximization. Then, the vascular structures are extracted through multiscale filtering based on Hessian eigenvalue analysis, which responds differently based on the shape (linear, convoluted, spherical) of the underlying structures. The final step is taken to ensure the extraction of only the wanted structure, by means of tracking with manual placed seed points.

4 Open Access Validation Tools

Algorithms for chamber quantification are commonly benchmarked against manual references by experts. In the case of ultrasound, MR is also considered as the gold standard to compare with. Clearly, this implies a substantial bias towards the clinical ground truth data used and the clinician producing the references. As a result, it becomes extremely hard to compare results from different groups. Head-to-head comparison on common ground truth data becomes essential given the multiplication of efforts in the same direction, moreover is important for a more coordinated technological advancement.

In this sense, there have been remarkable efforts in the research community towards to construction of open access databases of ground truth data. The release of such databases is often accompanied by the organization of "grand challenges", hosted by main conferences such as MICCAI and ISBI. To have an updated version of what available, we point therefore the reader to the site https://grand-challenge.org/. For what concerns cardiac chamber quantification, the more relevant resources available to the best of our knowledge are the following.

For what concerns LV assessment with 3D ultrasound, the CETUS database (https://www.creatis.insa-lyon.fr/Challenge/CETUS/index.html) provides segmented 3D LV volumes of 45 subjects spanning different pathophysiological conditions. The STRAUS dataset [20] provides 8 synthetic 3D US sequences with assigned ground truth geometry and motion (https://team.inria.fr/asclepios/data/straus/).

For what concerns LV segmentation from MR, the cardiac atlas project (http://www.cardiacatlas.org/) provides hundreds of segmented LV anatomies from healthy and ischemic subjects.

The left atrial segmentation challenge provides labelled atrial geometries from both MR and CT images (http://www.cardiacatlas.org/challenges/left-atrium-segmentation-challenge/).

Ground truth data for RV ventricle segmentation from MR is available at (http://www.litislab.fr/?projet=1rvsc).

5 Conclusions

We tried to provide a synthetic overview of the state of the art in the volumetric assessment of the heart with medical images. Due to the amount of work which has been and is constantly done in this field, this review is far from being exhaustive. Yet, we tried to provide, for each modality, an overview of the principal families of techniques employed and to point the key articles. For more exhaustive and voluminous reviews, expressively dedicated to specific modalities, we address the reader to the recent [74] by Peng et al. for what concerns CMR; to [40] by Leung et al. and [42] by Pedrosa et al. for what concerns cardiac ultrasound and to [41] by Noble and Boukerroui for more general applications of medical ultrasound. An assessment of the state of the art for heart segmentation with CT is provided in [64]. Finally, throughout this chapter we provide links to the principal open access databases of labelled cardiac data, which can be used for a more reproducible evaluation of new techniques.

Acknowledgements Martino Alessandrini received funding from the European Union's Horizon 2020 research and innovation programme under the Marie Skłodowska-Curie grant agreement No 659082.

References

1. Kass M, Witkin A, Terzopoulos D (1987) Snakes: active contour models. Int J Comput Vis 1(4):321–331
2. Terzopoulos D, Fleischer K (1988) Deformable models. Vis Comput 4:306–331
3. Terzopoulos D, Witkin A, Kass M (1988) Constraints on deformable models: recovering 3D shape and non-rigid motion. Artif Intell 36(1):91–123
4. Paragios N (2002) A variational approach for the segmentation of the left ventricle in cardiac image analysis. Int J Comput Vis 50(3):345–364
5. Corsi C, Lamberti C, Catalano O et al (2005) Improved quantification of left ventricular volumes and mass based on endocardial and epicardial surface detection from cardiac MR images using level set models. J Cardiovasc Magn Reson 7(3):595–602
6. Lynch M, Ghita O, Whelan PF (2008) Segmentation of the left ventricle of the heart in 3-D+T MRI data using an optimized nonrigid temporal model. IEEE Trans Med Imaging 27(2):195–205
7. Schaerer J, Casta C, Pousin J, Clarysse P (2010) A dynamic elastic model for segmentation and tracking of the heart in MR image sequences. Med Image Anal 14(6):738–774

8. Constantinides C, Chenoune Y, Kachenoura N et al (2009) Semi-automated cardiac segmentation on cine magnetic resonance images using GVF-Snake deformable models. MIDAS J-Cardiac MR Left Ventricle Segm Chall
9. Ringenberg J, Deo M, Devabhaktuni V et al (2012) Automated segmentation and reconstruction of patient-specific cardiac anatomy and pathology from in vivo MRI. Meas Sci Technol 23(12):125407
10. Wu Y, Wang Y, Jia Y (2013) Segmentation of the left ventricle in cardiac cine MRI using a shape-constrained snake model. Comput Vis Image Underst 117(9):990–100
11. Cordero-Grande L, Vegas-Sánchez-Ferrero G, Casaseca-dela-Higuera P et al (2011) Unsupervised 4D myocardium segmentation with a Markov random field based deformable model. Med Image Anal 15(3):283–301
12. Khalifa F, Beache GM, Farb GG et al (2012) Accurate automatic analysis of cardiac cine images. IEEE Trans Biomed Eng 59(2):445–457
13. Queirós S, Barbosa D, Heyde B, Morais P, Vilaça JL, Friboulet D, D'hooge J (2014) Fast automatic myocardial segmentation in 4D cine {CMR} datasets. Med Image Anal 18(7):1115–1131
14. Queirós S, Barbosa D, Engvall J, Ebbers T, Nagel E, Sarvari, SI, D'hooge J (2015) Multicentre validation of an automatic algorithm for fast 4D myocardial segmentation in cine CMR datasets. Eur Heart J Cardiovasc Imaging
15. Mitchell SC, Bosch JG, Lelieveldt BP et al (2002) 3-D active appearance models: segmentation of cardiac MR and ultrasound images. IEEE Trans Med Imaging 21(9):1167–117
16. Van Assen HC, Danilouchkine MG, Frangi A et al (2006) SPASM: a 3D-ASM for segmentation of sparse and arbitrarily oriented cardiac MRI data. Med Image Anal 10(2):286–305
17. Lekadir K, Merrifield R, Yang GZ (2007) Outlier detection and handling for robust 3-D active shape models search. IEEE Trans Med Imaging 26(2):212–224
18. Nambakhsh CM, Yuan J, Punithakumar K et al (2013) Left ventricle segmentation in MRI via convex relaxed distribution matching. Med Image Anal 17(8):1010–1024
19. Alba X, Ventura F, Rosa M et al (2014) Automatic cardiac LV segmentation in MRI using modified graph cuts with smoothness and interslice constraints. Magn Reson Med 72(6):1775–1784
20. Caiani EG, Colombo A, Pepi M et al (2014) Three-dimensional left ventricular segmentation from magnetic resonance imaging for patient-specific modelling purposes. Europace 16(Suppl 4):iv96–iv101
21. Qin X, Tian Y, Yan P (2015) Feature competition and partial sparse shape modeling for cardiac image sequences segmentation. Neurocomputing 149:904–915
22. Maier OM, Jiménez D, Santos A, Ledesma-Carbayo MJ (2012) Segmentation of RV in 4D cardiac MR volumes using region merging graph cuts. In: Computing in cardiology. IEEE, pp 697–702
23. Mahapatra D (2013) Cardiac image segmentation from cine cardiac MRI using graph cuts and shape priors. J Digit Imaging 26(4):721–732
24. Wang L, Lekadir K, Lee SR et al (2013) A general framework for context-specific image segmentation using reinforcement learning. IEEE Trans Med Imaging 32(5):943–958
25. Catalano O, Corsi C, Antonaci S et al (2007) Improved reproducibility of right ventricular volumes and function estimation from cardiac magnetic resonance images using level set models. Magn Reson Med 57(3):600–605
26. Liu Y, Captur G, Moon JC et al (2016) Distance regularized two level sets for segmentation of left and right ventricles from cine-MRI. Magn Reson Imaging 34(5):699–706
27. Grosgeorge D, Petitjean C, Dacher S et al (2013) Graph cut segmentation with a statistical shape model in cardiac MRI. Comput Vis Image Underst 117(9):1027–1037
28. Ou Y, Doshi J, Erus G et al (2012) Multi-atlas segmentation of the right ventricle in cardiac MRI. In: Proceedings of MICCAI RV segmentation challenge
29. Oghli MG, Dehlaghi V, Zadeh AM et al (2014) Right ventricle functional parameters estimation in arrhythmogenic right ventricular dysplasia using a robust shape based deformable model. J Med Signals Sens 4(3):211
30. Petitjean C, Zuluaga MA, Bai W, Dacher JN, Grosgeorge D, Caudron J, Yuan J (2015) Right ventricle segmentation from cardiac MRI: a collation study. Med Image Anal 19(1):187–202

31. Karim R, Housden RJ, Balasubramaniam M et al (2013) Evaluation of current algorithms for segmentation of scar tissue from late gadolinium enhancement cardiovascular magnetic resonance of the left atrium: an open-access grand challenge. J Cardiovasc Magn Reson 20(15):105
32. Tobon-Gomez C, Geers A, Peters J et al (2015) Benchmark for algorithms segmenting the left atrium from 3D CT and MRI datasets. IEEE Trans Med Imaging. https://doi.org/10.1109/TMI.2015.2398818
33. Tao Q, Ipek EG, Shahzad R et al (2016) Fully automatic segmentation of left atrium and pulmonary veins in late gadolinium-enhanced MRI: towards objective atrial scar assessment. J Magn Reson Imaging 44(2):346–354
34. Wachinger C, Fritscher K, Sharp G et al (2015) Contour-driven atlas-based segmentation. IEEE Trans Med Imaging 34(12):2492–2505
35. Kutra D, Saalbach A, Lehmann et al (2012) Automatic multi-model-based segmentation of the left atrium in cardiac MRI scans. Med Image Comput Comput Assist Interv 15(Pt 2):1–8
36. Veni G, Fu Z, Awate SP et al (2013) Bayesian segmentation of atrium wall using globally-optimal graph cuts on 3D meshes. Inf Process Med Imaging 23:656–667
37. Zhu L, Gao Y, Yezzi A et al (2013) Automatic segmentation of the left atrium from MR images via variational region growing with a moments-based shape prior. IEEE Trans Image Process 22(12):5111–5122
38. Valinoti M, Fabbri C, Turco D et al (2016) Development of 3D patient-specific models for left atrium geometric characterization to support ablation in atrial fibrillation patients, vol 43. IEEE Press, pp 77–80
39. Dewi EO, Abduljabbar HN, Supriyanto E (2014) Review on advanced techniques in 2-D fetal echocardiography: an image processing perspective. In: Advances in medical diagnostic technology. Springer Singapore, Singapore, pp 53–74
40. Leung KYE, Bosch JG (2010) Automated border detection in three-dimensional echocardiography: principles and promises. Eur Heart J Cardiovasc Imaging 11(2):97–108
41. Noble JA, Boukerroui D (2006) Ultrasound image segmentation: a survey. IEEE Trans Med Imaging 25(8):987–1010
42. Pedrosa J, Barbosa D, Almeida N et al (2016) Cardiac chamber volumetric assessment using 3D ultrasound—a review. Curr Pharm Design 22:105–121
43. Corsi C, Saracino G, Sarti A et al (2002) Left ventricular volume estimation for real-time three-dimensional echocardiography. IEEE Trans Med Imaging 21(9):1202–1208
44. Angelini ED, Homma S, Pearson G et al (2005) Segmentation of real-time three-dimensional ultrasound for quantification of ventricular function: a clinical study on right and left ventricles. Ultrasound Med Biol 31(9):1143–1158
45. Barbosa D, Dietenbeck T, Schaerer J et al (2012) B-spline explicit active surfaces: an efficient framework for real-time 3-D region-based segmentation. IEEE Trans Image Process 21(1):241–251
46. Orderud F, Rabben SI (2008) Real-time 3D segmentation of the left ventricle using deformable subdivision surfaces. In: IEEE conference on computer vision pattern recognition, pp 1–8
47. Hansegard J, Orderud F, Rabben SI (2007) Real time active shape models for segmentation of 3D cardiac ultrasound. In: Proceedings of the 12th international conference on computer analysis of images and patterns, pp 157–164
48. Cootes TF, Taylor CJ, Cooper DH (1995) Active shape models-their training and application. Comput Vis Image Underst 61(1):38–59
49. Yang L, Georgescu B, Zheng Y, Meer P, Comaniciu D (2008) 3D ultrasound tracking of the left ventricle using one-step forward prediction and data fusion of collaborative trackers. In: 2008 IEEE conference on computer vision and pattern recognition, Anchorage, AK, pp 1–8
50. Milletari F, Yigitsoy M, Navab N (2014) Left ventricle segmentation in cardiac ultrasound using hough-forests with implicit shape and appearance priors. Midas J 49–56. http://hdl.handle.net/10380/3485
51. Oktay O, Gomez A, Keraudren K et al (2015) Probabilistic edge map (PEM) for 3D ultrasound image registration and multi-atlas left ventricle segmentation. In: van Assen H, Bovendeerd P, Delhaas T (eds) Functional imaging and modeling of the heart. Proceedings of the 8th international conference, FIMH 2015, Maastricht, The Netherlands, 25–27 June 2015, pp 223–230

52. Lempitsky V et al (2009) Random forest classification for automatic delineation of myocardium in real-time 3D echocardiography. Lecture notes in computer science (including subseries Lecture notes artificial intelligence, Lecture notes bioinformatics), vol 5528, pp 447–456
53. Bernard O, Bosch JG, Heyde B et al (2016) Standardized evaluation system for left ventricular segmentation algorithms in 3D echocardiography. IEEE Trans Med Imaging 35(4):967–977
54. Engås A (2008) Segmentation of right ventricle in 3D ultrasound recordings. PhD thesis, NTNU, Trondheim, Norway
55. Almeida N, Friboulet D, Sarvari SI et al (2016) Left-atrial segmentation from 3-D ultrasound using B-spline explicit active surfaces with scale uncoupling. IEEE Trans Ultrason Ferroelectr Freq Control 63(2):212–221
56. Almeida N, Papachristidis A, Pearson P et al (2016) Left atrial volumetric assessment using a novel automated framework for 3D echocardiography: a multi-centre analysis. Eur Heart J Cardiovasc Imaging [Epub ahead of print]
57. Voigt I, Mansi T, Mihalef V et al (2011) Patient-specific model of left heart anatomy, dynamics and hemodynamics from 4D TEE: a first validation study. Lecture notes in computer science (including subseries Lecture notes artificial intelligence, Lecture notes bioinformatics), vol 6666, pp 341–349
58. Tsang W, Salgo IS, Zarochev L et al (2013) Fully automated quantification of left ventricular and left atrial volumes from transthoracic 3D echocardiography: a validation study. J Am Coll Cardiol 61(10):E904
59. Smith-Bindman R, Lipson J, Marcus R et al (2009) Radiation dose associated with common computed tomography exams and the associated lifetime attributed risk of cancer. Arch Intern Med 169(22):2078–2086
60. Greenland P, Bonow RO, Brundage BH et al (2007) Coronary artery calcium scoring: ACCF/AHA 2007 clinical expert consensus document on coronary artery calcium scoring by computed tomography in global cardiovascular risk assessment and in evaluation of patients with chest pain. J Am Coll Cardiol 49:378–402
61. Markham R, Murdoch D, Walters D et al (2016) Coronary computed tomography angiography and its increasing application in day to day cardiology practice. Intern Med J 46(1):29–34
62. Ecabert O, Peters J, Weese J, et al (2006) Automatic heart segmentation in CT: current and future applications. MedicaMundi. 50:12–13
63. Schoenhagen P, Halliburton SS, Stillman AE et al (2005) CT of the heart: Principles, advances, clinical uses. Clevel Clin J Med 72(2):127–138
64. Zhuang X (2013) Challenges and methodologies of fully automatic whole heart segmentation: a review. J Health Eng 4(3):371–408
65. Zheng Y, Barbu A, Georgescu B et al (2008) Fast automatic heart chamber segmentation from 3D CT data using marginal space learning and steerable features. IEEE Trans Med Imaging 27(11):1668–1681
66. Pluim JPW, Maintz JBA, Viergever MA (2003) Mutual-information-based registration of medical images: a survey. IEEE Trans Med Imaging 22(8):986–1004
67. Suri JS (2000) Computer vision, pattern recognition and image processing in left ventricle segmentation: the last 50 years. Pattern Anal Appl 3(3):209–242
68. Zhu L, Gao Y, Appia V et al (2013) Automatic delineation of the myocardial wall from ct images via shape segmentation and variational region growing. IEEE Trans Biomed Eng 60(10):2887–2895
69. Saruhassini K, Vanithamani R (2015) An efficient system for automatic heart wall segmentation from cardiac CT images. Int J Adv Res Comput Sci Manag Stud 3(4):316–326
70. European Carotid Surgery Trialists Collaborative Group (1999) Randomised trial of endarterectomy for recently symptomatic carotid stenosis: final results of the MRC european carotid surgery (ECST). Lancet 351:1379–1387
71. Dehkordi MT, Sadri S, Doosthoseini A (2011) A review of coronary vessel segmentation algorithms. J Med Signals Sens 1(1):49–54
72. Tian Y, Pan Y, Duan F, et al (2016) Automated segmentation of coronary arteries based on statistical region growing and heuristic decision method. BioMed Res Int. Article ID 3530251

73. Zhou C, Chan HP, Chughtai A et al (2012) Automated coronary artery tree extraction in coronary CT angiography using a multiscale enhancement and dynamic balloon tracking (MSCAR-DBT) method. Comput Med Imaging Graph Off J Comput Med Imaging Soc 36(1):1–10
74. Peng P, Lekadir K, Gooya A et al (2016) A review of heart chamber segmentation for structural and functional analysis using cardiac magnetic resonance imaging. Magma 29:155–195

Automated Techniques for Vessel Detection and Segmentation in Cardiovascular Images

Kristen M. Meiburger, Cristina Caresio, Massimo Salvi and Filippo Molinari

1 Introduction

Imaging plays a fundamental role in the assessment of the cardiovascular system and it aids clinicians and researchers in several fields and applications. As examples, from a clinical point of view, imaging is fundamental in the planning of surgical structural interventions [1], in functional studies (such as myocardial perfusion) [2], and in the monitoring of post-surgical patients [3]. In research, examples of imaging applications are the study of inflammatory processes [4], of atherosclerosis [5], and of biomarkers targeted for specific diseases [6–8].

In a recent review, Di Carli et al. [9] summarized which could be the future of cardiovascular imaging, both from the point of view of the technology advances and of the applications. They showed that to properly phenotype cardiovascular diseases, clinical, molecular, and genomic studies had to be associated. They also put emphasis on the critical role of functional and morphological imaging, which is capable of precise, organ-specific anatomic localization and quantification of disease traits.

A fundamental aspect of cardiovascular imaging is the capability of providing data from both invasive [10] and non-invasive (or minimally-invasive) [11] acquisitions. This characteristic, coupled with the several imaging devices adapted to cardiovascular imaging, led to the development of integrated examinations, known as multi-modality imaging [12].

Quantitative imaging is nowadays becoming more and more important. In fact, given the wide range of applications of cardiovascular imaging, there are specific studies or assessments that can be effectively performed only by relying on computer systems. Finer image details, global image parameters, and time-varying physiological phenomena can be accurately described only by a numerical analysis of the

K. M. Meiburger · C. Caresio · M. Salvi · F. Molinari (✉)
Biolab, Department of Electronics and Telecommunications, Politecnico di Torino, Turin, Italy
e-mail: filippo.molinari@polito.it

S. Golemati and K. S. Nikita (eds.), *Cardiovascular Computing—Methodologies and Clinical Applications*, Series in BioEngineering,
https://doi.org/10.1007/978-981-10-5092-3_7

acquired images. As an example, in atherosclerosis studies, the visualization and quantification of the cellular and molecular components involved in atherosclerotic plaque stability can be computed only by numerically processing the images [13]. More generally, when biological properties of the tissues must be explored, a numerical analysis of the images is required.

One of the fields of cardiovascular imaging in which computer systems proved their importance is the analysis of vessels and vascular structures. Apart from atherosclerosis, in which the accurate analysis of the vessel walls is fundamental [14], other pathologies require a precise analysis of vessels, such as diabetes [15], cancer [16], and neurological diseases [17].

In this chapter, we will present the most widely used techniques for the automated detection and segmentation of vessels in cardiovascular images. We will focus on the most clinically used imaging modalities (i.e., CT, MRI, and US) and will describe, for each modality, the most used and established techniques. Given the wide application spectrum, the non-invasivity, the portability, and the exceptional temporal resolution, ultrasound imaging will have emphasis in this chapter.

2 Automated Vessel Recognition

Typically, the first step in a completely automatic image analysis pipeline is the identification of the organ or tissue of interest. Occasionally, the specific organ or tissue may present a very distinct morphology and characteristics compared to the surrounding tissue, making the automatic detection a simpler phase. Such is the case of vessel recognition.

2.1 Vessel Structure and Blood Appearance

If we consider arteries, their geometry is quite well defined and repeatable: arteries, especially the bigger arteries of the human body, have a circular section, a three-layered wall, and lumen filled by blood. Therefore, geometry or blood aspect can be useful to automatically detect the vessel position in the image frame. Regarding blood, it must be remembered that:

- In ultrasound images, blood is anechoic (see Fig. 1). This means that the lumen of the vessels is theoretically black, since blood is not reflecting any portion of the ultrasound beam. The liquid part of the blood (plasma) is anechoic as all liquids are, whereas the erythrocytes (i.e., the corpuscular part) have dimension much lower than the resolution power of the ultrasound equipment.
- Blood shows a small linear absorption coefficient to X-rays. Since CT scanners map the linear coefficient of tissues into Hounsfield units (HU), being zero the HU of water, blood is usually mapped in the range [45, 65] HU [18]. Since blood can

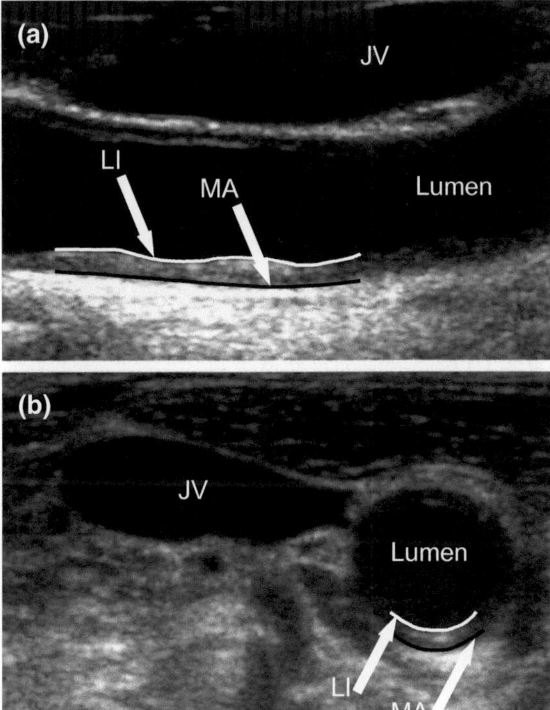

Fig. 1 Ultrasound image of a common carotid artery in **a** longitudinal and **b** transverse projection. The jugular vein (JV) is also visible in both projections. The vessel lumen is black, since blood has an anechoic aspect in ultrasound images. LI—lumen-intima interface. MA—media adventitia interface

have HU values like those of other tissues, often a contrast agent dye is injected when vascular examinations are performed. In this case, for example during a CT angiography (CTA), the contrast agent increases the HU values associated to blood, thus making the lumen of the vessels clearly distinguishable. Figure 2 reports a sample CT in which it is possible to observe the thoracic aorta (TA) before (Fig. 2a) and after (Fig. 2b) contrast agent injection. The HU value of the TA lumen raised from about 50 to 300.

- Since the MR maps a relaxation time (either T_1 or T_2), depending on the excitation sequence, blood can have a bright or dark appearance (i.e., it may have an increased or reduced radiofrequency signal). Bright-blood (Fig. 3a) is usually obtained through conventional gradient-echo sequences, whereas spin-echo sequences are used to acquire a better visualization of the myocardium and of the valvular structures, coupled with a black-blood appearance [19] (Fig. 3b). By using a contrast agent dye, it is possible to acquire a better description of the vascular structure and perform a MR angiography (MRA) (Fig. 3c).

The three-layered structure of the arterial wall is neatly observable in US images. In longitudinal projection (Fig. 1a), the arterial structure is characterized by a black lumen, which can be roughly considered as a black rectangle, surrounded by two bright stripes, which represent the adventitial layer of the walls. It has been demon-

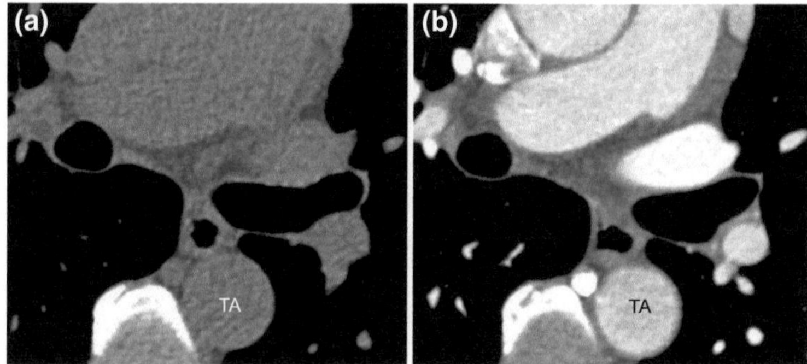

Fig. 2 CT representation of an axial slice of the thoracic aorta (TA). **a** CT without contrast agent. **B** CT with contrast agent. For both figures, the visualization parameters of the CT images were WL:34 and WW:890. In **a** the lumen of the TA had average HU of about 50; in **b** of about 300

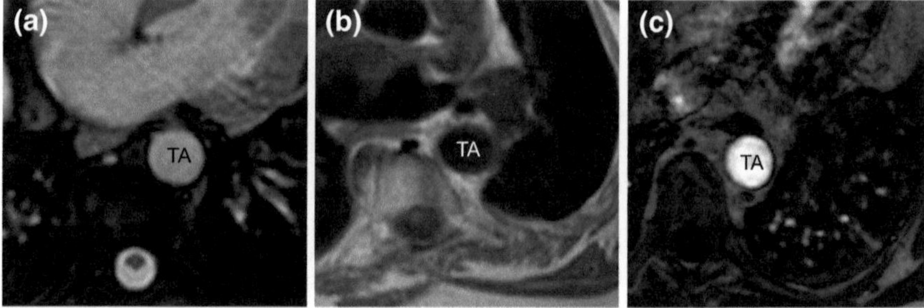

Fig. 3 MR representation of axial slices of the thoracic aorta (TA). **a** Bright-blood. **b** Black-blood. **c** MRA after the injection of a gadolinium-based contrast agent bolus

strated that the adventitial layers are usually the most hyperechoic structures in an arterial scan, when no calcium deposits are present [20]. Due to resolution limitations, the intima layer is usually merged with the media layer, leading to the definition of two interfaces: the lumen-intima (LI) and the media-adventitia (MA) interfaces. Some Authors prefer to name as "intima-media complex" the arterial wall portion that is comprised between the LI and MA interfaces [21, 22]. In transverse projection (Fig. 1b), the arteries appear as circular black regions delimited by an upper and a lower bright bound. The lateral portions of the wall are usually under-represented, due to poor reflection of the ultrasound wave.

In CTA and MRA, vessels are usually tracked to reconstruct their 3-D morphology. Compared to US, MR and, especially, CT have a lower resolution on the vessel wall, but offer the possibility of describing the 3-D architecture of the vessel and of its network. In MR images, it is possible to visualize the inner and outer boundaries of the artery, without distinguishing between the three layers. In CT images, the arterial wall is not clearly visible and, as aforementioned, CTA is usually performed in order to better delineate the vessel lumen. In both CT/CTA and MR/MRA 3-D acquisitions, vessels are recognized and segmented in slices that are orthogonal to the vessels' axis. Hence, in this projection, arteries are substantially circular. The method proposed by van't Klooster et al. is a good example of a semi-automated method for the tracking of arteries in axial MR images [23].

The recognition and segmentation of veins is still an open problem. The morphology of veins is very variable among subjects. Also, a specific vein can be opened or collapsed depending on several factors, including body position and pressure. Therefore, there are no standard and established methods for the processing of vein images. More specifically, no reviews have been published ever about vein processing techniques in US, MR, or CT images.

2.2 *Techniques for Vessels Localization*

In an automated analysis framework, the first step consists in the localization of the vessel in the image frame. Such localization can initially be coarse, since a more accurate segmentation will be performed in a subsequent step.

Automated techniques for the coarse localization of vessels can be divided into the following macro-areas:

- Shape priors techniques
- Texture and classification techniques
- Pixel intensity and/or local statistics based techniques.

2.2.1 Shape Priors

Anatomical shape prior methods are based on the a priori knowledge of the expected anatomical structure. As aforementioned, this knowledge can be easily exploited in the case of arteries recognition. These types of techniques can cope very well with suboptimal images; i.e., with images affected by noise, or with weak or under-represented edges. Models are typically built from a large database of training samples to determine the final shape prior.

The possible drawback of these techniques is represented by pathology. As an example, if a shape prior was built on the healthy common carotid artery morphology, it would be difficult to adapt it to the case of a diseased vessel possibly containing a plaque. In other words, shape priors are usually as good as the training samples.

2.2.2 Texture and Classification

These types of methods are based on finding the features of the microstructure of the tissue being imaged and consequently classifying the pixels or sections of the image into different regions based on these features. An advantage of texture techniques is that they are typically based on statistical patterns of the pixel intensities, so they are more independent of the physics of the imaging system. Many of these texture techniques are based on the calculation of Haralick's co-occurrence matrices [24] which, despite being computationally expensive, have performed well in a number of applications and studies [25–28].

In this category, we also find the so-called "superpixel" or "graph-based" techniques. These techniques are mainly based on the division of the original image into "superpixels" or patches, which are then labeled as belonging to either the vessel or background, using graph cuts [29]. A more detailed example of this technique, specifically tuned on carotid ultrasound images, is available in the work by Rosati et al. [30]. In this multi-scale approach, different patches of a pixel's neighborhood

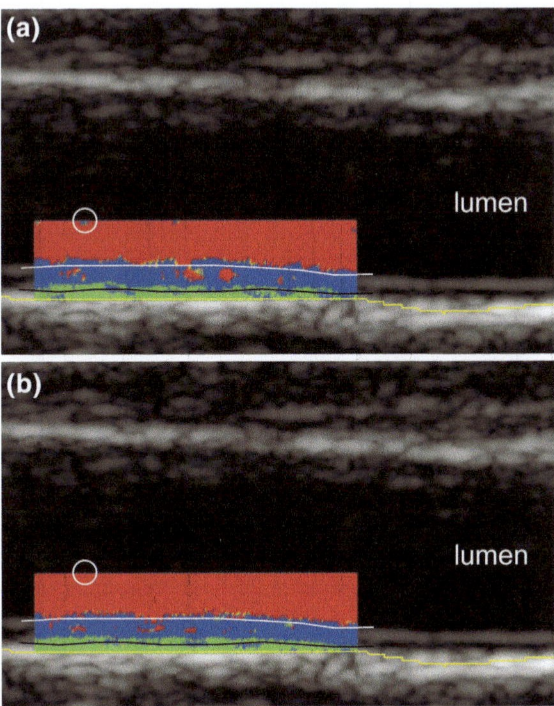

Fig. 4 Comparison between the first version of voting classifier, **a** trained with three datasets of 1500 pixels each and the final voting classifier, **b** trained with three datasets of 1800 pixels each. Red, blue, and green points mark the pixels classified as belonging to lumen, IM, and adventitia classes, respectively. Pixels not classified by the voting procedure are indicated with yellow points. The white circle highlights an example of pixels zone added to the initial datasets. These pixels are chosen among those pixels resulting in a wrong class from the first voting classification (**a**) and in the last classifier the same pixels result in correct class (**b**) The white line corresponds to the lumen-intima (LI) interface, the black line marks out the media-adventitia (MA) interface, and the yellow line delimits the far adventitia layer. (Reproduced from [30] with permission)

were considered, and up to 141 features were computed. Figure 4 shows the result of this work, in which pixels were assigned to either the lumen (red), the intima and media layers (blue), or the adventitia (green) layer. Such result was obtained after a feature selection and reduction step, followed by a voting classifier. In a first version (Fig. 4a), the Authors used three training datasets of 1500 pixels each, and then (Fig. 4b) three datasets of 1800 pixels each.

2.2.3 Pixel Intensity and/or Local Statistics

These approaches exploit the vessel appearance in a specific image modality (i.e., US, MR, CT). Vessel representation can be thought of as a mixture model with varying intensity distributions. This is because, as discussed in the previous section:

- pixels belonging to the vessel lumen are characterized by a given intensity (close to zero in US and black-blood MR images) and low standard deviation;
- pixels belonging to the adventitia layer of the carotid wall are characterized by different intensity (very bright in US images and black-blood MR) and low standard deviation;
- all remaining pixels should have different mean intensity and higher standard deviation.

Thus, it is possible to explore the neighborhood of a pixel and, based on its intensity value, of the mean intensity of the neighborhood, and of the standard deviation of the neighborhood, state if this pixel belongs to lumen, wall, or to other structures/tissues.

A complete description of such approach, specifically tuned for longitudinal carotid ultrasound images, can be found in the works by Molinari et al. [27, 31, 32]. With reference to Fig. 5, the pixels belonging to the arterial lumen (and, more in general, to blood) are easily detected because they are characterized by a low intensity value and low standard deviation of their neighborhood. Hence, by considering a bidimensional histogram (Fig. 5b) it is possible to mark all the pixels possibly corresponding to blood in the image (Fig. 5c). From that mask, by using simple conditions, it is possible to mark the center of the lumen (L) and the far adventitia wall (Fig. 5d). This completes the automated detection of the vessel in the image.

Once the vessel has been recognized in the image frame, its walls must be accurately segmented. This step is fundamental for several purposes, among which: atherosclerosis assessment, morphology visualization, analysis of wall alterations, intima-media thickness measurement, classification of stable/instable plaques, and subsequent strain imaging [33].

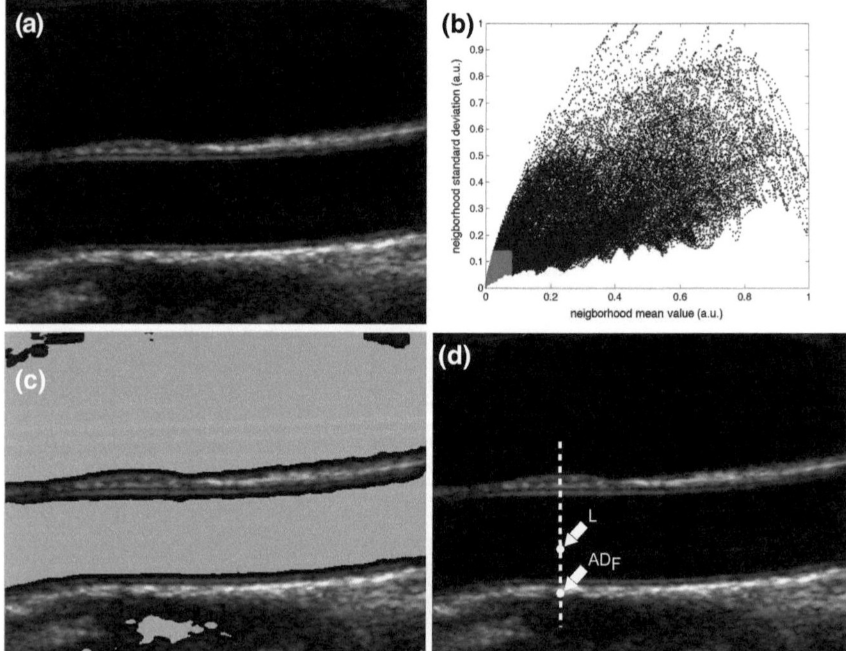

Fig. 5 Strategy for far wall adventitial tracing. **a** Original image. **b** 2DH. The gray portion of the 2DH denotes the region in which we suppose to find only lumen pixels. **c** Original image with lumen pixels overlaid in gray. **d** Sample processing of one column, with the marker points of the far (ADF) adventitia layer and of the lumen (L). (Reproduced from [27] with permission)

3 Wall Segmentation in MR Data

Most of the techniques that have been proposed for the segmentation of vessels in MR/MRA images consider axial slices. Often, such techniques produce a 3-D segmentation of the vessel, which is in fact obtained by a stack of 2-D processed axial images. There are, however, studies based on 3-D adjustable models.

3.1 Wall Thickness (WT) and Arterial Wall Area (AWA) Measurement in 1.5T 2-D Images

In this type of image, the most widely used segmentation technique is the level-sets method (LSM). Level-sets are active contours, also called geometric deformable models. The basic idea is to represent the contours as the zero-level of a higher-order implicit function, which is the level-set function. Then the level-set function evolves according to imposed partial differential equations (PDEs). One of the most widely used implementations of the LSM is the one by Li et al. which is also known as variational LSM without re-initialization [34].

If we consider a 2-D contour and name it as C, then it can be thought as the zero-level of a 3-D level-set φ, so that:

$$C = \{(x, y)|\varphi = 0$$

Being the LSM an active and deformable method, the contour C can be made time-varying, so that its definition can be written as:

$$C(t) = \{(x, y)|\varphi(\mathrm{t}) = 0$$

In the proposal by Li et al. the variation of the level-set is obtained by the following equation:

$$\frac{\partial \varphi}{\partial t} = \mu\left[\nabla\varphi - div\left(\frac{\nabla\varphi}{|\nabla\varphi|}\right)\right] + \lambda\,\delta\varphi\,div\left(g\frac{\nabla\varphi}{|\nabla\varphi|}\right) + \upsilon\,g\,\delta\varphi$$

where:

- $\mu > 0$ is a parameter that controls the effect of penalizing the level-set from getting too distant from a signed distance function;
- $\lambda > 0$ is a parameter that controls and regularizes the length of the curve C;
- υ is a parameter controlling the speed of motion of the level-set;
- $\delta\varphi$ is the univariate Dirac function applied to the level-set;
- g is an edge-map, used to communicate to the level-set which are the edges to be tracked in the image. If we name as I the input image, and if we call as G a specific Gaussian smoothing kernel, then:

$$g = \frac{1}{1 + |\nabla G * I|^2}$$

An example of segmentation obtained by this method is reported by Fig. 6. Saba et al. applied this segmentation strategy to MRI carotid images [35]. Proton-density weighted (PDW) images were used for plaque segmentation. The parameters for PDW sequence were: flip angle 180°, field of view (FOV) 16 × 16 cm, TR 700 ms, TE 10 ms, number of excitations 2, slice thickness 2 mm, matrix size 640 × 640. They examined 10 patients coming from their Stroke Unit (7 males; age: 67 ± 6 years) with stenosis to the internal carotid artery. The longitudinal coverage for each carotid artery was 72 mm. By using the above descripted LSM technique, they traced the inner and outer boundaries of each slice of the artery, and then computed the wall thickness (WT) and arterial wall area (AWA), by measuring the geometric distance between the inner and outer border (for WT) and the area comprised between the two borders (for AWA). Numerical results obtained by LSM were compared to those manually measured by three independent observers. Observers manually traced the inner/outer

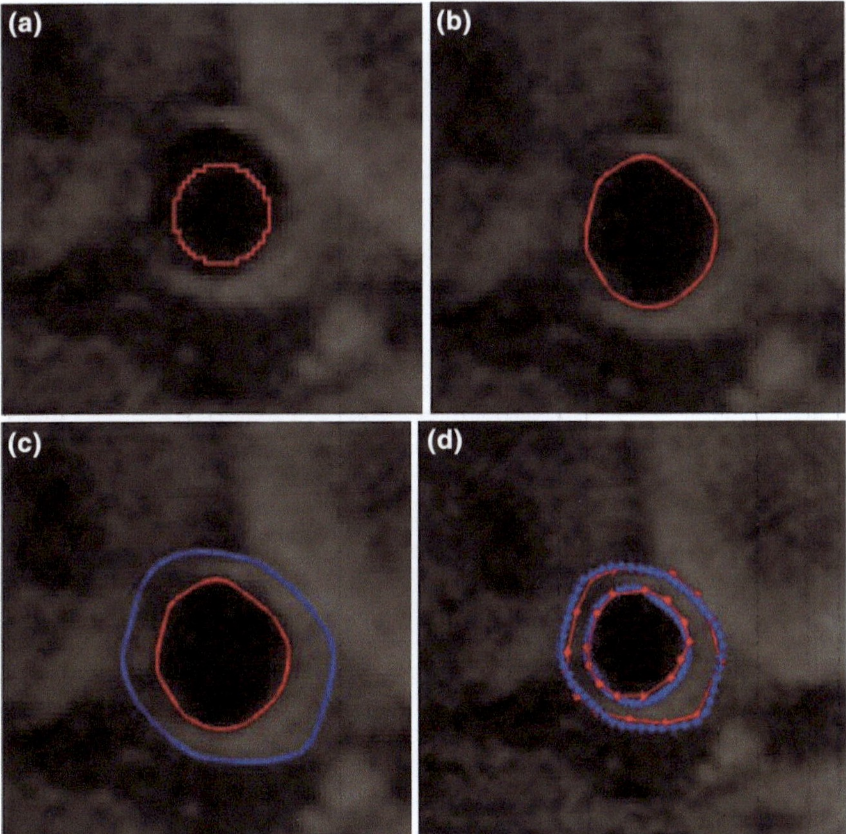

Fig. 6 Segmentation results from LSM. **a** Initial contour for lumen boundary; **b** lumen boundary from LSM; **c** lumen/outer wall boundary from LSM; **d** overlay with manual segmentation (dotted lines). (Reproduced from [35] with permission)

borders of the artery in each image frame, then WT and AWA were measured in the same way as for LSM obtained boundaries. The average positioning error of the inner boundary for LSM compared to the observers was 0.34 ± 0.2 mm, and that for the outer boundary was 0.47 ± 0.2 mm. The average WT error was approximately 0.10 ± 0.2 mm. The overall absolute AWA error between the LMS and observers was lower than 10%, with a correlation index close to 0.8.

3.2 *Wall Thickness (WT) and Arterial Wall Volume (AWV) in 3T 3-D Images*

van't Klooster et al. proposed a segmentation method based on non-uniform rational B-spline surfaces (NURBS). Conceptually, by using NURBS, they developed a deformable cylindrical 3-D model of the carotid artery [23]. This model could adapt to the data under analysis by a very simple and user-friendly interaction between the model and the MR images. Such interaction had to be driven by an operator. From the computer-generated boundaries of the artery, the WT and arterial wall volume (AWV) were computed and compared to those obtained by manual measurements by experts. They studied 45 subjects (56% males; mean age = 52 years; age range = [19, 79] years) and acquired images by using a 3 T scanner. Black-blood images were obtained by using a time-of-flight MRA sequence, with these parameters: flip angle 20°, field of view (FOV) 300 mm, TR 7.7 ms, TE 3.8 ms, pixel sixe 1 mm × 1.23 mm × 5.0 mm. The WT measurement error was 0.12 ± 0.21 mm and that of the AWV was 45.4 ± 80.2 mm^3. The correlation between manual and computer-based measurements of WT and AWV were approximately equal to 0.7 and 0.8, respectively.

4 Discussion

The segmentation of the arterial walls in MR images cannot be considered a closed problem. First of all, as documented in the work by Saba et al. [35], the segmentation techniques currently available are often user-driven and lack full automation. This is mainly because it has been shown that automated vessel detection techniques are less robust in MRI than in other imaging modalities. Secondly, often the 3-D profile of the vessel is obtained only through the independent processing of the 2-D slices.

Moreover, some further considerations should be made.

- **Measurement accuracy**. When the vessel segmentation is performed to measure some morphological parameters, the measurement accuracy must be considered. The WT is usually measured with a bias of about 0.1 ± 0.2 mm. Such value is statistically higher than that obtained by WT measurement performed on ultrasound images. Even though some studies documented a high sensitivity of the MRI in detecting the focal arterial wall thickening (see [36] as an example), usually US are used as gold-standard for the validation of MRI measurement algorithms [37].
- **2-D versus 3-D techniques**. Typically, 2-D techniques showed higher accuracy in segmenting the vessel walls, compared to 3-D methods. The deformable contours are among the most used approaches to process 2-D images, whereas modelling approaches are preferred in a 3-D scenario. If 3-D techniques offer a greater robustness to local noise, 2-D techniques are more sensible to localized alterations of the vessel wall. Therefore, global parameters like the AWV and AWA are better estimated by 3-D techniques.

- **Noise sources**. MRI vascular images may be affected by some noise sources that lower the performance of computer systems for vessel segmentation. One of the most important is the partial volume effect, which can cause blurring in the wall edges [35]. In presence of blurred edges, the segmentation techniques may misplace the wall contours, thus increasing the WT measurement error. In 3T scans, several studies reported an increase of the signal-to-noise and contrast-to-noise ratio compared to the same scans performed at 1.5T [38]. Nowinski et al. also showed that vascular reconstructions made at 3T and 7T showed more vessels than the same scans at 1.5T, thus revealing an increased resolution of the MRI techniques in presence of a higher magnetic field [39].

5 Wall Segmentation in US Images

Ultrasound imaging is the most used diagnostic tool to assess the arterial wall. In clinical practice, ultrasounds offer several advantages such as: (i) use of non-ionizing radiations, (ii) safety and quick examination of the patient, (iii) absence of documented biological effects, (iv) low-cost equipment (if compared to other medical imaging devices), (v) wide availability of the ultrasound scanners, and (vi) ultrasounds can effectively visualize the components of the arterial wall. Unfortunately, ultrasound images have a signal-to-noise ratio (SNR) that is lower than other imaging modalities.

Computer methods for segmenting the ultrasound arterial images mainly aim at tracing the LI and MA boundaries. The IMT, in fact, can be computed by measuring the distance of the LI from the MA boundary. In some studies, the media and intima thicknesses were measured separately [40].

5.1 Edge-Tracking and Gradient-Based Techniques

Pignoli et al. were the first to apply a computer-based technique to perform the IMT measurement of the carotid artery [41]. Considering a carotid image in longitudinal projection, they measured the distal wall IMT by considering the intensity profile of a section of the image when moving from the centre of the vessel to the borders. Being the vessel lumen ideally black (i.e., zero-mean), they tracked the increase in the intensity profile that occurs in proximity of the LI interface [42].

A similar approach was adopted in 2001 by Liguori et al. [43]. They proposed a segmentation technique based on edge-detection that used image gradients. They considered the artery as horizontally placed in the B-Mode image. For each column of the image they calculated the gradient of the intensity profile. In order to facilitate edge detection, Liguori et al. adopted a statistical thresholding to reduce noise before computing the image gradient.

Edge-tracking and gradient-based methods may suffer from the problem of the superimposed noise. In fact, noise may preclude the proper detection of the LI and MA interfaces. Faita et al. adopted a gradient-based approach which is more noise robust than the traditional ones [43, 44]. The core of the method is the first-order absolute moment (FOAM):

$$FOAM(x,y) = \frac{1}{A_\theta}\int\limits_{\theta} \left|I_1(x,y) - I_2\left(x-x',y-y'\right)\right| * G\left(x',y',\sigma\right)\,dx'dy'$$

where:

- $I_1(x,y) = I(x,y) * G_1(x,y,\sigma_1)$, is a Gaussian low-pass filtered version of the input image $I(x,y)$;
- $I_2(x,y) = I(x,y) * G_2(x,y,\sigma_2)$, is a Gaussian low-pass filtered version of the input image $I(x,y)$, with different standard deviation;
- $G\left(x',y',\sigma\right)$ is a regularization term, and third version of Gaussian low-pass filter.

Conceptually, this operator computes the average dispersion of the image pixels in a circular domain called A_θ. The FOAM is null when the image has no intensity changes in the domain θ. In correspondence of a neat intensity transition, the FOAM has a high value. The overall performance of this methodology was very high: IMT measurement error was equal to 10.0 ± 38.0 μm. Moreover, FOAM operator and intelligent procedures to discover maxima ensured a good robustness to noise. This technique is real-time; hence, it is suited to clinical application.

5.2 *Dynamic Programming Techniques*

Dynamic programming techniques were introduced starting from early 90s to reduce the variability in ultrasound measurements [45]. Wendelhag et al. first introduced a dynamic programming procedure for the automatic detection of echo interfaces [46]. This technique combined multiple measurements of echo intensity, intensity gradient, and boundary continuity. The system also included optional interactive modification by the human operator. An initial set of ultrasound images was manually segmented by expert operators and served as reference (ground truth). The estimated values of the three boundary features (echo intensity, intensity gradient, and boundary continuity) were linearly combined to create a cost function. Each image point was associated with a specific cost that in turn correlated with the likelihood of that point being located at the echo interface. Therefore, points being located at the interfaces between different artery layers were expected to be associated with a low cost, whereas points located far from the interfaces was associated with a high cost. The weights of the linear combination originating the cost function were determined by training the system, considering the ground truth as reference. Dynamic programming was used to reduce the computational cost given by the need of inspecting all the points of the image. The IMT measurement error of this technique was better than 40 ± 36 μm.

Dynamic programming techniques can be applied also in a multi-resolution framework: starting from the image in a low-resolution scale, the image features are computed; then, a refinement procedure is applied and the features are computed at each step [47]. The artery detection can therefore be obtained in the coarse scale image, whereas the accurate detection of the LI/MA interfaces can be made in the fine scale image.

5.3 *Active Contours (Snakes)*

Active parametric contours, also called *snakes*, have been widely used in segmentation of medical images. The snake can be thought as a set of vertices connected by line segments, which can evolve under the action of different forces. The popularity of the snake-based segmentation methodology relies on the fact that the artery LI and MA boundaries can be well distinguished in the image. Therefore, a straight deformable model could be able to adapt to such interfaces after a proper tuning of its parameters. Most of the studies adopted the traditional formulation of a snake as proposed by Williams and Shah [48]. From a geometrical point of view, a two-dimensional snake is a parametric contour represented by $v(s) = [x(s), y(s)]$, where (x, y) denotes the spatial coordinates of an image and $s \in [0, 1]$ represents the parametric domain. The snake adapts itself by a dynamic process that minimizes a global energy function:

$$E[v(s)] = E_{int}[v(s)] + E_{ext}[v(s)]$$

where:

- $E_{int}[v(s)]$ is called "internal energy" and constrains the shape of the curve. Usually, such energy term is proportional to the curve derivatives, in order to regularize the curvature and elasticity of the curve. When snakes are used to segment the LI/MA interfaces in longitudinal US images, the internal energy is kept to a high value, since such interfaces look almost linear.
- $E_{ext}[v(s)]$ is called "external energy" and is used to drive the curve towards the image edges. Hence, often this energy term is modeled by image gradients.

The snake points should move towards the features of the image while remaining constrained by the internal forces. The equilibrium condition is met when the internal forces counterbalance the external ones. Therefore, fine tuning of the snake is fundamental for an accurate segmentation.

A complete and thorough summary of the snake performances in carotid segmentation was given in 2007 by Loizou et al. [49]. The same research team further improved their snake-based system and made it fully automated [50] and suitable also to the processing of arteries with plaques [51] (Fig. 7).

In 2012, Molinari et al. proposed a dual-snake system consisting of two different active contours (one for the LI and one for the MA interface) evolving together [52].

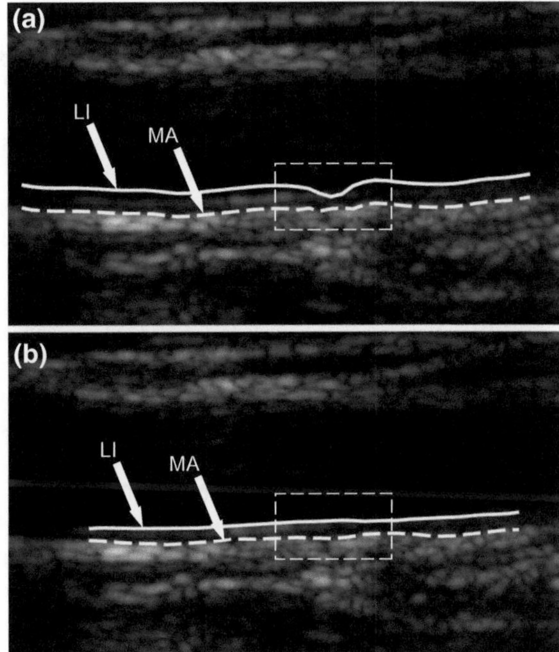

Fig. 7 Performance difference between unconstrained (panel a) and constrained (panel b) dual-snake segmentation system. The dashed box in panel a indicates an image region in which the unconstrained LI snake is almost collapsed on the MA snake. The constrained snakes are prevented from bleeding or collapsing, hence in panel b the inaccuracy is solved

In their implementation, they added a "mutual energy" term in order to prevent the LI snake from diverging or collapsing on the MA snake. The authors demonstrated that dual-snake systems have superior performance in IMT measurement compared to conventional snakes [53].

5.4 Transform-Based and Modelling Approaches

Often, the layers of the vessel can be recognized and accurately segmented by relying on modelling techniques or mathematical transformations.

One of the most used transformation approaches is the Hough transform [54]. This tool allows for an efficient detection of shapes in an image, if a description of the shape is mathematically provided and a scale parameter is selected. The Hough transform is mostly used to detect lines and circles. Some authors exploited the properties of the Hough transform and developed a technique that could automatically segment both longitudinal and transverse B-Mode images [55, 56]. The appearance of an artery is straight in longitudinal projections and circular in transverse projection. Hence, by using the Hough transform it is possible to detect straight lines in longitudinal images (corresponding to the LI/MA interfaces) and circles in transverse images. This method is fairly robust also to small morphological changes of the vessel wall, thus it can be used also in presence of small atherosclerotic plaques. It was shown that, compared to the pixel classification performed by human tracings, by using the Hough transform it is possible to segment the carotid artery with a sensitivity of about 96% in longitudinal images and 82% in transverse images, with specificity of about 96% in both cases.

In modelling approaches, the image is considered as the combination of the intensity typical of the vessel structures layers plus noise. Hence, an image region containing a portion of the vessel lumen, the wall, and some surrounding tissues could be characterized by the specific distributions mimicking the intensity distributions of the three components. The most used models, in vascular ultrasounds, are the Gaussian mixture model and the Nakagami modelling.

In 2014, Veronese et al. performed the IMT measurement of the abdominal aorta of foetuses by using a technique based on the Gaussian mixture model [57]. Considering a relatively large range of aorta IMT (spanning from 0.4 mm to more than 1 mm), they obtained a IMT measurement error lower than 19% when compared to human measurements. This error was of the same order of magnitude of the inter-observer variability of independent readers (about 14%).

The Nakagami distribution proved effective in modelling the radiofrequency ultrasound signal that was scattered by the artery wall layers [58]. Destrempes et al. proposed a segmentation strategy based on Nakagami mixture modelling and stochastic optimization [59]. This technique proved very performing in the segmentation of the common carotid artery in longitudinal projection: using the mean absolute distance metric the authors obtained LI and MA segmentation errors equal to 21.0 ± 13.0 μm and 0.16 ± 7.0 μm, respectively.

5.5 Data Mining Techniques

Recently, due to growing interest in the fields of data mining and, more generally, in big data analysis, non-linear and innovative techniques have been applied in the field of vascular ultrasounds. Most of these techniques have in common the following architecture [60]:

- *Step 1: feature extraction*. The image is analysed in order to extract as many descriptors (i.e., features) as possible to characterize the content of the image itself. Some authors stick to conventional and first-order descriptors (i.e, analysis of the gray scale distribution of the image or of a portion of the image) [31, 61], whereas others tend to include higher-order texture descriptors [24, 62].
- *Step 2: feature reduction/selection*. Given the high number of extracted features and the risk of having collinear variables that could lead to an over-constrained system, the features are usually selected and their number is reduced. Collinear and strongly correlated variables are taken out, whereas variables with negligible variance are ignored. The most performing and widely used reduction and selection techniques for vascular ultrasound images have recently been revised by Rosati et al. [30].

- *Step 3: classification.* The features associated to each pixel are classified in order to assign the pixel to a specific image component (i.e., the lumen, the intima, the media, the adventitia, etc). Pixels with borderline conditions are usually kept in a "uncertainty" class/cluster and ignored. Several methods have been used to accomplish this step, even though often fuzzy classifiers or artificial neural networks are used [60].
- *Step 4: vessel boundaries refinement.* Due to intrinsic data variability and to classification errors, the output of the classifier is usually not accurate enough to be considered as the final segmentation.

This approach has been used not only for IMT measurement and image segmentation, but also for the assessment of the cardiovascular risk score based on the analysis of the arterial layer [60], for the assessment of the subjects' vascular age [63], and for the characterization of the atherosclerotic plaque [25].

6 Discussion

Greater space has been allocated, in this chapter, to the discussion of the vessel segmentation in ultrasound images, since, as aforementioned, echographic examinations are of paramount importance in clinical routine and in research projects. Moreover, ultrasound images are the more challenging to process.

In fact, it is well known that noise represents perhaps the most prominent problem in ultrasound imaging. Speckle noise is an interference caused by multiple scattering of the sound waves. It reduces the overall quality of the image by creating a "pixelated" effect that is detrimental both to human perception and to numerical processing algorithms.

Ultrasound images also have overall quality that is dependent on the scanner used and on its settings. In fact, being ultrasound imaging a human-dependent scanning technique, different operators may render the same object in different fashions.

Specifically referring to CCA images, another complication is given by the high variability in normal vessel morphology and in vessel appearance under pathology.

If combined, all these challenges justify why, currently, the segmentation of vessels in ultrasound images is often still an open problem.

7 Final Remarks

The development of automated solutions for the detection and segmentation of vessels in cardiovascular images requires the adoption of specific approaches and techniques. As discussed in the chapter, given the different types of images (MRI, CT, US, etc…) and the variability caused by physiology and by pathological conditions, it is not possible to pick an "optimal" technique.

Robustness is certainly a key point. When facing the problem of vessel segmentation, it is important to remember that vessels are different for several parameters, including shape, size, orientation, and composition. Also, noise is another important challenge, mainly for ultrasound images.

Even though in this chapter only studies regarding the segmentation of arteries have been shown, it must be remembered that also approaches for the segmentation of veins have been developed. Vein segmentation, however, is still not well established, and the developed techniques are, up to now, mostly proof-of-concept researches. In fact, the physiological shape variability of the venous network is very high and it could preclude the performance of all the techniques relying on models, transforms, and active contours. Often, veins are of undetermined diameter, since their size depends on posture, physio/pathological conditions, and by the surrounding tissue.

References

1. Carminati M, Agnifili M, Arcidiacono C, Brambilla N, Bussadori C, Butera G et al (2013) Role of imaging in interventions on structural heart disease. Expert Rev Cardiovasc Ther 11(12):1659–1676
2. Qayyum AA, Kastrup J (2015) Measuring myocardial perfusion: the role of PET. MRI and CT Clin Radiol 70(6):576–584
3. Ferguson TB, Buch AN (2016) Improving quality and outcomes of coronary artery bypass grafting procedures. Expert Rev Cardiovasc Ther 14(5):617–631
4. Castañeda S, Nurmohamed MT, González-Gay MA (2016) Cardiovascular disease in inflammatory rheumatic diseases. Best Pract Res Clin Rheumatol 30(5):851–869
5. Ladeiras-Lopes R, Agewall S, Tawakol A, Staels B, Stein E, Mentz RJ et al (2015) Atherosclerosis: recent trials, new targets and future directions. Int J Cardiol 192:72–81
6. Jalalzadeh H, Indrakusuma R, Planken RN, Legemate DA, Koelemay MJW, Balm R (2016) Inflammation as a predictor of abdominal aortic aneurysm growth and rupture: a systematic review of imaging biomarkers. Eur J Vasc Endovasc Surg 52(3):333–342
7. Sharifi M, Rakhit RD, Humphries SE, Nair D (2016) Cardiovascular risk stratification in familial hypercholesterolaemia. Heart 102(13):1003–1008
8. Tehrani DM, Wong ND (2016) Integrating biomarkers and imaging for cardiovascular disease risk assessment in diabetes. Curr Cardiol Rep 18(11):105
9. Di Carli MF, Geva T, Davidoff R (2016) The future of cardiovascular imaging. Circulation 133(25)
10. Pison L, Proclemer A, Bongiorni MG, Marinskis G, Hernandez-Madrid A, Blomstrom-Lundqvist C et al (2013) Imaging techniques in electrophysiology and implantable device procedures: results of the European heart rhythm association survey. Europace 15(9):1333–1336
11. Blankstein R (2012) Introduction to noninvasive cardiac imaging. Circulation 125(3)
12. Cardim N, Galderisi M, Edvardsen T, Plein S, Popescu BA, D'Andrea A et al (2015) Role of multimodality cardiac imaging in the management of patients with hypertrophic cardiomyopathy: an expert consensus of the European association of cardiovascular imaging endorsed by the Saudi heart association. Eur Heart J Cardiovasc Imaging 16(3)
13. McAteer MA, Choudhury RP (2015) Noninvasive molecular imaging of mouse atherosclerosis. Methods Mol Biol 1339:61–83
14. Labropoulos N, Leon LR, Brewster LP, Pryor L, Tiongson J, Kang SS et al (2005) Are your arteries older than your age? Eur J Vasc Endovasc Surg 30(6):588–596
15. Kianoush S, Al Rifai M, Whelton SP, Shaya GE, Bush AL, Graham G et al (2016) Stratifying cardiovascular risk in diabetes: the role of diabetes-related clinical characteristics and imaging. J Diabetes Complicat 30(7):1408–1415

16. Laking GR, West C, Buckley DL, Matthews J, Price PM (2006) Imaging vascular physiology to monitor cancer treatment. Crit Rev Oncol Hematol 58(2):95–113
17. Dake MD (2012) Chronic cerebrospinal venous insufficiency and multiple sclerosis: history and background. Tech Vasc Interv Radiol 15(2):94–100
18. Buzug TM (2008) Computed tomography: from photon statistics to modern cone-beam CT. Springer
19. Krishnamurthy R, Cheong B, Muthupillai R (2014) Tools for cardiovascular magnetic resonance imaging. Cardiovasc Diagn Ther 4(2):104–25
20. Molinari F, Krishnamurthi G, Acharya UR, Sree SV, Saba L, Nicolaides A et al (2012) Hypothesis validation of far-wall brightness in carotid-artery ultrasound for feature-based IMT measurement using a combination of level-set segmentation and registration. IEEE Trans Instrum Meas 61(4):1054–1063
21. Rocha R, Campilho A, Silva J, Azevedo E, Santos R (2010) Segmentation of the carotid intima-media region in B-mode ultrasound images. Image Vis Comput 28(4):614–625
22. Touboul P-J, Hennerici MG, Meairs S, Adams H, Amarenco P, Bornstein N et al (2012) Mannheim carotid intima-media thickness and plaque consensus (2004–2006–2011). In: An update on behalf of the advisory board of the 3rd, 4th and 5th watching the risk symposia, at the 13th, 15th and 20th European stroke conferences, Mannheim, Germany, 2004. Cerebrovasc Dis 34(4):290–296
23. van't Klooster R, de Koning PJH, Dehnavi RA, Tamsma JT, de Roos A, Reiber JHC et al (2012) Automatic lumen and outer wall segmentation of the carotid artery using deformable three-dimensional models in MR angiography and vessel wall images. J Magn Reson Imaging 35(1):156–65
24. Molinari F, Caresio C, Acharya UR, Mookiah MRK, Minetto MA (2015) Advances in quantitative muscle ultrasonography using texture analysis of ultrasound images. Ultrasound Med Biol [Internet] 41(9):2520–32. http://www.ncbi.nlm.nih.gov/pubmed/26026375. Accessed 26 Nov 2015
25. Acharya RU, Faust O, Alvin APC, Sree SV, Molinari F, Saba L et al (2012) Symptomatic vs. asymptomatic plaque classification in carotid ultrasound. J Med Syst 36(3):1861–1871
26. Kakkos SK, Griffin MB, Nicolaides AN, Kyriacou E, Sabetai MM, Tegos T et al (2013) The size of juxtaluminal hypoechoic area in ultrasound images of asymptomatic carotid plaques predicts the occurrence of stroke. J Vasc Surg 57(3):609–618
27. Molinari F, Meiburger KM, Zeng G, Acharya UR, Liboni W, Nicolaides A et al (2012) Carotid artery recognition system: a comparison of three automated paradigms for ultrasound images. Med Phys 39(1):378
28. Tegos TJ, Mavrophoros D, Sabetai MM, Elatrozy TS, Dhanjil S, Karapataki M et al (2001) Types of neurovascular symptoms and carotid plaque ultrasonic textural characteristics. J Ultrasound Med 20(2):113–21
29. Mahapatra D (2014) Automatic cardiac segmentation using semantic information from random forests. J Digit Imaging 27(6):794–804
30. Rosati S, Balestra G, Molinari F, Rajendra Acharya U, Suri JS (2014) A selection and reduction approach for the optimization of ultrasound carotid artery images segmentation. Mach Learn Healthc Inf 309–32
31. Molinari F, Zeng G, Suri JS (2010) Intima-media thickness: setting a standard for a completely automated method of ultrasound measurement. IEEE Trans Ultrason Ferroelectr Freq Control 57(5):1112–1124
32. Molinari F, Liboni W, Giustetto P, Badalamenti S, Suri JS (2009) Automatic computer-based tracings (ACT) in longitudinal 2-D ultrasound images using different scanners. J Mech Med Biol [Internet] 9(4):481–505. http://www.worldscientific.com/doi/abs/10.1142/S0219519409003115. Accessed 6 May 2016
33. Sifakis EG, Golemati S (2014) Robust carotid artery recognition in longitudinal B-mode ultrasound images. IEEE Trans Image Process 23(9):3762–3772
34. Li C, Xu C, Gui C, Fox MD (2005) Level set evolution without re-initialization: a new variational formulation. In: 2005 IEEE computer society conference on computer vision pattern recognition. IEEE, pp 430–436

35. Saba L, Gao H, Raz E, Sree SV, Mannelli L, Tallapally N et al (2014) Semiautomated analysis of carotid artery wall thickness in MRI. J Magn Reson Imaging 39(6):1457–1467
36. Boussel L, Serusclat A, Skilton M, Vincent F, Bernard S, Moulin P et al (2007) The reliability of high resolution MRI in the measurement of early stage carotid wall thickening. J Cardiovasc Magn Reson 9(5):771–776
37. Underhill HR, Kerwin WS, Hatsukami TS, Yuan C (2006) Automated measurement of mean wall thickness in the common carotid artery by MRI: a comparison to intima-media thickness by B-mode ultrasound. J Magn Reson Imaging 24(2):379–387
38. Nael K, Krishnam M, Nael A, Ton A, Ruehm SG, Finn JP (2008) Peripheral contrast-enhanced MR angiography at 3.0T, improved spatial resolution and low dose contrast: initial clinical experience. Eur Radiol 18(12):2893–2900
39. Nowinski WL, Puspitasaari F, Volkau I, Marchenko Y, Knopp MV (2013) Comparison of magnetic resonance angiography scans on 1.5, 3, and 7 tesla units: a quantitative study of 3-dimensional cerebrovasculature. J Neuroimaging 23(1):86–95
40. Loizou CP, Pattichis CS, Nicolaides AN, Pantziaris M (2009) Manual and automated media and intima thickness measurements of the common carotid artery. IEEE Trans Ultrason Ferroelectr Freq Control 56(5):983–994
41. Pignoli P, Longo T (1988) Evaluation of atherosclerosis with B-mode ultrasound imaging. J Nucl Med Allied Sci 32(3):166–173
42. Molinari F, Rajendra Acharya U, Zeng G, Meiburger KM, Suri JS (2011) Completely automated robust edge snapper for carotid ultrasound IMT measurement on a multi-institutional database of 300 images. Med Biol Eng Comput [Internet] 49(8):935–45. http://www.ncbi.nlm.nih.gov/pubmed/21509593. Assessed 22 Sept 2015
43. Liguori C, Paolillo A, Pietrosanto A (2001) An automatic measurement system for the evaluation of carotid intima-media thickness. IEEE Transactions on instrumentation and measurement 50(6):1684–1691
44. Faita F, Gemignani V, Bianchini E, Giannarelli C, Ghiadoni L, Demi M (2008) Real-time measurement system for evaluation of the carotid intima-media thickness with a robust edge operator. J Ultrasound Med 27(9):1353–1361
45. Wendelhag I, Gustavsson T, Suurküla M, Berglund G, Wikstrand J (1991) Ultrasound measurement of wall thickness in the carotid artery: fundamental principles and description of a computerized analysing system. Clin Physiol 11(6):565–577
46. Wendelhag I, Liang Q, Gustavsson T, Wikstrand J (1997) A new automated computerized analyzing system simplifies readings and reduces the variability in ultrasound measurement of intima-media thickness. Stroke 28(11):2195–2200
47. Quan Liang Q, Wendelhag I, Wikstrand J, Gustavsson T (2000) A multiscale dynamic programming procedure for boundary detection in ultrasonic artery images. IEEE Trans Med Imaging 19(2):127–142
48. Williams DJ, Shah MA (1992) Fast algorithm for active contours and curvature estimation. CVGIP Image Underst 55(1):14–26
49. Loizou CP, Pattichis CS, Pantziaris M, Tyllis T, Nicolaides A (2007) Snakes based segmentation of the common carotid artery intima media. Med Biol Eng Comput 45(1):35–49
50. Loizou CP, Nicolaides A, Kyriacou E, Georghiou N, Griffin M, Pattichis CS (2015) A Comparison of ultrasound intima-media thickness measurements of the left and right common carotid artery. IEEE J Transl Eng Health Med 3:1–10
51. Loizou CP, Pattichis CS, Pantziaris M, Nicolaides A (2007) An integrated system for the segmentation of atherosclerotic carotid plaque. IEEE Trans Inf Technol Biomed 11(6):661–667
52. Molinari F, Meiburger KM, Saba L, Zeng G, Acharya UR, Ledda M et al (2012) Fully automated dual-snake formulation for carotid intima-media thickness measurement. J Ultrasound Med 31(7):1123–1136
53. Molinari F, Meiburger KM, Saba L, Acharya U Rajendra, Ledda M, Nicolaides A et al (2012) Constrained snake vs. conventional snake for carotid ultrasound automated IMT measurements on multi-center data sets. Ultrasonics 52(7):949–961
54. Paul VCH (1960) Method and means for recognizing complex patterns

55. Golemati S, Stoitsis J, Sifakis EG, Balkizas T, Nikita KS (2007) Using the hough transform to segment ultrasound images of longitudinal and transverse sections of the carotid artery. Ultrasound Med Biol 33(12):1918–1932
56. Golemati S, Tegos TJ, Sassano A, Nikita KS, Nicolaides AN (2004) Echogenicity of B-mode sonographic images of the carotid artery: work in progress. J Ultrasound Med 23(5):659–669
57. Veronese E, Tarroni G, Visentin S, Cosmi E, Linguraru MG, Grisan E (2014) Estimation of prenatal aorta intima-media thickness from ultrasound examination. Phys Med Biol 59(21):6355–6371
58. Shankar PM (2003) A compound scattering pdf for the ultrasonic echo envelope and its relationship to K and Nakagami distributions. IEEE Trans Ultrason Ferroelectr Freq Control 50(3):339–343
59. Destrempes F, Meunier J, Giroux M-F, Soulez G, Cloutier G (2009) Segmentation in ultrasonic B-mode images of healthy carotid arteries using mixtures of nakagami distributions and stochastic optimization. IEEE Trans Med Imaging 28(2):215–229
60. Rosati S, Meiburger KM, Balestra G, Acharya UR, Molinari F (2016) Carotid wall measurement and assessment based on pixel-based and local texture descriptors. J Mech Med Biol [Internet] 16(1):1640006. http://www.worldscientific.com/doi/abs/10.1142/S0219519416400066. Accessed 16 Jan 2017
61. Delsanto S, Molinari F, Giustetto P, Liboni W, Badalamenti S, Suri JS (2007) Characterization of a completely user-independent algorithm for carotid artery segmentation in 2-D ultrasound images. IEEE Trans Instrum Meas [Internet] 56(4):1265–74. http://ieeexplore.ieee.org/lpdocs/epic03/wrapper.htm?arnumber=4277021. Accessed 22 Sept 2015
62. Pazinato D, Stein B, Almeida W, Werneck R, Mendes Junior P, Penatti O et al (2014) Pixel-level tissue classification for ultrasound images. IEEE J Biomed Health Inform [Internet]. http://www.ncbi.nlm.nih.gov/pubmed/25561598. Accessed 28 Nov 2015
63. Meiburger KM, Rosati S, Balestra G, Acharya UR, Molinari F (2016) Ultrasound B-mode descriptors and their association to age and automated IMT and IMT variability. J Mech Med Biol 16(1):1640007

Intrinsic Cardiovascular Wave and Strain Imaging

Elisa Konofagou

Abstract Cardiovascular diseases remain America's primary killer by a large margin, claiming the lives of more Americans than the next two main causes of death combined (cancer and pulmonary complications). In particular, coronary artery disease (CAD) is by far the most lethal, causing 17% of all (cardiac-related or not) deaths every year. One of the main reasons for this high death toll is the severe lack of effective and accessible imaging tools upon anomaly detected on the electrocardiogram (ECG), especially at the early stages when CAD can be stabilized with appropriate pharmacological regimen. Arrhythmias refer to the disruption of the natural heart rhythm. Cardiac arrhythmias lead to a significant number of cardiovascular morbidity and mortality. This irregular heart rhythm causes the heart to suddenly stop pumping blood. Atrial pathologies are the most common arrhythmias with atrial fibrillation and atrial flutter being the most prevalent. In this chapter, we introduce ultrasound-based methodologies that are based on inferring to the mechanical and electrical properties of the myocardium in order to better image the onset and progression of the aforementioned diseases.

1 Myocardial Elastography

1.1 Introduction

According to the latest report on Heart Disease and Stroke Statistics by the American Heart Association [6], more than 2150 Americans die of cardiovascular disease each day, an average of 1 death every 40 s. Cardiovascular disease currently claims more lives each year in both men and women than the next two most deadly diseases combined, i.e., cancer and chronic lower respiratory disease. Among the cardiovascular diseases, coronary artery disease (CAD) is by far the most deadly causing approximately 1 of every 6 deaths in the United States in 2010. Approximately every 34 s,

E. Konofagou (✉)
Columbia University, 1210 Amsterdam Ave, ET351, MC 8904, New York, NY 10027, USA
e-mail: ek2191@columbia.edu

S. Golemati and K. S. Nikita (eds.), *Cardiovascular Computing—Methodologies and Clinical Applications*, Series in BioEngineering,
https://doi.org/10.1007/978-981-10-5092-3_8

experienced exponential growth in new procedures, the progress in the development of novel diagnostic techniques has stalled by comparison.

1.2 Mechanical Deformation of Normal and Ischemic or Infarcted Myocardium

Detection of cardiac dysfunction through assessment of the mechanical properties of the heart, and more specifically, the left-ventricular muscle, has been a long-term goal in diagnostic cardiology. This is because both ischemia [8], i.e., the reduced oxygenation of the muscle necessary for its contraction, and infarction [2], i.e., the complete loss of blood supply inducing myocyte death, alter the mechanical properties and contractility of the myocardium. In the ischemic heart, the diastolic left-ventricular pressure-volume or pressure-length curve slope is typically increased, suggesting increased chamber stiffness. Regional myocardial stiffness has also been reported to increase as a result of ischemia [1, 5, 39, 40]. The increased stiffness could be due to myocardial remodeling, including elevated collagen and desmin expression as well as the titin isoform switch. Acute myocardial infarction caused by partial or total blockage of one or more coronary arteries can cause complex structural alterations of the left-ventricular muscle. These alterations may lead to collagen synthesis and scar formation, which can cause the myocardium to irreversibly change its mechanical properties. Holmes et al. [10] reported that this myocardial stiffening can be measured within the first 5 min following ischemic onset. As reported by Gupta et al. (1994), in vitro mechanical testing showed that the stiffness of the infarcted region increases within the first 4 h, and continues to rise by up to 20 times, peaking 1–2 weeks following the infarct and decreasing 4 weeks later (down to 1–10 times the non-infarcted value). The fact that the mechanical properties induced by the ischemia change right at the onset, continue changing thereafter and peak two weeks later, indicate the potential for a mechanically-based imaging technique to detect the ischemia and infarct extent early. Regarding its conduction pattern, ischemia or infarction will alter the normal pattern and result into reduced and complete lack of conduction, respectively, at the region of abnormality since the myocytes no longer properly conduct the action potential.

1.3 Myocardial Elastography

Our group has pioneered the technique of Myocardial Elastography that it has been developing for more than a decade [13, 16–18, 19, 20, 21, 23]. This technique encompasses imaging of mechanical (cumulative or systolic; Fig. 1) or electromechanical (incremental or transient) strain or activation times to respectively highlight the mechanical or electrical function of the myocardium, Myocardial Elastography benefits from the development of techniques be used for high precision 2D time-shift based strain estimation [14] and high frame rates available in echocardiography scanners [17] to obtain a detailed map of the transmural strain in normal [23, 27, 32], ischemic [27] and infarcted [3] cases in vivo. These strain imaging techniques aim at achieving high precision estimates through recorrelation techniques [14] and customized cross-correlation methods [15] and are thus successful in mapping the full 2D and 3D strain tensors [23, 26, 42].

2D strain estimation and imaging—A fast, normalized cross-correlation function is first be used on RF signals from consecutive frames to compute two-dimensional motion and deformation [14, 30]. The cross-correlation function uses a 1-D kernel (length = 5.85 mm, overlap = 90%) in a 2D (or, 3D) search to estimate both axial and lateral (and elevational) displacements (Eq. 1; Figs. 1 and 2). The correlation kernel size is approximately 10 wavelengths, which has been found to be the optimal length using cross-correlation [29]. It should also be noted that the elastographic resolution has been shown to depend mainly on the kernel shift (not the kernel size) [37], which in our studies is 10%, or 0.6 mm. When searching in the lateral (or, elevational) direction, the RF signals are linearly interpolated by a factor of 10 in order to improve lateral (or, elevational) displacement [14, 25, 27]. Recorrelation techniques are applied in two iterations that aim at increasing the correlation coefficient of each strain component by correction or shifting the RF signals by the displacements estimated in the other (two) orthogonal direction(s) [14, 25]. A least-squares kernel [12] is finally applied to compute the axial and lateral strains in 2D-PBME (Parallel Beamforming Myocardial Elastography) and axial, lateral and elevational strains in 3D-PBME. The estimated displacements use a reference point of the first frame in each estimation pair, yielding incremental (inter-frame) strains that are then accumulated over the entire systolic phase. Radial, circumferential and longitudinal strains is then be calculated. For **2D**, radial and circumferential strains are estimated in a short-axis view (Fig. 2b, c). In 2D-PBME, a rotation matrix, **R**, for each material point within the myocardium in a 2D short axis view are written as

$$\mathbf{R} = \begin{bmatrix} \cos\theta & \sin\theta \\ -\sin\theta & \cos\theta \end{bmatrix}, \tag{1}$$

where θ are the angle relative to the origin of the Cartesian coordinates in the FE models. Strains in cardiac coordinates are therefore obtained by

$$\hat{\mathbf{E}} = \mathbf{RER}^T, \tag{2}$$

where $\hat{\mathbf{E}}$ is the 2D radial-circumferential strain tensor. The diagonal components of $\hat{\mathbf{E}}$ are radial ($\mathbf{E}_{rr}$) and circumferential ($\mathbf{E}_{cc}$) strains. Positive and negative radial strains indicate myocardial thickening and thinning, respectively, while myocardial stretching and shortening are represented by positive and negative circumferential strains, respectively. A standard B-mode image (Fig. 2a) is reconstructed from the RF data, allowing for manually initialized segmentation of the myocardial border

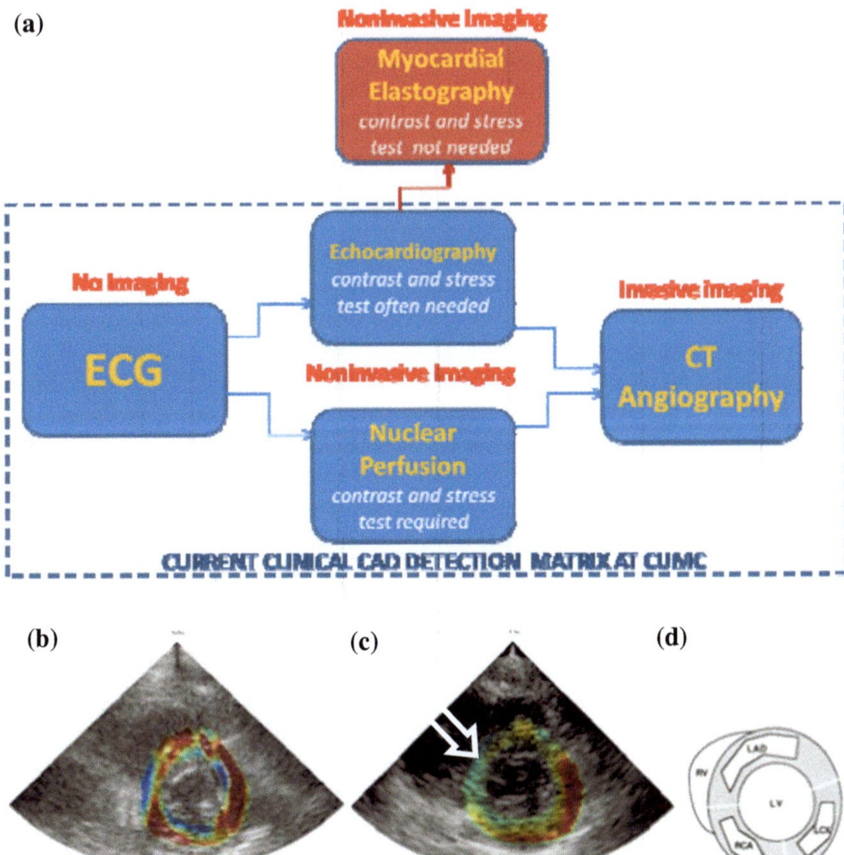

Fig. 1 a Envisioned role and b, c initial findings of Myocardial Elastography in the current clinical routine to avoid false positives and/or thus unnecessary invasive procedures and false negatives by the currently used techniques; **b** Normal short-axis radial strain image (largely red (thickening) myocardium) in an echocardiography **false positive case** where CT angiography was administered only to confirm normal function; **c** Abnormal short-axis radial strain image containing an ischemic region (in blue or thinning; arrow) in a nuclear perfusion and subsequently CT angiography confirmed Myocardial Elastography findings regarding two occluded territories (64-year-old female, 40% LAD and 30% RCA occlusion); **d** Coronary territories given for reference [24]. CUMC: Columbia University Medical Center. LAD: Left anterior descending artery. LCx: Left-circumflex artery. RCA: right coronary artery. **Myocardial Elastography was capable of detecting normal function and identifying both compromised territories**

which are subsequently automatically tracked throughout the cardiac cycle based on the estimated displacements as previously developed by our group [30].

3D strain estimation and imaging—3D will include the estimation of longitudinal strains. The MATLAB function interp3 is used to interpolate all three orthogonal components (axial, lateral, radial and circumferential) between each of the 16 slices.

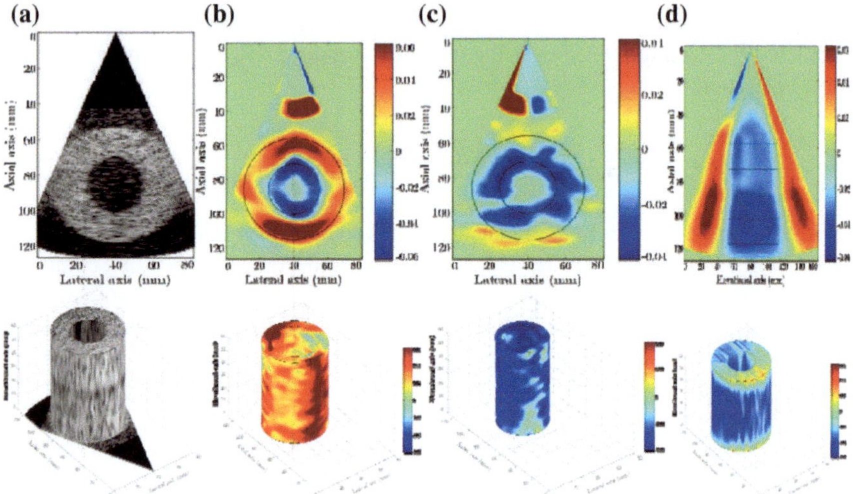

Fig. 2 **a** B-mode, **b** radial, **c** circumferential and **d** longitudinal strain images of a cylindrical model undergoing radial deformation using PBME in phased array configuration in FIELD II for 2D (Top panel) and 3D (Bottom panel) Myocardial Elastography. In the proposed study, the canine LV geometry and electromechanical simulation model (Fig. 3) are used. The black boundaries in the top panel represent where the simulated myocardium. Strains outside the tissue are not taken into account

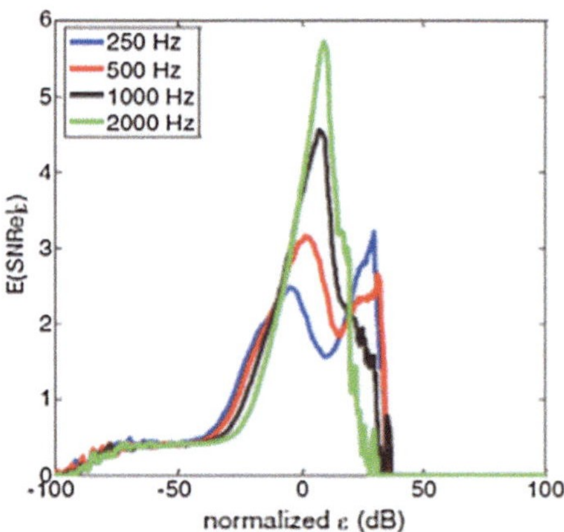

Fig. 3 E(SNRe|ε) transverse strain curves increase with frame rate

The interpolated data set is depicted in 3D, on two surfaces: one located near the endocardium, the other located near the epicardium. The frame rate is lower by a 16-fold compared to 2D, i.e., 344 frames/s in 3D (from 5500 frames/s in 2D) but is tested whether it can be sufficient to estimate strain at high SNR as predicted by preliminary findings (Fig. 3).

PBME performance assessment—A probabilistic framework has been developed by our group in order to compare the strain estimation quality between conventional and parallel beamforming [3, 35]. The elastographic signal-to-noise-ratio (SNR_e) are calculated for each sequence over the phase of systole. SNR_e is computed for every point in an image using

$$SNR_e = \frac{\mu(\varepsilon)}{\sigma(\varepsilon)} \tag{3}$$

where $\mu(\varepsilon)$ and $\sigma(\varepsilon)$ refer to the mean and standard deviation of the strain (ε) magnitude within a small 2D ROI (3.0 × 3.2 mm). Since both strain and SNR_e are computed for each point in the myocardium throughout systole, a large number (>600,000) of strain-SNR_e pairs are generated for each sequence [3]. The conditional expected value of SNR_e for each strain is calculated using [3, 35].

$$E(SNR_e|\varepsilon) = \int_0^{+\infty} SNR_e \frac{f(SNR_e, \varepsilon)}{f(\varepsilon)} dSNR_e \tag{4}$$

E(SNRe|ε) curves are generated for each sequence, which allows for a relatively easy comparison to be performed between different sequences for a wide range of strain values. Example of E(SNRe|ε) curves for radial strain estimation is provided in Fig. 3. The SNR_e of both 2D-PBME and 3D-PBME are computed with respect to the strain (equivalent to frame rate) and compared to focused (standard 2D and 3D Myocardial Elastography) to perform a quality comparison with parallel beamforming techniques. Both inter-frame (electromechanical) and cumulative (mechanical) strain SNRe are quantified.

Compounding—A compounding technique that the PI's group has developed for strain imaging for the first time are applied to determine increase in SNR when parallel beamforming is applied. Plane waves are electronically steered and transmitted at three different angles separated by 20° (−20°, 0°, 20°) and the resulting RF frames are combined into a compounded image. The received radiofrequency (RF) frames are reconstructed by applying a delay-and-sum method on GPU-based parallel computing to accelerate reconstruction processing [35]. In preliminary studies, we have found that compounding in human hearts in vivo decreases the frame rate from 5500 fps to 1375 fps, which is sufficiently high for Myocardial Elastography (Fig. 3) while SNR increases by a 4-fold.

1.4 Simulations

A phased array simulation model for the quality assessment of PBME. Field II, an established and publicly available ultrasound field simulation program [11] (Jensen and Svendsen 1992) are used to simulate the RF signals of the myocardium. The simulated mesh, including the myocardium, cavity and background are loaded into FIELD II (Luo et al. 2008a, 2009b). Instead of a focused wave, a diverging wave sequence is employed for transmit by placing the focus 6.75 mm (half the size of the aperture) behind the array surface to achieve a 90° angle insonification [35]. For 2D-PBME, the RF signals are obtained from 192 elements and 3.5-MHz center frequency with 60% bandwidth (at −6 dB) phased-array similar to what are used in the canine study. Hanning apodization are applied both during transmit and receive to reduce grating lobes. The width and height of the phased array are 43 and 7 mm, respectively. The RF signals are reconstructed by coherent summation of the signals received by all the elements using a delay-and-sum algorithm. For 3D-PBME, RF signals are obtained from a 2-D array with 16×16, 32×32 and 64×64 elements and 3-MHz center frequency, similar to what are used in experiments (aims 1–3).

1.5 Myocardial Ischemia and Infarction Detection in Canines in Vivo

1.5.1 Ischemic Model

In order to test Myocardial Elastography in the assessment of ischemia by depicting the change in both mechanical and electrical properties, twelve (n = 12) adult male dogs (20–25 kg) were used according to well-established anesthetized canine models. The flow in that artery was continuously controlled via pressure-flow curves: *Step 1 (control)*: Mongrel dogs with normal/healthy myocardium, as verified using standard echocardiography, are used for control measurements. Channel data with both 2D- and 3D-PBME are continuously acquired during 5 min in sets of three cardiac cycles each taken 20 s apart, i.e., approximately15 sets total. This established the strain baseline; *Step 2 (mild to acute ischemia)*: The dogs undergo a left thoracotomy followed by gradual constriction of the mid-proximal left anterior descending coronary artery (LAD) using the Ameroid constrictor by 0–100% of baseline, at intervals of 20% for 15 min each. Strain images are shown in Fig. 4a. The slope of the coronary pressure-flow curves (using Millar catheters and sonomicrometry) are used to monitor the ischemic onset at each occlusion step. RF data in the same views as in Step 1 were continuously acquired during the full 15 min in sets of three cardiac cycles (10 s apart), i.e., approx. 70 sets total (Fig. 4).

1.5.2 Infarct Model

Mongrel dogs underwent similar surgical procedure as in the ischemia model but survived for four days after complete ligation only in order to develop a fully-developed infarct.

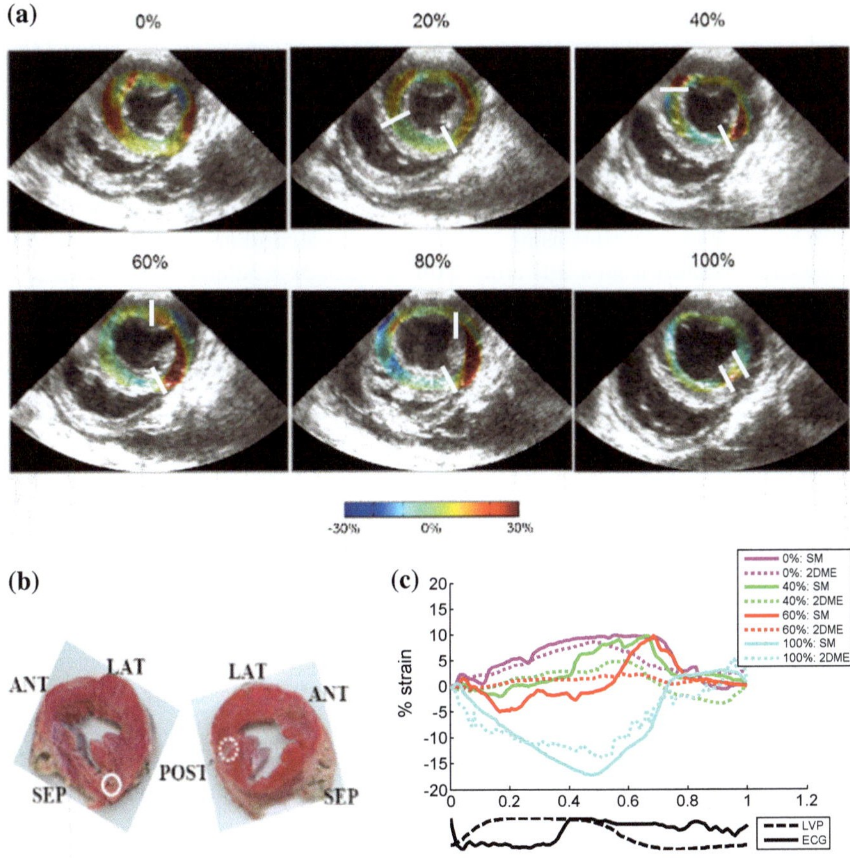

Fig. 4 **a** Progression of ischemia (in 'blue' or thinning systolic strain as indicated compared to the surrounding 'red' or non-ischemic (thickening) strain) from 0 to 100% occlusion in the same dog using **2D-PBME** and identifying the region and extent of ischemia in each case (shown with the R0I); **b** TTC pathology showing pale (unstained by TTC; ischemic) versus red (stained by TTC; normal) myocardium. **c** Temporal radial strain profiles in the anterior wall region of 3×3 mm^2 at 0, 40, 60, and 100% occlusion levels with sonomicrometry (SM) and 2DME [27]

1.6 Validation of Myocardial Elastography Against CT Angiography

CT angiography is an established technique used for reliable detection of a coronary occlusion and were used to confirm the occlusion and validate the location of the ischemia or infarct as detected by Myocardial Elastography. The objectives of this study were to show that 2-D myocardial strains can be imaged with diverging wave imaging and are different in average between healthy subjects and coronary artery disease (CAD) patients. In this study, 15 CAD patients and 8 healthy subjects

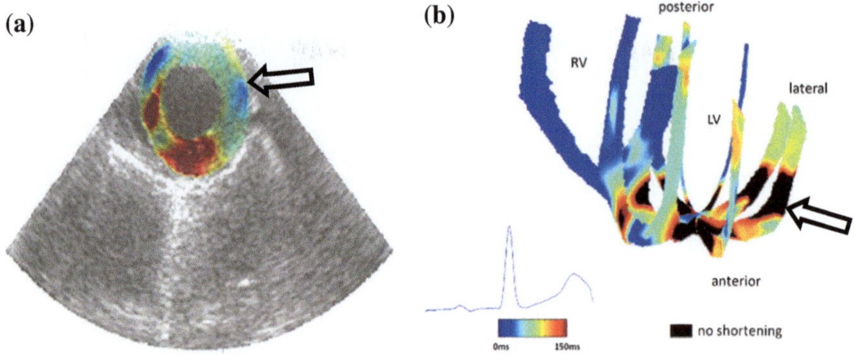

Fig. 5 **a** Transthoracic systolic radial strain image of a **canine left ventricle in vivo. Thinning (blue) strain region clearly indicates the extent of infarction. b Electromechanical isochrones in 3D identifying spatial extent of MI. Arrow denotes MI region**

were imaged with ME. Patients with more than 50% occlusion in one of the main coronary arteries were considered to have obstructive CAD. Incremental axial and lateral displacements were estimated using normalized 1-D cross-correlation and then accumulated during systole. Axial and lateral cumulative strains were then estimated from the displacements and converted to radial cumulative strains (Fig. 6). The end-systolic radial strain in the total cross-section of the myocardium in healthy subjects ($14.9 \pm 8.2\%$) was significantly higher than obstructive CAD patients ($-0.9 \pm 7.4\%$, $p < 0.001$) and in non-obstructive CAD patients ($3.7 \pm 5.7\%$, $p < 0.05$). End-systolic radial strain in the left anterior descending (LAD) territory was found to be significantly higher in healthy subjects ($16.9 \pm 12.9\%$) than in patients with obstructed LAD ($2.2 \pm 7.0\%$, $p < 0.05$) and patients with non-obstructed LAD ($1.7 \pm 10.3\%$, $p < 0.05$) (Fig. 7). These preliminary findings indicate that end-systolic radial strain measured with Myocardial Elastography is higher on average in healthy subjects compared to CAD patients and indicates that Myocardial Elastography has the potential to be used for non-invasive, radiation free early detection of CAD.

2 Electromechanical Wave Imaging

2.1 Cardiac Arrhythmias

Cardiac arrhythmias can be separated into atrial (or, supraventricular) and ventricular. While ventricular arrhythmias, such as ventricular fibrillation (chaotic rhythm), ventricular tachycardia (rapid rhythm) and ventricular bradycardia (slow rhythm), incur the most episodes of sudden death, they are less common and easier to diagnose than atrial arrhythmias. Atrial arrhythmias include atrial fibrillation (Afib or AF) and atrial flutter (AFL), are the most common. Similar to the ventricular def-

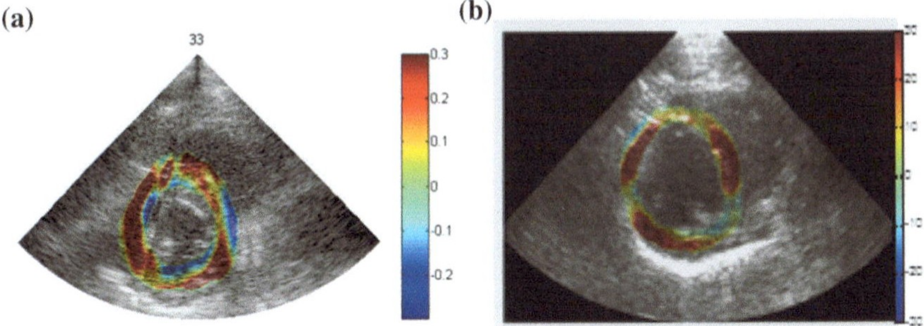

Fig. 6 Comparison between **a** 2DME (conventional (focused) beamforming) using ECG gating and **b** 2D-PBME (parallel beamforming) systolic radial strain image in a normal patient. The quality is comparable without the artifacts from sector matching and ECG gating in the former (**a**)

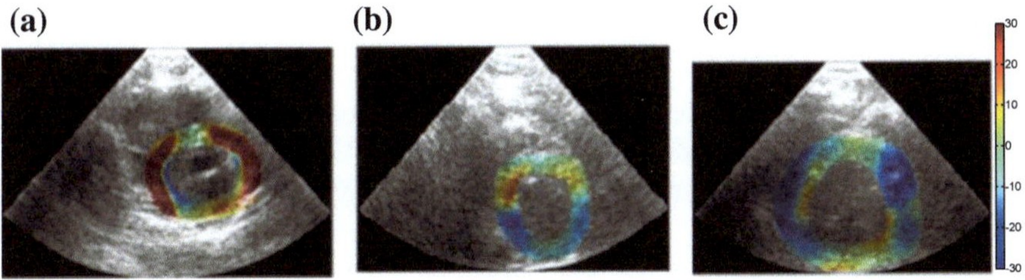

Fig. 7 2D-PBME showing progression of coronary disease in three different patients: **a** Normal, **b** (RCA: 90%; LAD: 20%, LCX: 20%) occlusions and **c** (RCA: 99%; LAD: 100%, LCX: 100%) occlusions. Figure 1d can be used for reference of coronaries

inition, atrial fibrillation denotes the chaotic rhythm while atrial flutter denotes the regular but abnormal (rapid or slow) rhythm. The number of individuals with atrial fibrillation in the United States is expected to reach 12 million by 2050 (Lloyd-Jones et al. 2009) with the atrial flutters, often a result of treatment, also expected to rise as more of these treatments are administered. The methodology has the dual purpose of both enhancing the diagnosis and treatment planning and guidance of arrhythmias that are the most common and most difficult to diagnose, i.e., the atrial arrhythmias. Below a short overview of the state-of-the-art diagnostic and treatment techniques is provided.

2.2 *Clinical Diagnosis of Atrial Arrhythmias*

ECG recordings and no imaging modality is typically used for the noninvasive identification of atrial arrhythmias. If ECG recordings indicate atrial flutter or fibrillation, Radio-frequency (RF) ablation (see next section) is warranted that allows for catheterized cardiac mapping during its procedure. Cardiac mapping involves the insertion of a catheter containing a small number of electrodes in the heart chamber to contact the endocardium and measure times of activation. The procedure is minimally invasive and ionizing since it uses Computed Tomography (CT) guidance, but it can be a lengthy procedure requiring topical or general anesthesia and is warranted only when the ECG recordings indicate that RF ablation is the appropriate course of treatment. Limitations include some inaccessible endocardial sites and the inability to map the mid-myocardium and epicardium. More importantly, potentials in only one or a few locations in the atrium are measured per heartbeat, it can be used only to study stable, repeatable arrhythmias.

2.3 *Treatment of Atrial Arrhythmias*

Radio-frequency ablation is a minimally invasive technique rapidly emerging as the most commonly used therapeutic modality for atrial flutter and atrial fibrillation. For this treatment, a catheter, whose tip carries an electrode, is inserted through the femoral vein and the tip of the electrode is positioned at the arrhythmic origin. The tip causes a frictional heat generated by intracellular ions moving in response to an alternating current. The electrode is connected to a function generator and the electrical current flows and raises the local temperature up to 95 °C maintaining it for about 15 min, generating thermal lesions in the vicinity of the ablating catheter. The treatment consists thus in modifying or in blocking the circuits of electrical conduction in heart. Current surgical procedures are invasive and have a moderate efficiency in the persistent forms of atrial fibrillation. AF in some patients may be due to focal activity originating in the pulmonary veins and 70% of these patients can be successfully treated by RF ablation of the focus inside the pulmonary veins. However, the treatment of AF using RF ablation can often lead to the development of other arrhythmias. For example, a sizeable increase of atypical flutter is due to catheter ablation of atrial fibrillation.

2.4 *Electromechanical Wave Imaging (EWI)*

2.4.1 The Cardiac Electromechanics

The heart will not adequately contract unless it is electrically activated via a very specific route (Fig. 8; green arrows). In sinus rhythm (or, natural contraction), the path of activation originates at the sinoatrial (SA) node (right before the ECG's P-wave), from which the electrical signal in the form of an action potential spreads to both right and left atria causing their contraction (during the P-wave). The wave then propagates to the atrioventricular (AV) node (right after the P-wave), through the Bundle of His and along the left and right bundles on the interventricular septum (during the Q-R segment) to the Purkinje fibers (S-wave) finally causing both

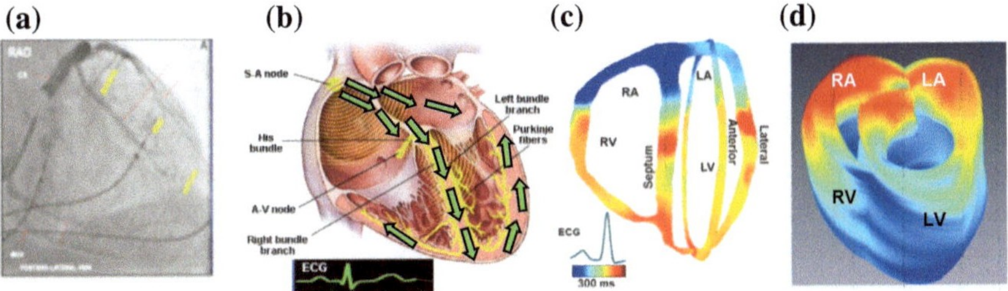

Fig. 8 **a** State-of-the-art CT angiography of the CRT leads. The ablation catheters and coronaries are clearly visible but not the heart or the myocardium. A similar system is used to guide electroanatomic mapping. **b** Illustration of the cardiac conduction system. The green arrows indicate the path of activation as the action potential propagates from the sinoatrial node (SA node) in the right atrium along the Purkinje fiber network (in yellow). **c** Current (2D) 4-chamber EWI activation map with conventional beamforming in a normal human heart obtained transthoracically; **d** 3D-rendered, 4-chamber EWI activation map (reversed color map used compared to (**c**) in vivo

ventricles to synchronously contract, starting at the apex towards their lateral and posterior walls (Fig. 8). The heart is thus an electromechanical pump that requires to first be electrically activated in order to contract. Propagating electrical waves of excitation result into localized contractions. Each electrical activation in Fig. 8b is followed by an electromechanical one, i.e., the depolarization of a cardiac muscle cell, or, myocyte, is followed by an uptake of calcium, which triggers contraction (Bers 2002) after a certain electromechanical delay of a few milliseconds (Ashikaga et al. 2007; Cordeiro et al. 2004). In the presence of arrhythmia, electrical and electromechanical patterns are disrupted.

2.4.2 Electromechanical Wave Imaging (EWI)

Our group has pioneered a unique noninvasive and direct (as opposed to inverse problem) imaging technique that could reliably map the conduction wave in the heart in all of its four cardiac chambers. Electromechanical Wave Imaging [22, 32, 41] (Pernot and Konofagou 2005; Konofagou et al. 2006, 2007; Provost et al. 2011b, d) has been shown capable of noninvasively mapping the conduction wave during propagation. We identified that high frame rate (>500 frames/s (fps)) and precise 2D imaging of the cardiac deformation is feasible so that the transient cardiac motion resulting from the fast electromechanical wave can be mapped in murine [22]. Canine and human [34, 41] hearts in vivo. Through a R21 study, we were also capable of demonstrating that EWI is angle-independent [34], has excellent correlation with electrical activation measurements in canines in vivo [34]; slope of 0.99 and r^2 = 0.88; Figs. 9 and 10) and is in excellent agreement with electromechanical simulations [7, 33]. More importantly, our group was capable of recently showing that EWI was feasible in the atria of human hearts in vivo undergoing sinus rhythm [34]. There is simply no other modality that can directly map the conduction of the atria under sinus rhythm noninvasively in the clinic. An important additional advantage of this methodology is that it can be routinely applied in the clinic through straightforward integration with any echocardiography system. It could thus be used both at the diagnostic and at the treatment guidance levels, either off- or on-line. Despite the fact that EWI can map both the atria and the ventricles, we chose to focus on the atrial arrhythmias in this study given that they are far more common, more salvageable and completely lacking of any noninvasive imaging modality that can map their conduction properties.

EWI can be useful in a number of diseases that can be treated with ablation therapy: e.g., atrial fibrillation, atrial flutter, ventricular tachycardia, Wolff-Parkinson-White (WPW) syndrome, etc. WPW is a heart condition where an additional electrical pathway links the atria to the ventricles. It is the most common heart rate disorder in infants and children and is preferably treated using catheter ablation. EWI could be used in predicting the location of the accessory pathway, thus reducing the overall time of the ablation procedure. Since a sizeable increase of atypical flutter is due to catheter ablation of atrial fibrillation, the prevalence of atrial flutter is also expected to rise. However, the relationship between AF and AFL is still not fully understood. Atrial flutter, a type of atrial tachycardia, has historically been defined exclusively from the ECG recordings. More specifically, differentiation between flutter and other tachycardias was based on the atrial rate and the presence or absence of isoelectric baselines between atrial deflections. Since then, electrophysiological studies and RF ablation brought new understanding into the atrial tachycardia mechanisms, which did not correlate well with these ECG-based definitions. In other words, ECG recordings offer only a limited value in the determination of specific atrial tachycardia mechanisms, and, ultimately, for the selection of the appropriate course of treatment. Cardiac mapping allowed different mechanisms of macroreentrant atrial tachycardia to be identified, such as typical flutter, reverse typical flutter, left atrial flutter, etc., although a significant number of atypical flutters are still poorly understood. While mapping the right atrium is routinely undertaken successfully using this procedure, mapping the left atrium is riskier since it requires a transseptal puncture. However, as it currently stands in the clinic, right-atrium arrhythmia cannot be distinguished from left-atrium one prior to treatment and only the latter warrants transseptal puncture, which is a riskier procedure. In some cases, the left atrium arrhythmia is not diagnosed until the entire right atrium is ablated (which may involve several unproductive hours of intervention), posing further risk to the patient. Consequently, left atrial activation sequences are not well characterized in many atrial tachycardia cases. Moreover, the surface ECG is insufficiently specific to distinguish left from right atrial flutters. EWI could thus offer an important step for the localization of the right versus left atrial arrhythmia as well as localize the origin(s) at the treatment planning stage, i.e., prior to the catheterization of the patient rendering the treatment to be more efficient, much shorter in duration with unnecessary ablations in the wrong chamber or avoiding unnecessary transseptal punctures.

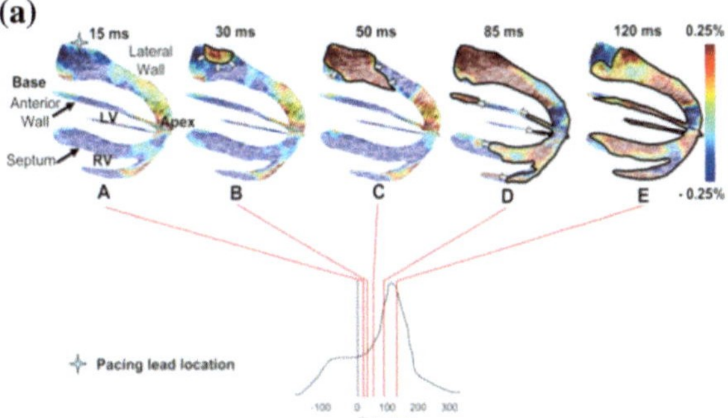

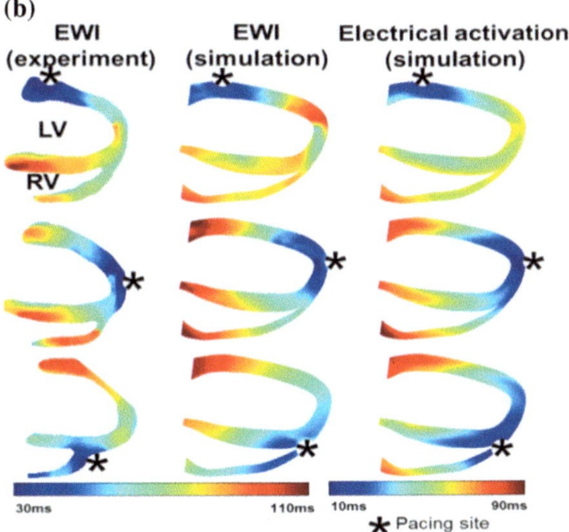

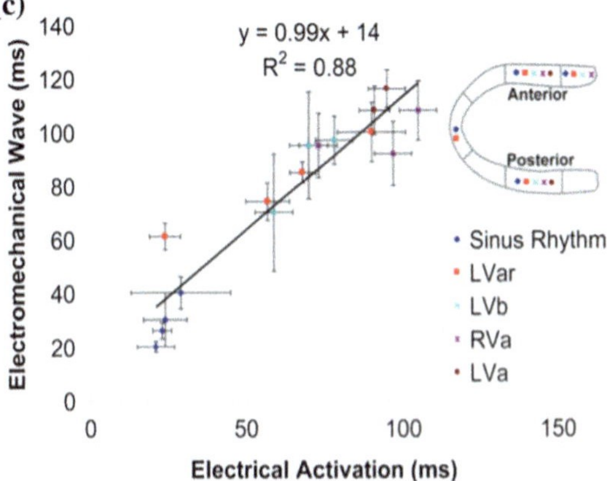

Fig. 9 **a** Propagation of the electromechanical wave when paced from the lateral wall, near the base. Activation in this view corresponds to thickening of the tissue (red). Activated regions are traced at (A) 15 ms, (B) 30 ms, (C) 50 ms (D) 85 ms and (E) 120 ms and indicated on the (F) electrocardiogram. 0 ms corresponds to the pacing stimulus. (A–C) The EW propagates from the basal part of the lateral wall towards the apex. (D) Note that in the apical region, a transition from lengthening to shortening is observed rather than a transition from thinning to thickening. (D–E) In the anterior wall, the EW propagates from both the base and apex. The scale shows inter-frame strains. **b** Correlation of EWI with simulation findings of electromechanical and electrical activation (Provost et al. 2011); **c** Electrical and electromechanical activation times during the four pacing protocols and sinus rhythm in four different heart segments in the posterior and anterior walls

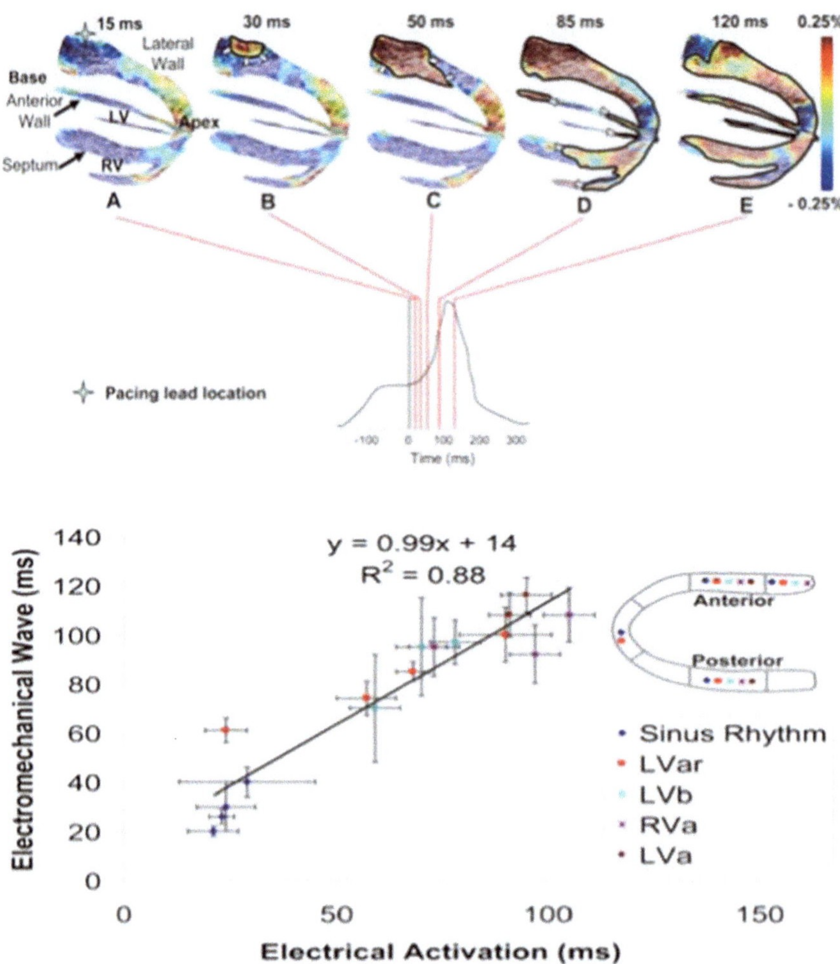

Fig. 10 **Top**: Propagation of the electromechanical wave when paced from the lateral wall, near the base. Activation in this view corresponds to thickening of the tissue (red). Activated regions are traced at (A) 15 ms, (B) 30 ms, (C) 50 ms (D) 85 ms and (E) 120 ms and indicated on the (F) electrocardiogram. 0 ms corresponds to the pacing stimulus. (A–C) The EW propagates from the basal part of the lateral wall towards the apex. (D) Note that in the apical region, a transition from lengthening to shortening is observed rather than a transition from thinning to thickening. (D–E) In the anterior wall, the EW propagates from both the base and apex. The scale shows inter-frame strains. **Bottom**: Electrical and electromechanical activation times during the four pacing protocols and sinus rhythm in four different heart segments in the posterior and anterior walls

2.4.3 Treatment Guidance Capability of EWI

Currently, there is simply no noninvasive electrical conduction mapping techniques of the heart that can be used in the clinic. In addition, apart from being the currently available clinical electrical mapping methods are all catheter-based, and limited to mapping the endocardial or epicardial activation sequence; they are also time-consuming and costly. Even in a laboratory setting, mapping the 3D electrical activation sequence of the heart can be a daunting task (Nash and Pullan 2005). Studies of transmural electrical activation usually require usage of a large number of plunge electrodes to attain sufficient resolution, or are applied to small regions of interest in vivo. Non-contact methods to map the electrical activation sequence have also emerged but are not used in the clinic. Optical imaging techniques use voltage-sensitive dyes that bind to cardiac cell membranes and, following illumination, fluoresce if the cell undergoes electrical activation. Optical imaging methods can map the activation sequence of ex vivo tissue on the endo- an epicardial surfaces and transmurally [9] but cannot be applied in the clinic since they require the use of an electromechanical decoupler that inhibits cardiac contraction during imaging. Other newly developed methods to map the local electrical activity of the heart based on inverse problems are available: electrocardiographic imaging (ECGI) [36] and non-contact mapping [38]. The former is based on body surface potentials and CT or MRI scans and provides reconstructed epicardial action potentials, including the atria. The latter consists in reconstructing the transmural potentials from potentials measured in the heart chamber based on specific assumptions that may be susceptible to inverse problem errors.

2.5 Imaging the Electromechanics of the Heart

As of today, no imaging method currently used in the clinic has been capable of mapping the electromechanics of the heart. Initial measurements to determine the correlation between the electrical and electromechanical activities have been reported (Badke et al. 1980; Wyman et al. 1999). These results suggest that the electrical activation sequence could be deduced from the electromechanics. Clinically available imaging modalities such as standard echocardiography or MRI cannot adequately detect the electromechanical wave (EW) since they are too slow, i.e., the time required to acquire a single image is similar to the duration of the entire ventricular depolarization. The electrical activation lasts approximately 60–100 ms and requires a resolution of a few milliseconds (e.g., 2–5 ms) to generate precise activation maps. Moreover, the regional inter-frame deformation to be measured at these frame rates is very small (~0.25% at a 2-ms temporal resolution and requires a highly accurate strain estimator. We have shown that EWI is capable of reaching high frame rates (up to 2000 frames/s) as well attain the precision of the incurred strains (up to 0.25%) which result from an electromechanical activation and therefore fulfill the requirements of both high temporal and spatial resolution unique to our technology.

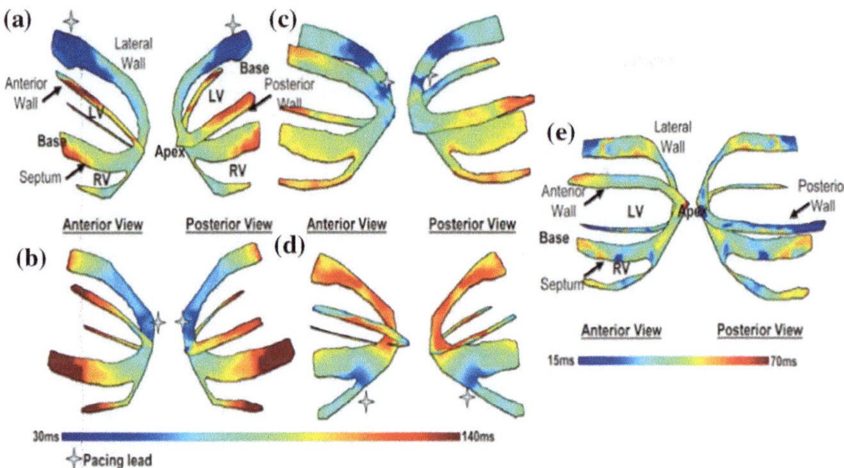

Fig. 11 Isochrones showing the activation sequence under different pacing protocols as shown. Arrow indicates the pacing origin. **a** Pacing from the basal region of the lateral wall. **b** Pacing from the apex. **c** Pacing from the apical region of the lateral wall. **d** Pacing from the apical region of the right-ventricular wall. **e** Isochrones showing the EW activation sequence during sinus rhythm. The activation sequence exhibits early activation at the median level and late activation at the basal and apical levels. Activation of the right ventricular wall occurred after the activation of the septal and lateral walls. The blue cross indicates the pacing lead location

2.6 EWI Sequences

A block diagram of EWI is shown in Fig. 11. Two imaging sequences, the automated composite technique (ACT) [41] and the temporally-unequispaced acquisition sequences (TUAS) (Provost et al. 2011d) have been developed and implemented (Provost et al. 2008b, 2009, 2010b, 2011d) as well as the single-heartbeat sequence [4, 35] (Provost et al. 2015; Costet et al. 2015).

The ACT sequence—An Ultrasonix RP system with a 3.3 MHz phased array was used to acquire RF frames from 390 to 520 frames/s (fps) using an automated composite technique (ACT) [41]. Briefly, to increase the resulting frame rate, the image is divided into partially overlapping sectors corresponding to separate cardiac cycles (Fig. 11a). The axial incremental displacements are obtained with a RF-based cross-correlation method (Fig. 11b) (window size: 4.6 mm, 80% overlap). Briefly, this method consists in dividing every ultrasound beam in a large number of overlapping, one-dimensional, 4.6-mm-long windows. Then, the following process is applied to each window and each sampled time t. A reference window at time t_1 is compared with all the windows contained in the same beam at sampled time t_2. The axial location of the window providing the highest correlation determines the axial displacement between two consecutive sampled times. After repeating this process for every available window and every available sampled time, we obtain axial displacements at multiple locations along the ultrasound beam and for every sampled time. The full-view image is then reconstructed using the motion-matching technique (Fig. 11c) (Provost et al. 2010b). Briefly, this method consists of comparing, through a cross-correlation method, the incremental displacements measured in the overlapping line of two sectors obtained at different heartbeats to synchronize the sectors. More specifically, the acquisition sequence is designed such that each sector contains at least one ultrasound beam that is also part of the following sector. Therefore, this overlapping beam is expected to result in identical (or highly similar) axial displacements whether they corresponds to heartbeat h that occurred when sector s was acquired or to heartbeat h + 1 that occurred when sector s + 1 was acquired. By comparing, over time, the displacements obtained in the overlapping beams, the time delay corresponding to the maximum cross-correlation coefficient are obtained to synchronize each set of neighboring sectors. The procedure is repeated for each pair of sectors, allowing the reconstruction of the full-view of the heart, hence ensuring the continuity of the transition incremental displacements across sectors. This method does not rely on the ECG. Therefore it is especially useful in cases where the ECG may be unavailable or too irregular to perform ECG gating (Provost et al. 2010b). The axial incremental strains were then obtained by taking the spatial derivative of incremental strains in the axial direction using a least-squares estimator [12] with a kernel equal to 6.75 mm (Fig. 11d). The myocardium was segmented using an automated contour tracking technique [28] and displacement and strain maps were then overlaid onto the corresponding B-mode images (Fig. 11e). Isochrones were generated by mapping the first time occurrence at which the incremental strains crossed zero following the Q-wave. More specifically, the absolute value of the incremental strains was minimized in a temporal window following the Q-wave in up to a hundred manually-selected regions. Noisy data were excluded. Subsample resolution was obtained through spline interpolation and Delaunay interpolation was used to construct continuous isochronal maps. Two echocardiographic planes, identical to the planes imaged in the standard apical four- and two-chamber views, were imaged across the long axis of the heart. These two views were temporally co-registered using the ECG signals, spatially co-registered by an echocardiography expert, and displayed in a three-dimensional biplane view in Amira 4.1 (Visage Imaging, Chelmsford, MA) (Figs. 12 and 2).

The TUAS sequence—We have developed and implemented in an Ultrasonix MDP system a temporally-unequispaced acquisition sequence (TUAS) (Fig. 12), which is a sector-based sequence, adapted to optimally estimate cardiac deformations. In TUAS, it is possible to simultaneously achieve a wide range of frame rates for motion estimation, large beam density, and a large field of view in a single heartbeat, thus avoiding the motion-matching and reconstruction steps in EWI (Fig. 8), with little dependence on depth and beam density. Consequently, for a given set of imaging parameters, motion can be estimated at frame rates varying from a few Hz to kHz. The prior knowledge, in this case, is the minimum sampling rate, i.e., the Nyquist rate, of the motion over time at a given pixel. The conventional way to construct an ultrasound image using a phased array is to acquire a finite number of beams, typically 64 or 128, over a 90° angle. These beams are acquired sequentially, and the process is repeated for each frame. For example, a given beam, e.g., beam 3 (Fig. 12),

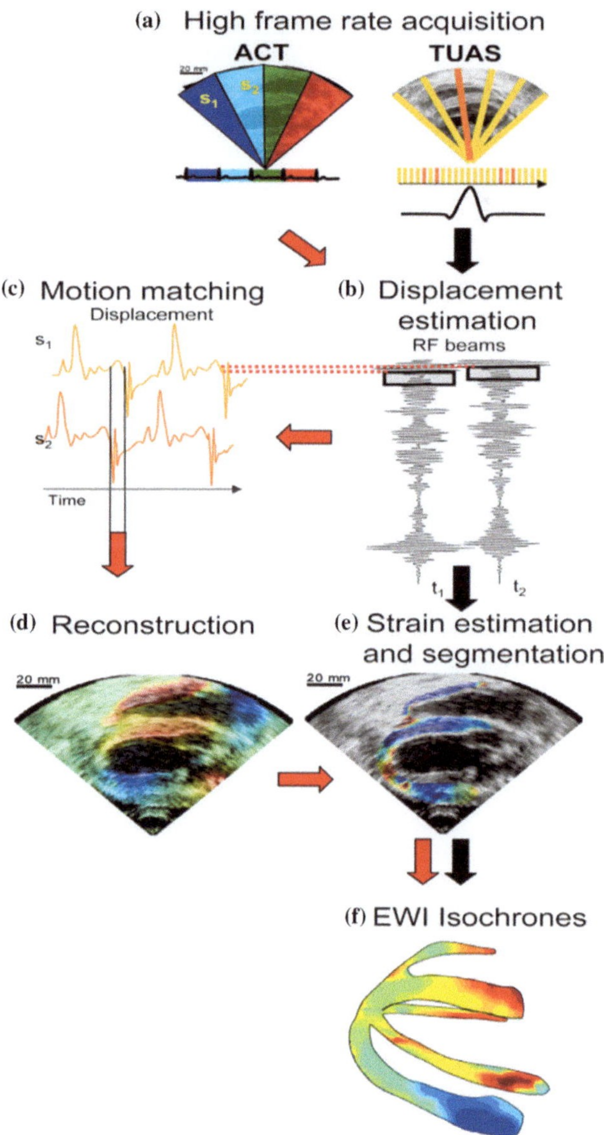

Fig. 12 Block diagram of the EWI technique. **a** High frame-rate acquisition is first performed using either ACT (follow red arrows) or TUAS (black arrows). **b** High precision displacement estimation between two consecutively acquired RF beams (t1, t2) is then performed using very high frame rate RF speckle tracking. **c** In ACT only, a region of the heart muscle, common to two neighboring sectors, is then selected. By comparing the temporally varying displacements measured in neighboring sectors (s1, s2) via a crosscorrelation technique, the delay between them is estimated. **d** In ACT only, a full-view ciné-loop of the displacement overlaid onto the B-mode can then be reconstructed with all the sectors in the composite image synchronized. **e** In ACT and TUAS, the heart walls are then segmented, and incremental strains are computed to depict the EW. **f** By tracking the onset of the EW, isochrones of the sequence of activation are generated

are acquired at a fixed rate (Fig. 12, conventional sequence). In TUAS, the beam acquisition sequence is reordered to provide two distinct rates, defined as follows (Fig. 12): the motion-estimation rate and the motion-sampling rate. The motion-estimation rate r_{me} is defined as the inverse of the time, i.e., T_{me}, lapsing between the two RF frames used to estimate motion. The motion-sampling rate r_{ms} is defined as the inverse of the time, i.e., T_{ms}, lapsing between two consecutive displacement maps. In conventional imaging sequences, these two rates are equal, because a given frame is typically used for two motion estimations (u_n and u_{n+1} in Fig. 12). In TUAS, the operator can adjust the motion-estimation rate. As shown in Fig. 12, a frame in the TUAS case is used only once for motion estimation, thus halving the motion-sampling rate relative to the conventional method. For example, an acquisition performed at a 12-cm-depth with 64 beams with a conventional sequence corresponds to a frame rate of 100 Hz. However, while 100 Hz may suffice to satisfy the Nyquist sampling criterion of cardiac motion, it is usually insufficient for accurate motion tracking using RF cross-correlation. Therefore, to reach a higher frame rate of, e.g., 400 Hz typically used for EWI, the conventional sequence requires to divide the number of beams by four, and thus reduces either the beam density, the field of view, or both. At the same depth and beam density, TUAS provides a motion-sampling rate of 50 Hz and a motion-estimation rate that can be varied, as shown in the following section, within the following group: {6416, 3208, 1604, 802, 401, 201, 100} Hz. This has numerous advantages. For example, both the beam density and the field of view can be maintained while estimating the cardiac motion with an optimal frame rate, which could be, e.g., either 401 or 802 Hz, depending on the amplitude of the cardiac motion. This results into halving of the motion-sampling rate; however, the motion-sampling rate has only little effect on the motion estimation accuracy. Theoretically, if this rate remains above the Nyquist rate of the estimated cardiac motion, it will have no effect. We estimated that at a motion-sampling rate above 120 Hz, the effect of the motion-sampling rate became negligible compared to the effect of the motion-estimation rate (Provost et al. 2011e).

Single-heartbeat EWI and optimal strain estimation—In TUAS, a wide range of frame rates can be achieved, including very high frame rates, independently of other imaging parameters. Therefore, by maintaining a set of imaging parameters (e.g., field of view, imaging depth), and varying the frame rate, it is possible to identify an optimal frame rate by studying the link between the strain signal-to-noise ratio (SNRe) and the EW. Previous report (Varghese and Ophir 1997) on the strain-filter indicates that the SNRe depends mostly on the value of the strains to be measured, when the imaging parameters are fixed. This theoretical framework allows the construction of an upper limit on the SNR_e as a function of the strain amplitude (k., the strain filter). The strain filter corresponds, in this case, to the Ziv-Zakai Lower Bound (ZZLB) on the variance. The ZZLB is a combination of the Cramér-Rao Lower Bound (CRLB) and the Barankin bound (BB). The ZZLB transitions from the CRLB to the BB when decorrelation becomes important to the point that only the envelope of the signal contains information on the motion (Weinstein and Weiss 1984). In the correlation model used here, this transition occurs only at very large strains. Since the amplitude of strains to be measured is directly related to

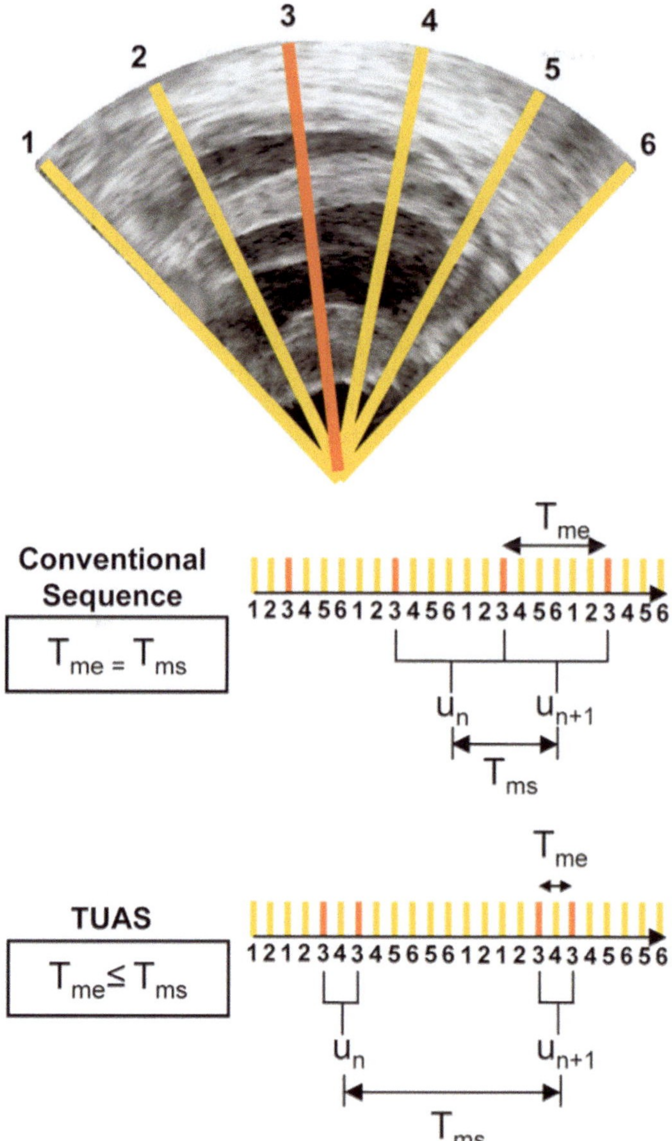

Fig. 13 Illustration of an acquisition sequences in a simple case where only 6 lines form an image with each sector using two lines. In a conventional acquisition sequence, the time separating two acquisitions of the same line is the same. In TUAS, the time separating two acquisitions of the same line are modulated to optimize motion-estimation

the motion-estimation rate (a large motion-estimation rate will result in small inter-frame strains), finding an optimal strain value is equivalent to finding an optimal motion-estimation rate. The strain filter was calculated with the imaging parameters used in this study as a reference; however, it was developed for the analysis of strains occurring in static elastography, and is not adapted to the more complex motion of the heart. We have therefore developed a new probabilistic framework based on experimental data acquired in a paced canine in vivo to not only establish an upper bound on the SNR_e, but to estimate the probability of obtaining a given SNR_e for a given strain amplitude (Provost et al. 2011e). Since the motion-estimation rate can be used as a means to translate and narrow the strain distribution), the optimal motion-estimation rate can be found by studying the link between the strains and the SNR_e. More specifically, a conditional probability density function spanning a large range of strains values was constructed (Fig. 13B) and was found in agreement with the strain-filter theory, which provides a higher bound on the SNRe. The ZZLB predicts a sharp transition between the CRLB and BB when decorrelation becomes important to the point that the phase of the signal does not contain information about motion. Figure 13 shows that the conditional probability density function is comprised within the CRLB up to approximately 4% before it becomes comprised within the BB. A sharp decrease in the expected value of the SNRe is also observed at 4% strain, underlining the importance of using the phase information of the RF signal for accurate strain measurements. A distortion in the strain distribution may indicate that while a high SNRe can be maintained, the accuracy of the strain estimator is strongly impaired at low motion-estimation rates, i.e., less than 350 Hz in this case (Fig. 13B). Finally, we showed that TUAS is capable of accurately depicting non-periodic events at high temporal resolution. Therefore, the optimal frame rate will need to be between 389 and 3891 Hz according to the strains estimated (Fig. 13). Strain patterns expected during such a phenomenon were depicted, such as a disorganized contraction, leading to little to no large scale motion of the heart. Regions of the myocardium were oscillating rapidly from thinning to thickening and thickening to thinning over time. Studying the frequencies of these oscillations could be useful in understanding the mechanisms of fibrillation and we plan to use Fourier based analysis and principal component analysis in order to identify those components in fibrillation and better identify the arrhythmic origin(s).

2.7 *Characterization of Atrial Arrhythmias in Canines in Vivo*

2.7.1 Electrical Mapping

Data from the St. Jude EnSite system was exported to a workstation for co-registration with EWI isochrones. Comma-separated-value (CSV) files containing the coordinates of the 3D mesh as well as the data from each acquired point (activation time and spatial coordinates) were retrieved. The 3D mesh was recreated in Maya (Maya 2016, Autodesk, San Rafael, CA, USA) and the open-source software MeshLab (Visual Computing Lab – ISTI, CNR, meshlab.sourceforge.net). 3D co-registration was performed by aligning the isochrones with the 3D mesh using anatomical landmarks such as the location of the apex, the mitral valve annulus, the lateral wall, or the septum. Once both the isochrones and the mesh were aligned, positions of the acquired points on the EnSite system were projected onto the isochrones and times of activation were compared. This process provided pairs of electrical and electromechanical activation times which were then plotted against each other. Linear regression was then performed and slope, intercept and R^2 values were obtained.

2.7.2 Validation

The objective of this study was to validate EWI against electrical mapping using an electroanatomical mapping system, in all four chambers of the heart. Six (n = 6) normal adult canines were used in this study. The electrical activation sequence was mapped in all four chambers of the heart, both endocardially and epicardially using a

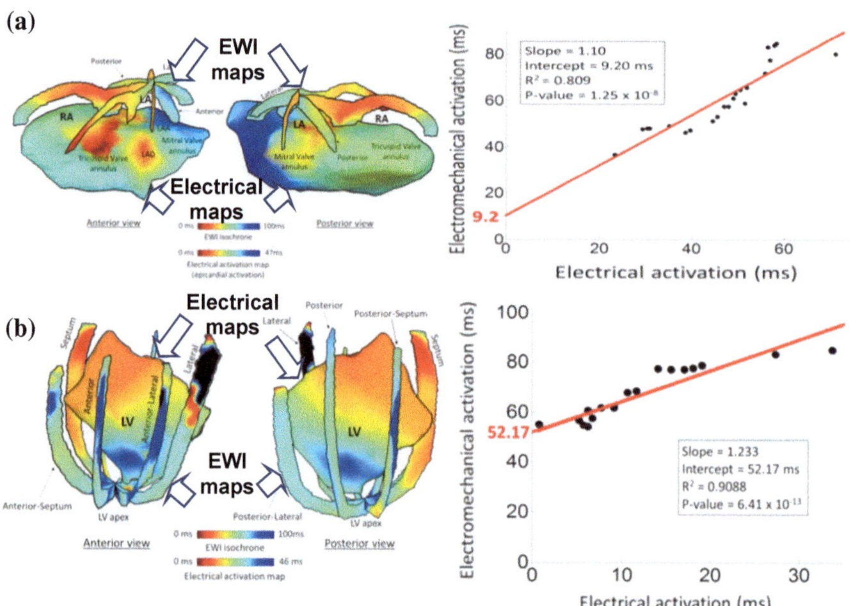

Fig. 14 Comparison of EWI against electroanatomic mapping. Anterior and posterior views in the **a right (RA)** and **left (LA) atria** and **b** entire canine **left ventricle (LV)** using EWI noninvasively and electroanatomic mapping with the proposed clinical system (Ensite, St. Jude Medical). Linear regression analysis shows excellent correlation between the electromechanical and electrical activation with the intercept indicating the electromechanical delay (Costet et al. 2016c)

St. Jude EnSite mapping system (St. Jude Medical, Secaucus, NJ). EWI acquisitions were performed during normal sinus rhythm and pacing and isochrones of the electromechanical activation were generated. Electromechanical and electrical activation times were plotted against each other and linear regression was performed for each pair of activation maps. Electromechanical and electrical activations were found to be highly correlated with slopes of the correlation ranging from 0.77 to 1.83, electromechanical delays between 9 and 58 ms and R^2 values from 0.71 to 0.92 (Fig. 14). The excellent linear correlation between electromechanical and electrical activation and good agreement between the activation maps indicate that the electromechanical activation follows the pattern of propagation of the electrical activation. This suggests that EWI could be used to accurately characterize arrhythmias and localize its source.

2.8 EWI in Normal Human Subjects and with Arrhythmias

The objectives of the clinical studies [3, 35] (Provost et al. 2011, 2015) were (1) to determine the potential for clinical role of EWI, by predicting activation patterns in normal subjects, (2) to determine the feasibility of EWI to identify the site of origin in subjects with tachyarrhythmia, and (3) to identify the myocardial activation sequence in patients undergoing CRT. In normal subjects (Figs. 15 and 16), the EW propagated, in both the atria and the ventricles, in accordance with the expected electrical activation sequences based on reports in the literature. In subjects with CRT, EWI successfully characterized two different pacing schemes, i.e., LV epicardial pacing and RV endocardial pacing versus sinus rhythm with conducted complexes. In two subjects with AFL (Fig. 17), the propagation patterns obtained with EWI were in agreement with results obtained from invasive intracardiac mapping studies, indicating that EWI may be capable of distinguishing LA from RA flutters transthoracically. Finally, we have shown the feasibility of EWI to describe the activation sequence during a single heartbeat in a patient with AFL and RBBB (Provost 2012; Fig. 17). The results presented demonstrate for the first time that mapping the transient strains occurring in response to the electrical activation, i.e., the electromechanical wave

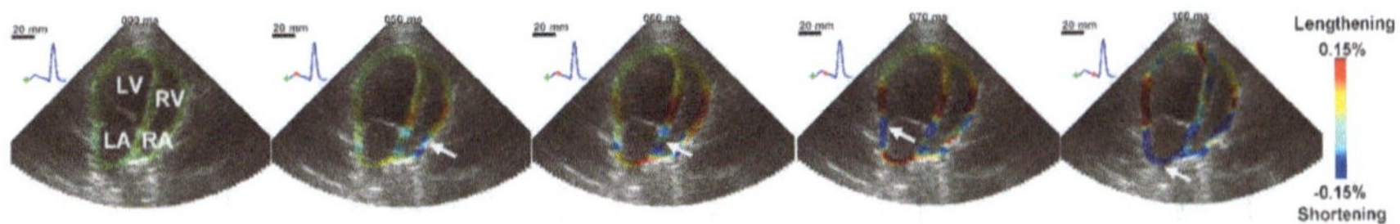

Fig. 15 EWI using a flash sequence for motion estimation (motion sampling rate: 2000 Hz, motion estimation rate: 500 Hz) overlaid on a standard 128-beams, 30-fps B-mode. All four chambers are mapped but only atrial activation is shown here. Activation (shortening, in blue) was initiated in the right atrium (RA) (50 ms) and propagated towards the atrial septum (60 ms), the left atrium (LA) (70 ms) until complete activation of both atria (100 ms). RV: right ventricle, LV: left ventricle

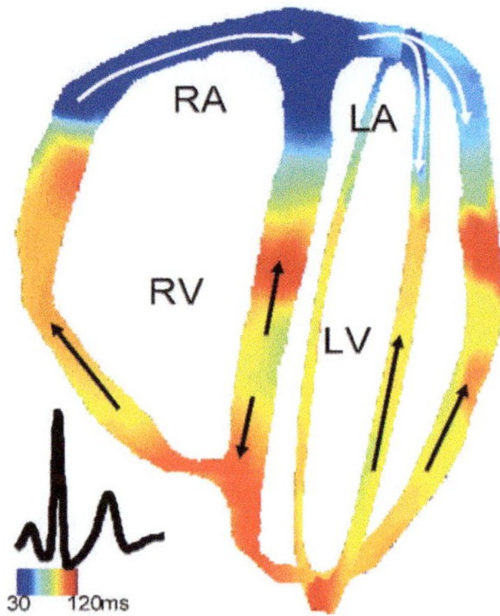

Fig. 16 EWI isochrone in all four chambers in a healthy, 23-year-old male subject. Activation in this view corresponds to shortening of the tissue (blue). Activation is initiated in the right atrium and propagates in the left atrium. After the atrio-ventricular delay, activation is initiated in the ventricles from multiple origins, which are possibly correlated with the Purkinje terminals locations. Arrows (both white and black) indicate the direction of propagation

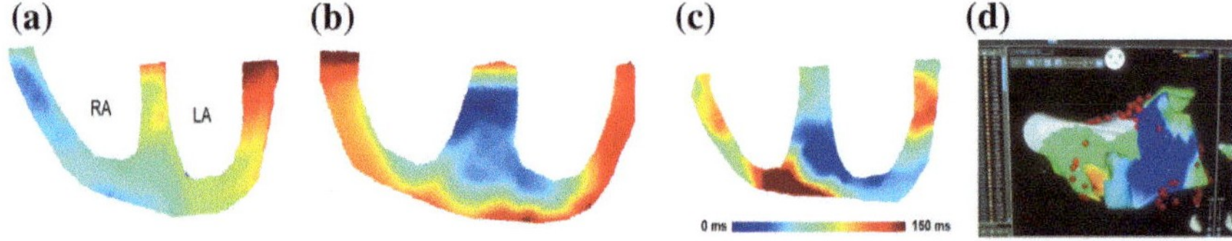

Fig. 17 Noninvasively detecting and characterizing atrial flutter with EWI in three human subjects (RA: right atrium, LA: left atrium). **a** Normal subject (Activation is initiated in the right atrium and propagates towards the left atrium); **b** Unknown atrial flutter in a flutter patient with a prosthetic mitral valve, which was believed to cause the atrial flutter from the left side. Since the patient could not sustain the long procedure needed to construct a full activation map using cardiac mapping, ablation was attempted without complete information in two locations in the left atrium, which did not lead to cardioversion, i.e., did not return to sinus rhythm. The patient was sent home and a second ablation is scheduled in the near future. **This case exemplifies the need for a faster mapping method**, which could have led to the proper identification of the ablation site and potentially limit the number of ablation procedures needed to treat this patient. Indeed the EWI isochrones shown here display the initial activation in the left atrium, close to the septum; **c** Atypical left atrial flutter patient confirmed by cardiac mapping. EWI isochrones also show early activation is initiated in the left atrium. See **Appendix 1** for the corresponding EWI cine-loops. **d** CARTO map of a left-sided flutter case

propagation, can be used to characterize both normal rhythm and arrhythmias in humans, in all four cardiac chambers transthoracically using multiple and single-heartbeat methodologies. EWI has the potential to noninvasively assist in clinical decision-making prior to invasive treatment, and to aid in optimizing and monitoring response to CRT. Some more recent endeavors are using multi-2D rendering for reconstruction of the ventricular (Fig. 8(d); [31]) and atrial surfaces.

Acknowledgements The results presented herein were produced by current and previous members of the Ultrasound and Elasticity Imaging Laboratory: Ethan Bunting, Ph.D., Alexandre Costet, Ph.D., Julien Grondin, Ph.D., Wei-Ning Lee, Ph.D., Pierre Nauleau, Ph.D. and Jean Provost, Ph.D. The studies were in part supported by R01 EB006042 and R01 HL114358.

References

1. Amano J, Thomas JX, Lavallee M, Mirsky I, Glover D, Manders WT, Randall WC, Vatner SF (1987) Effects of myocardial-ischemia on regional function and stiffness in conscious dogs. Am J Physiol 252(1):H110–H117
2. Bertrand ME, Rousseau MF, Lefebvre JM, Lablanche JM, Asseman PH, Carre AG, Lekieffre JP (1978) Left-ventricular compliance in acute transmural myocardial-infarction in man. Eur J Cardiol 7:179–193
3. Bunting EA, Provost J, Konofagou EE (2014) Stochastic precision analysis of 2D cardiac strain estimation in vivo. Phys Med Biol 59(22):6841–6858. Epub 2014/10/22. NIHMS638316. PMCID: PMC Journal—In Process
4. Costet A, Provost J, Gambhir A, Bobkov Y, Danilo P Jr, Boink GJ, Rosen MR, Konofagou EE (2014) Electromechanical wave imaging of biologically and electrically paced canine hearts in vivo. Ultrasound Med Biol 40(1):177–87. PMCID: PMC3897195
5. Edwards CH, Rankin JS, Mchale P, Ling D, Anderson RW (1981) Effects of ischemia on left-ventricular regional function in the conscious dog. Am J Physiol 240(3):H413–H420
6. Go S et al (2014) Heart disease and stroke statistics–2014 update: a report from the American Heart Association. Circulation 129:e28–e292
7. Gurev V, Constantino J, Rice JJ, Trayanova N (2009) Three-dimensional activation sequence determines transmural changes in electromechanical delay
8. Haga JH, Beaudoin AJ, White JG, Strony J (1998) Quantification of the passive mechanical properties of the resting platelet. Ann Biomed Eng 26:268–277
9. Hillman EMC, Bernus O, Pease E, Bouchard MB, Pertsov A (2007) Depth-resolved optical imaging of transmural electrical propagation in perfused heart. Opt Express 15:17827–17841
10. Holmes JW, Borg TK, Covell JW (2005) Structure and mechanics of healing myocardial infarcts. Annu Rev Biomed Eng 7:223–253
11. Jensen J (1996) Field: a program for simulating ultrasound systems. Paper presented at the 10th Nordic-Baltic conference on biomedical imaging, Published in Medical & Biological Engineering & Computing 34:1351–1353
12. Kallel F, Ophir J (1997) A least-squares strain estimator for elastography. Ultrason Imaging 19:195–208
13. Konofagou E, D'hooge J, Ophir J (2000) Cardiac elastography—a feasibility study. Proc IEEE Ultrason Symp 1273–1276
14. Konofagou E, Ophir J (1998) A new elastographic method for estimation and imaging of lateral displacements, lateral strains, corrected axial strains and Poisson's ratios in tissues. Ultrasound Med Biol 24:1183–1199
15. Konofagou EE (1999) Estimation and imaging of three-dimensional motion and Poisson's ratio in elastography. PhD dissertation, University of Houston, TX
16. Konofagou EE, Harrigan T, Solomon S (2001) Assessment of regional myocardial strain using cardiac elastography: distinguishing infarcted from non-infarcted myocardium. Proc IEEE Ultrason Symp 1589–1592
17. Konofagou EE, D'Hooge J, Ophir J (2002) Myocardial elastography—a feasibility study in vivo. Ultrasound Med Biol 28:475–482

18. Konofagou EE, Manning W, Kissinger K, Solomon SD (2003) Myocardial elastography-comparison to results using MR cardiac tagging. Proc IEEE Ultrason Symp 130–133
19. Konofagou EE, Fung-Kee-Fung S, Luo J, Pernot M (2006a) Imaging the mechanics and electromechanics of the heart. Proc IEEE EMBS Conf 6648–6651
20. Konofagou EE, Luo J, Fujikura K, Cervantes D, Coromilas J (2006b) Imaging the electromechanical wave activation of the left ventricle in vivo. Proc IEEE Ultrason Symp 985–988
21. Konofagou EE, Lee W-N, Luo J (2008) Cardiovascular elasticity imaging. In: Fatemi M, Al-Jumaily A (eds) Biomedical applications of vibration and acoustics in imaging and characterizations. Chapter 6, 93-117. ASME Press, New York, NY
22. Konofagou EE, Luo J, Saluja D, Cervantes DO, Coromilas J, Fujikura K (2010) Noninvasive electromechanical wave imaging and conduction-relevant velocity estimation in vivo. Ultrasonics 50(2):208–215. [Invited] PMCID: PMC4005418
23. Konofagou EE, Provost J (2012) Electromechanical wave imaging for noninvasive mapping of the 3D electrical activation sequence in canines and humans in vivo. J Biomech 45(5):856–864. [Invited] PMCID: PMC4005422
24. Lauerma K et al (1997) Multislice MRI in assessment of myocardial perfusion in patients with single-vessel proximal left anterior descending coronary artery disease before and after revascularization. Circulation 96:2859–2867
25. Lee WN, Ingrassia CM, Fung-Kee-Fung SD, Costa KD, Holmes JW, Konofagou EE (2007) Theoretical quality assessment of myocardial elastography with in vivo validation. IEEE Trans Ultrason Ferroelectr Freq Control 54:2233–2245
26. Lee WN, Konofagou EE (2008) Angle-independent and multi-dimensional myocardial elastography—from theory to clinical validation. Ultrasonics 48:563–567
27. Lee WN, Provost J, Fujikura K, Wang J, Konofagou EE (2011) In vivo study of myocardial elastography under graded ischemia conditions. Phys Med Biol 56(4):1155–72. PMCID: PMC4005801
28. Luo J, Konofagou EE (2008) High-frame rate, full-view myocardial elastography with automated contour tracking in murine left ventricles in vivo. IEEE Trans Ultrason Ferroelectr Freq Control 55:240–248
29. Luo J, Lee W-N, Konofagou EE (2009) Fundamental performance assessment of 2-D myocardial elastography in a phased array configuration. IEEE Trans Ultrason Ferroelectr Freq Control (in press)
30. Luo J, Konofagou E (2010) A fast normalized cross-correlation calculation method for motion estimation. IEEE Trans Ultrason Ferroelectr Freq Control. 57(6):1347–57. PMCID: PMC4123965
31. Nauleau P, Melki L, Wan E, Konofagou E (2017) A 3-D rendering algorithm for electromechanical wave imaging of a beating heart. Med Phys 44(9):4766–4772
32. Provost J, Lee WN, Fujikura K, Konofagou EE (2010) Electromechanical wave imaging of normal and ischemic hearts in vivo. IEEE Trans Med Imaging 29(3):625–635. PMCID: PMC3093312
33. Provost J, Gurev V, Trayanova N, Konofagou EE (2011) Mapping of cardiac electrical activation with electromechanical wave imaging: an in silico-in vivo reciprocity study. Heart Rhythm 8(5):752–759. PMC3100212
34. Provost J, Nguyen VT, Legrand D, Okrasinski S, Costet A, Gambhir A, Garan H, Konofagou EE (2011) Electromechanical wave imaging for arrhythmias. Phys Med Biol 56(22):L1–L11 PMID: 22024555
35. Provost J, Thiebault S, Luo J, Konofagou EE (2012) Single-heartbeat electromechanical wave imaging with optimal strain estimation using temporally unequispaced acquisition sequences. Phys Med Biol 57(4):1095–1112. NIHMS375306 [PMCID in Process]
36. Ramanathan C, Ghanem RN, Jia P, Ryu K, Rudy Y (2004) Noninvasive electrocardiographic imaging for cardiac electrophysiology and arrhythmia. Nat Med 10:422–428
37. Righetti R, Ophir J, Ktonas P (2002) Axial resolution in elastography. Ultrasound Med Biol 28(1):101–113

38. Schilling RJ, Peters NS, Davies W (1998) Simultaneous endocardial mapping in the human left ventricle using a noncontact catheter—comparison of contact and reconstructed electrograms during sinus rhythm. Circulation 98:887–898
39. Varma N, Eberli FR, Apstein CS (2000) Increased diastolic chamber stiffness during demand ischemia—response to quick length change differentiates rigor-activated from calcium-activated tension. Circulation 101(18):2185–2192
40. Varma N, Eberl FR, Apstein CS (2001) Left ventricular diastolic dysfunction during demand ischemia: rigor underlies increased stiffness without calcium-mediated tension. Amelioration by glycolytic substrate. J Am Coll Cardiol 37(8):2144–2153
41. Wang SG, Lee WN, Provost J, Luo J, Konofagou EE (2008) A composite high-frame-rate system for clinical cardiovascular imaging. IEEE Trans Ultrason Ferroelectr Freq Control 55:2221–2233
42. Zervantonakis IK, Fung-Kee-Fung SD, Lee WN, Konofagou EE (2007) A novel, view-independent method for strain mapping in myocardial elastography: eliminating angle and centroid dependence. Phys Med Biol 52:4063–4080

Image-Based Motion and Strain Estimation of the Vessel Wall

Spyretta Golemati, Eleni Patelaki and Konstantina S. Nikita

Abstract The estimation of vessel wall motion is valuable for characterising vessel status in health and disease. Following the periodic movement of the heart and the resulting blood pressure variations during the cardiac cycle, the vascular wall performs a complex three-dimensional motion. Wall motion can be quantified through the calculation of a number of kinematic parameters, including displacements, velocities, and accelerations, as well as strain, which has gained attention for characterising tissue function. To estimate vascular motion from images, different imaging modalities can be used, including ultrasound, magnetic resonance imaging (MRI) and computed tomography (CT). Among these, ultrasound imaging is the most widely used technique for vascular motion estimation, due to its wide availability, easy use, high temporal resolution, and possibility to access various central and peripheral vessels. Offering lower temporal but higher spatial resolutions than ultrasound, MRI and CT have been used mostly in aortic kinematics. In parallel to the development of sophisticated imaging and analysis methods, which will allow to reveal unexplored aspects of the complex kinematic phenomena of vascular tissue, the systematic application of image-based motion indices to clinical practice is crucial towards improving clinical decision making and ultimately public health.

1 Introduction

Blood vessels, including arteries, veins and capillaries, form part of the cardiovascular system, and are responsible for transporting blood and nutrients between the heart and all cells of the body [1]. The vast system of blood vessels is over 60,000 miles long. As they move away from the heart, vessels branch repeatedly into branches

S. Golemati (✉)
Medical School, National Kapodistrian University of Athens, Athens, Greece
e-mail: sgolemati@med.uoa.gr

E. Patelaki · K. S. Nikita
School of Electrical and Computer Engineering,
National Technical University of Athens, Athens, Greece

S. Golemati and K. S. Nikita (eds.), *Cardiovascular Computing—Methodologies and Clinical Applications*, Series in BioEngineering,
https://doi.org/10.1007/978-981-10-5092-3_9

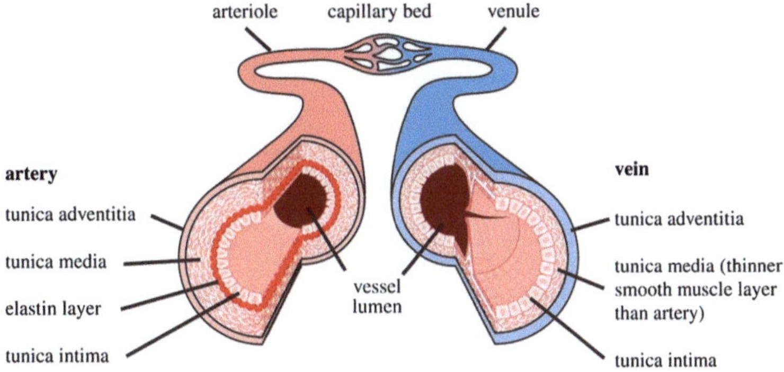

Fig. 1 Schematic representation of vessel structure

with decreasing diameters. Anatomically, the vessel wall is composed of three distinct layers, namely an inner *tunica intima*, a middle *tunica media* and an outer *tunica adventitia*. Figure 1 illustrates a schematic representation of vascular structure. Vessel wall layers are parallel and contiguous and their main components include elastin, collagen and smooth muscle cells [2]. The relative proportion, geometric configuration and spatial arrangement of these components determine the stability, resilience and mechanical behaviour of the vessel wall. Following the periodic movement of the heart and the resulting blood pressure variations during the cardiac cycle, the vessel wall performs a complex three-dimensional (3D) motion [3]. All wall layers are involved in vascular motion, and relative movement between them is often observed.

The estimation of vessel wall motion in both health and disease is a task of considerable importance. Objective assessment of normal motion patterns is important for understanding the local mechanical phenomena, which are useful in the study of blood vessel function under normal conditions. Assessment of motion patterns in disease, injury, following treatment, as well as with ageing, is also valuable for characterising and monitoring vessel pathophysiology. Motion estimation allows the calculation of a number of kinematic parameters, among which strain has gained attention for characterising the mechanical properties of tissue. An important feature of motion estimation is that the related kinematic indices are indicative of the function of the underlying tissue, which, compared to anatomical indices, are more sensitive to tissue structural changes accompanying physiological or pathological processes. Quantitative estimation of vessel wall motion has remained particularly challenging in clinical practice and prone to significant variability [4].

Different physical principles can be utilised to view and assess vascular motion. Ultrasound-based techniques are the most widely used, due to a number of advantages, including low cost, bedside availability and, also importantly, high temporal resolution, which allows recording of the fast vascular phenomena. Magnetic resonance imaging (MRI), which yields high-contrast images, and computed tomography (CT), which allows for high spatial resolution, have also been used for this task [4]. The basic principles of these modalities are described in Chap. 2.

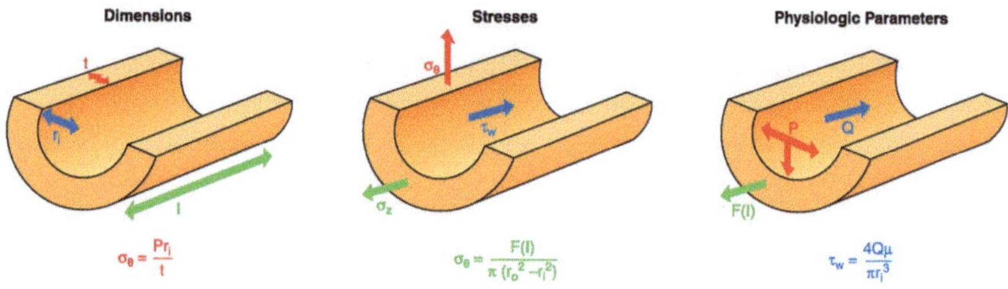

Fig. 2 Relationships between the vessel wall dimensions, stresses, and physiological parameters. The dimensions include inner radius (r_i), length (l), and thickness (t). The stresses include wall shear stress (τ_W), longitudinal stress (σ_Z), and average circumferential stress (σ_Θ). The physiological parameters include volumetric blood flow (Q), longitudinal tethering forces [F(l)], and blood pressure (P). The viscosity of blood (μ) is also included in the wall shear stress equation. The equations show how changes in the vessel wall dimensions and/or physiological parameters can alter the wall stresses. (Reprinted from [2] with permission)

This chapter provides an overview of the field of vessel wall motion and strain estimation from images. In this context, some basic principles of wall motion are described, and pathophysiological and clinical implications are highlighted, derived mostly from applications in real data. It is pointed out that the great majority of works in this field involves motion of arteries, mainly due to their increased resilience and higher tolerance of stresses, which facilitate motion tracking and analysis; veins often collapse, which is quite challenging for reliable motion estimation.

2 Basic Principles of Vessel Wall Movement

2.1 Physiology and Pathophysiology of Vessel Wall Movement

During systole, blood is ejected from the left ventricle into the aorta, which increases in diameter and the expansion travels down the arterial system in the form of a wave, known as the 'pressure wave'. Blood is brought back to the heart through two major veins, namely the superior vena cava, which serves the head and arms, and the inferior vena cava, which serves the abdomen and legs.

Vessel movement during the cardiac cycle is due to the effect of stresses applied on the wall, which in turn originate from forces caused by blood pressure, blood flow and tethering to surrounding tissues. Stress is defined as the force applied to an object divided by the surface area over which this force is applied. The stresses take place in circumferential directions, i.e. along the vessel radius, and in longitudinal directions, i.e. along the vessel axis (Fig. 2). The so called shear stress, namely the relative stress of two surfaces lying parallel to each other, also takes place in the longitudinal direction.

Most blood vessels are thin-walled tubes deforming axisymmetrically [3], and can therefore be treated as membranes. Under the effects of the different stresses, these membrane-like structures are constantly moving (deforming) in a complex 3D pattern. Vascular deformations include inflation, longitudinal stretching and shear, and torsion. Arteries transport blood under higher pressures than veins, are more resilient than veins, and when stretched they keep their shape and elongate, whereas small veins cannot tolerate such distortion without collapsing. Arterial deformations consist of rapid distension following ventricular systole, whereby 50% or more of the stroke volume is transiently accommodated, and of retraction during diastole. The largest motion and derived strains have been reported in the direction of vessel diameter changes, and the lowest in the direction corresponding to wall thickness changes. Specifically, most conduit arteries undergo 8–10% oscillation in external diameter or about 15% oscillation in internal diameter.

Similar to stresses, arterial strains occur in circumferential and longitudinal directions. Strain is defined as the change in position (or deformation) with respect to an initial position. Stresses and strains in the longitudinal direction are tensile because the vessel tends to distend in this direction with pressurisation. Strains and stresses in the circumferential direction are compressive as the wall tends to be narrowed with pressurisation.

In the course of the vessel lifetime, its wall motion is altered due to changes in its anatomical, morphological and mechanical properties. Ageing is responsible for reduced elastin and smooth muscle cell content within the arterial wall, in favour of collagen, and this is reflected in decreased wall mobility and elasticity [5]. The presence of a number of diseases, including not only cardiovascular disorders, like hypertension, but also other diseases, such as metabolic, respiratory and neurological diseases, may also have adverse effects on vessel wall alterations. In addition to these diffuse diseases, atheromatous plaque, which is a focal lesion specific to the arterial wall, and consists in the build-up of fatty material in the inner arterial wall, also affects wall mechanics, in addition to its anatomical and morphological properties.

2.2 *Indices of Vessel Wall Movement*

The motion of the vascular wall can be described by its displacements along the circumferential and longitudinal directions. Displacements, measured in mm (or other distance units), are commonly represented by waveforms (vectors) over one or more cardiac cycles. A number of indices can be extracted from these waveforms, including maximal/minimal values, amplitudes, frequencies, etc. Displacement waveforms are usually acquired from small vessel areas. Given the high complexity and inhomogeneity of motion along the vascular wall, such displacements can be significantly different within small tissue regions. Velocities and accelerations can also be determined from the first and second derivatives of displacements, respectively. Inverse calculations, namely integration of velocities to obtain displacements, are also often encountered in MRI and CT modalities.

Strain is often used to describe vascular motion and deformation. Similar to displacement, strain is also represented by waveforms over one or more cardiac cycles, from which quantitative indices can be extracted. Strain tensors can also be used, consisting in multi-dimensional arrays of numerical values which describe the different components of strain. Strain rate, derived from the first derivative of strain, can also characterise tissue kinematics. Strain is a dimensionless feature, whereas strain rate is measured in s^{-1}.

Displacement- and strain-based indices, as well as those calculated from their derivatives, characterise the kinematic properties of the underlying tissue. To estimate tissue mechanical properties, namely its elasticity, an estimate of pressure or stress is required in addition to kinematic features. A number of formulae exist to estimate tissue elasticity indices from displacement/strain and pressure measurements, including distensibility, compliance, etc. [6]. Additionally, the stress-strain relationship is a widely used method to describe tissue mechanical properties. Stress-strain relationships in blood vessels are nonlinear, i.e. they do not obey Hooke's law; vascular tissue creeps under constant stress and relaxes under constant strain [3]. The Young's modulus, derived from the stress-strain relationship, is commonly used to characterise tissue stiffness.

3 Image-Based Estimation of Motion and Strain of the Vessel Wall

Vascular tissue motion can be estimated through the analysis of image sequences acquired using ultrasound, MR and CT modalities. The application of a variety of image analysis methods on these sequences allows the identification of a number of indices, according to the principles outlined in the previous section, towards characterising different phenomena of tissue motion. A major application of motion analysis is elastography, consisting in the calculation and mapping of local tissue strain [7]. The major modalities allowing elastography in vessels are ultrasound and magnetic resonance imaging. In the following subsections, the most important findings and implications are outlined derived from the application of imaging modalities to estimation vascular motion.

3.1 Ultrasound Imaging

Ultrasound-based tissue motion can be estimated in one dimension (1D), using M(otion)-mode or Tissue Doppler Imaging (TDI). This dimension lies along the direction of the ultrasound beam, which usually coincides with the radial direction of vascular motion. It is also possible to measure vessel wall motion in 2D and 3D using B(brightness)-mode or radio-frequency (RF) data [8]. B-mode images provide lower spatial and temporal resolutions than RF data, but are more widely (commercially) available. The various modalities of ultrasound elastography allow mapping of tissue strains (e.g. conventional elastography) and elasticity in terms of the Young's modulus (e.g. shear wave elastography) [9]. Temporal resolution in ultrasound imaging ranges from around 25 frames per second in commercial devices to frame rates higher than 1,000 frames per second in ultrafast imaging systems [10].

Speckle tracking methods have been widely used to estimate vascular tissue motion from ultrasound images [11]. These methods rely on tracking the intensity or the interference patterns produced by the so called speckle, the characteristic pattern of ultrasound images. Speckle is derived by interfering echoes of a transmitted waveform that originate from tissue heterogeneities, and carries useful information about the underlying tissue activity. Speckle tracking encompasses a number of approaches, including block matching and differential methods. Image registration methods estimate motion by frame-to-frame or group-wise registering successive ultrasound frames with a deformable shape tracking approach. The deformation field is parameterised using smooth basis functions, such as B-splines. To regularise the motion, the energy function is optimised, by adding extra cost terms. The more recently suggested phase-based approaches consist in processing the information carried by the phase of the images, namely in the frequency domain.

Applications of ultrasound-based vascular tissue motion estimation in real image data include (a) the central vessels, namely the aorta and the coronary arteries, and (b) peripheral vessels, namely the carotid, brachial, femoral and popliteal arteries, as well as the jugular vein.

Description of aortic wall kinematics is important not only for understanding its physiological functioning but also for early detection of pathophysiological changes such as aortic stiffening, aneurysm formation, and aortic dissection. Using four-dimensional ultrasound and speckle tracking, it was shown that the ascending aorta undergoes a more complex deformation than the abdominal aorta, consisting in alternating clockwise and counterclockwise twist, and length and diameter changes of the same order of magnitude with a phase shift between both [12]. A fast calculation of the normalised correlation coefficient in ultrasound-based motion estimation was proposed in [13] and used to demonstrate that wall motion and blood flow were uniform and synchronous in normal murine aortas, but reduced, spatially varied and less synchronous in aneurysmal aortas. Ultrasound-based displacements of abdominal aortic aneurysms were recently utilised in combination with finite element analysis to determine wall stresses, in an attempt to improve stratification of rupture risk [14].

In coronary arteries, intravascular ultrasound (IVUS) has been used to estimate vascular wall motion, with the major endpoint being the identification of vulnerable plaque, i.e. plaque that is prone to rupture and cause cardiac symptoms. The application of methods, including optical flow and nonrigid registration, has yielded strain and elasticity maps of vessel areas, and the term IVUS elastography is widely used. The feasibility of in vivo IVUS elastography was demonstrated in [15], yielding higher strain values in non-calcified plaque than in calcified plaque. With the use of optical flow, radial and shear strain distributions were generated, yielding high and low values in soft and hard plaque tissue, respectively [16]. To estimate the apparent

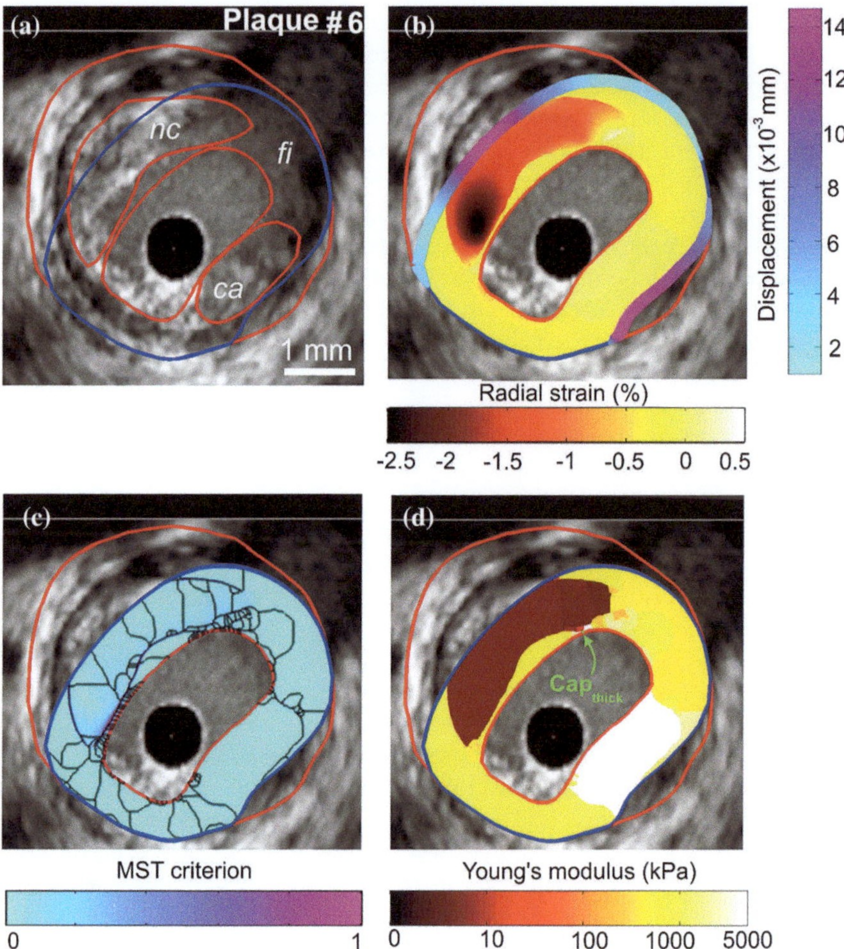

Fig. 3 Performance of the proposed modulography technique to detect a vulnerable plaque with a large calcified inclusion. **a** Intravascular ultrasound image of plaque with plaque contours. **b** Radial strain-elastogram and displacement applied on the intraplaque outer endoluminal boundary. **c** Spatial distribution of the normalised modified Sumi's transform criterion and extracted inclusions contours (n = 150). **d** Computed modulogram. nc: necrotic core; fi: fibrous region; ca: calcified inclusion. Reprinted from [18] with permission from Elsevier

stress-strain modulus of arterial tissue, the IVUS elasticity palpography technique has been suggested [17]. IVUS modulography allows reconstruction of elasticity maps (or modulograms) from strain estimations. A recent update of the modulography technique for high-definition IVUS has allowed quantification of necrotic core areas and identification of Young's moduli of the necrotic cores and fibrous tissue (Fig. 3) [18].

The motion of the normal and diseased carotid artery wall has been interrogated in a number of studies and associated with different clinical manifestations, including the risk for cerebrovascular complications, such as strokes or transient ischaemic attacks [19]. These studies demonstrated the existence of a longitudinal component of wall motion, which had not been investigated as commonly as the radial component [20]. This longitudinal component exhibited a distinct multiphasic pattern of motion during the cardiac cycle, of the same magnitude as the diameter change in the common carotid artery of healthy humans, and was useful for detecting the presence of shear strain within the wall [21]. In pathological conditions, such as diabetes, it was shown that the amplitudes of diameter change and of longitudinal displacements of the near and far arterial walls of the left common carotid were significantly lower compared to those of healthy volunteers [22]. Carotid artery longitudinal displacements were shown to reflect cardiovascular status and predict short-term event-free survival in medium- to high-risk patients [23]. In a group of subjects with symptomatic and asymptomatic atheromatous plaque, symptomatic ones showed decreased amplitude of radial and longitudinal motion of the wall, higher motion amplitude of the plaque top surface, and higher relative movement between the plaque top and bottom surfaces [24] (Fig. 4). Although healthy individuals were found to have a retrograde wall motion pattern, a distinct anterograde pattern was noted with plaque presence [25]. Importantly, patients with severe plaque stenosis had greater anterograde motion than those with moderate stenosis, likely owing to high wall shear stresses associated with greater peak systolic velocities at the site of stenosis [25]. Recently, an association was demonstrated between carotid plaque strain and cognitive function. Specifically, the degree of strain instability measured within the atherosclerotic plaque directly predicted vascular cognitive decline [26]. This behaviour might be due to the presence of micro-emboli, which may lead to cognitive impairment, possibly as a result of the rupture of vulnerable plaque associated with increased strain, because higher strain is indicative of larger deformation and increased probability of plaque rupture.

The analysis of motion of the brachial and popliteal arteries has revealed a bidirectional pattern of longitudinal motion and shear strain between intima-media and adventitia, similar to those in the carotid artery [21].

Estimation of the pulse of the jugular vein from B-mode ultrasound has been recently reported and is useful in assessing the function of the internal jugular vein [27].

3.2 *Magnetic Resonance Imaging*

In addition to yielding high-contrast images, MRI also allows tissue motion estimation. The spatial and temporal resolution of MRI is 1–2 mm and 20–50 ms, respectively. Gradient echo techniques, such as cine MRI or balanced steady-state free-precession (SSFP), can be used for this task. In a standard scenario, to estimate tissue motion from MRI, segmentation of the interrogated area is first performed, followed by the application of strain tensors (Green-Lagrange), and pressure or disten-

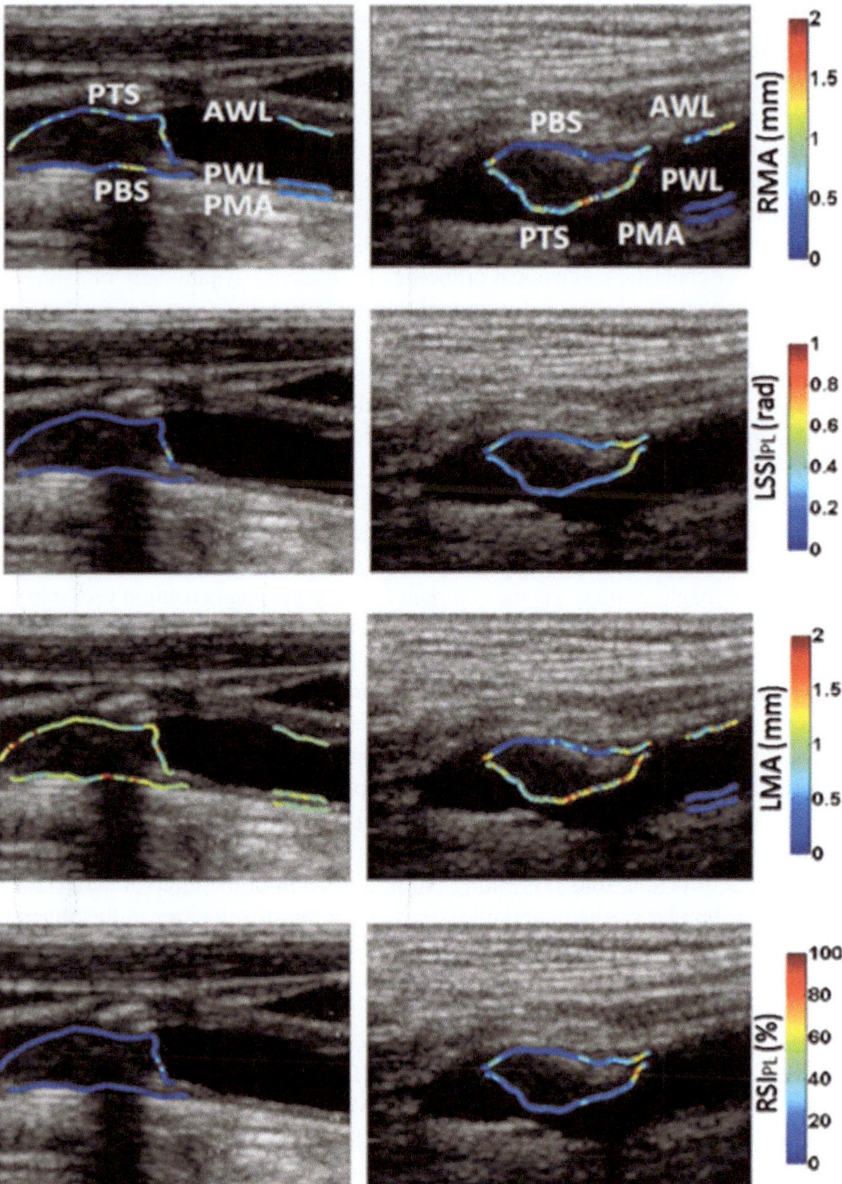

Fig. 4 Examples of color-coded distributions of various motion-derived indices for an asymptomatic (left column) and a symptomatic (right column) patient with an atherosclerotic plaque on the posterior and the anterior wall, respectively. White labels indicate the selected ROIs for each case. RMA/LMA: radial/longitudinal motion amplitude; $LSSI_{PL}$: longitudinal strain index at plaque; RSI_{PL}: radial strain index at plaque. (© Institute of Physics and Engineering in Medicine. Reproduced from [24] by permission of IOP Publishing. All rights reserved)

sibility formulae [28–30]. This scheme has been implemented and tested on different types of vessels, including the aorta [28], the carotid artery [29], as well as veins [30]. More recent MRI techniques allowing direct (i.e. without a segmentation step) tissue tracking and motion analysis, include tagged MRI, phase-contrast (PC) MRI, and pulse field gradient based MRI methods, such as harmonic-phase-imaging (HARP) and displacement-encoding-with-stimulated-echoes (DENSE) [31]. MR elastography (MRE) has emerged as a sensitive method for noninvasively evaluating the mechanical properties of biological tissues [32]. MRE enables direct quantification of the viscoelastic mechanical properties of tissue by dynamically imaging the propagation of cyclical shear deformations that are induced in a material. Such deformations are due to shear waves caused by mechanical excitations at frequencies of 50–100 Hz.

In MRI tagging, cine MR images are acquired with a superimposed parallel grid of dark saturation lines, which are induced by a special pre-pulse sequence immediately following the R-wave of the ECG and can subsequently be followed over the cardiac cycle [33]. Dedicated computer algorithms can subsequently be used to track the intersection points of the tagging lines automatically over the cardiac cycle, towards quantifying tissue deformations. In contrast to the tagging technique that images longitudinal magnetisation, i.e. the component of the net magnetisation vector in the direction of the static magnetic field, the PC method obtains information about tissue dynamics by phase encoding the velocity of transverse magnetisation [34]. Then, tissue displacement can be measured through integration of the velocity field. MR tagging is easy to visualise and implement, but it suffers from low spatial resolution, whereas velocity-encoded PC provides high spatial resolution, but is prone to phase distortion, when large gradient moments are applied to encode low velocities within a voxel. Pulsed gradient stimulated echo (PGSTE) techniques, which are a popular variation of the PFG techniques, store a part of the tissue magnetisation along the longitudinal direction, thus preventing phase distortion in the interval between the lobes of the bipolar gradient, and allowing integration of velocities in this interval. Based on this principle, DENSE [35] and FastHARP (Fig. 5) [36] have been proposed. In these techniques, a standardised PGSTE sequence is induced in the tissue and, subsequently, its impact is measured, in terms of tissue motion.

PC and DENSE have been applied to estimate vessel wall motion, due to their adequate spatial resolution. Using cine PC MRI of thoracic and abdominal healthy human aortas, Wedding et al. reported that PC-MRI can successfully quantify vessel wall cyclic strains [37]. Using DENSE MRI, Lin et al. found that strain estimation results from DENSE with a balanced SSFP readout in human carotid arteries agreed with the corresponding results derived from cine MRI, thus proving the feasibility of DENSE for mapping carotid artery strains [38]. Krishnan et al. applied DENSE MRI to patients with ascending thoracic aortic aneurysm (<5 cm) and showed that zero-pressure geometry and patient-specific material properties should be considered for designing an accurate model for ascending thoracic aortic aneurysm prediction [39]. HARP methodologies suffer from limited signal-to-noise ratio, which limits their applicability to vessel wall motion estimation.

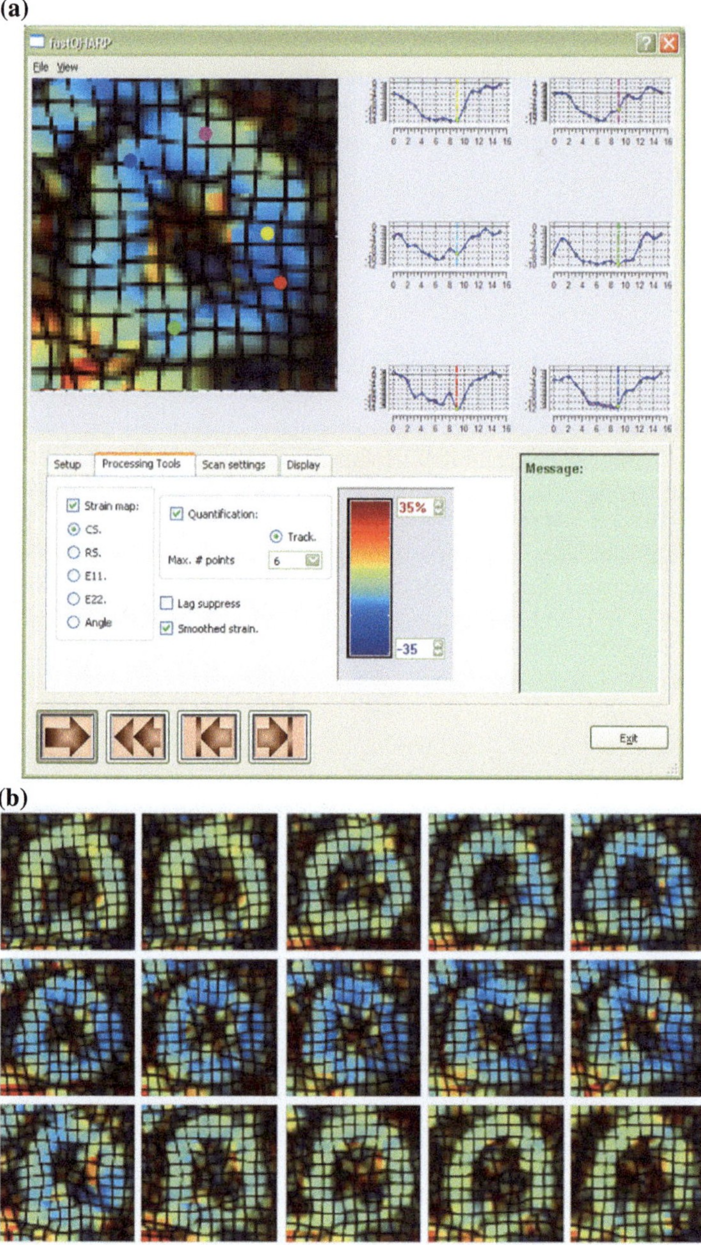

Fig. 5 **a** Processing/visualisation tool during a typical real-time strain quantification experiment. (Top left) Magnitude image of ROI at end systole with synthetic tags and Eulerian circumferential strain superimposed. The colour bar shows that a large negative strain has taken place over the myocardium, indicating a strong, healthy contraction. (Top left) Time profiles showing the circumferential strain over the previous cardiac cycle of six material points. The horizontal axes correspond to cardiac phase. **b** Real-time strain CINE map of 15 consecutive cardiac phases as were displayed in the visualisation tool. (© 2007 IEEE. Reprinted, with permission, from [36])

The feasibility of MRE to estimate arterial stiffness in vivo has been demonstrated for the aorta [40, 41]. Xu et al. used the pulse-gated cine MRE technique to study wave propagation along the aorta throughout the cardiac cycle, and reported good wave visualisation in diastole but not in systole [40]. It has also been found that hypertensive subjects presented significantly higher MRE-based aortic stiffness than normotensives [41].

3.3 Computed Tomography

CT allows imaging of anatomical areas of the cardiovascular system and the detection of malfunction or lesions [42]. CT is robust to motion artifacts, due to ECG-gating, and it offers relatively short scan times, although its use entails exposure to X-ray radiation [43]. Its spatial resolution is superior to that of MRI (0.5–0.6 mm) but its temporal resolution is inferior (83–135 ms) [44]. CT has been used in clinical practice for motion and strain estimation of vessels, mostly of the aorta. To achieve such task, segmentation is often performed prior to motion or strain estimation, to locate the vessel wall. For purposes of increased contrast of the blood vessels, CT angiography (CTA) can be used, consisting an injection with a contrast agent before the scan.

A number of methods have been used to estimate strain from CT images. These include the Green-Lagrange strain tensor [45], the stress-strain curve ([46, 49]), the pressure-strain modulus [47] and the Laplace (also known as Lamé) equation, for the calculation of the stress of the vessel wall [46, 47]. Lee et al. computed the dynamic, frequency-dependent local elastic modulus of porcine aortic specimens, as a function of the harmonics of the physiological pressure waveform and as a function of the angular position around the vessel circumference [49]. Other methods perform simpler calculations of the percent change in vessel circumference [47] or cross-sectional area [46]. It has been pointed out that using the aortic circumference for strain estimation is preferable to the diameter or the cross-sectional area, so as to avoid the assumption of circular vessel geometry, which may be misleading [45].

The issue of through-plane motion has been addressed in a number of studies [45, 48]. Morrison et al. implemented the Lagrangian reference frame technique, according to which the frame is fixed onto a specific region of the vessel, in order to track it throughout the cardiac cycle, even if its though-plane position changes [45]. Weber et al. proposed a four-dimensional approach designed for the aortic wall, which achieved tissue motion estimation in three spatial directions plus time [48]. This work introduced through-plane tracking, i.e. tracking along the vessel centerline of a specific location, using intensity-based matching.

The application of the previously described methodologies has revealed interesting findings for the motion of the aortic wall. Morrison et al. reported that the thoracic aorta enlarges circumferentially and axially, and deforms significantly less in the circumferential direction, with increasing age [45]. Schlicht et al. constructed two aortic models from polydimethylsiloxane with different elastic properties and

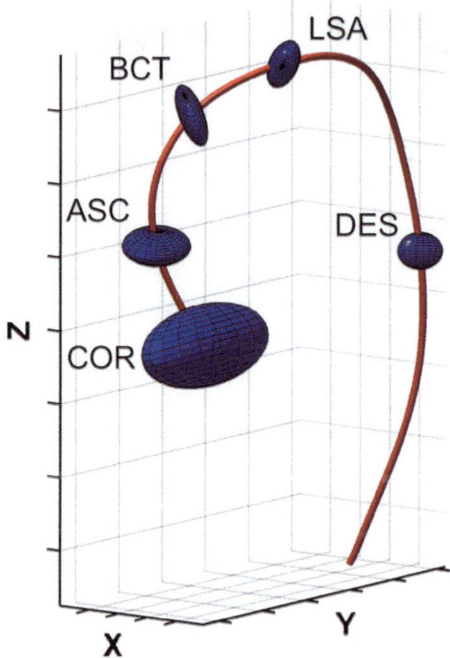

Fig. 6 Both displacement magnitude (size of ellipsoids) and predominant displacement direction (orientation of ellipsoids) at selected aortic locations. Sizes of ellipsoids represent 97.5% (two standard deviations) of displacements comprising mean aortic coordinates at each location and reconstruction interval. Orientation of ellipsoid axes are determined using a principal component analysis. Ellipsoids are scaled by a factor of 8 for better visibility. COR: left coronary artery, ASC: mid-ascending aorta, BCT: braciocephalic trunk, LSA: left subclavian artery, DES: descending aorta (Reprinted by permission from Springer Customer Service Centre GmbH: Springer Nature International Journal of Cardiovascular Imaging [48], 2013)

showed that the ECG-gated multi-detector CT Angiography protocol that they proposed was feasible for measuring the elastic properties of the aortic models and, potentially, of the in vivo functioning aorta [46]. In a group of ascending aortas of 45 male patients, Martin et al. came to similar conclusions as Morrison et al. [45], namely that the ascending aorta dilates and stiffens with aging [47]. Also, this study showed that the ascending aortic wall undergoes more tension with increasing age, a phenomenon likely associated with aneurysm and aortic dissection. Moreover, Weber et al. studied 4D displacements and wall distensions at different aortic locations using CT Angiography, and reported highest values in the ascending aorta (Fig. 6) [48]. They also found that the highest vessel wall displacement and distention among all examined locations was observed in the ascending aortic segment, including the aortic root. Finally, the feasibility of 3D dynamic CT for the quantification of the arterial elastic modulus was substantiated by Lee et al., through the comparison with corresponding results from standard uniaxial tensile testing and volumetric measurements [49].

4 Future Perspectives and Concluding Remarks

This chapter provided an outline of methodologies for estimating vascular wall motion from imaging modalities, including ultrasound, MR and CT. Different aspects of vascular motion can be estimated using imaging modalities in combination with advanced image analysis algorithms, towards extracting valuable functional information useful for the study of vascular physiology and pathophysiology, as well as for diagnosis and decision-making.

Appropriate utilisation and combination of the particular characteristics and possibilities of the different modalities for vascular imaging will allow a novel all-around characterisation of vascular tissue. At a local, i.e. vessel-specific, level, such combination is promising for an overall consideration of vascular kinematics and mechanics. At a global level, it will allow the investigation of spatial variability of kinematic and elastic vascular properties, namely their variability along the entire vascular tree.

A crucial issue in the development and implementation of motion analysis methods is their application in clinical practice. Many vascular kinematic and mechanical properties have been quantified and a large number of indices are currently available. The inclusion of these indices in large-scale clinical trials will allow to identify those indices that are most robust towards improved clinical decision making.

In conclusion, numerous aspects of vascular motion can be estimated using imaging and image analysis. In parallel to the development of sophisticated imaging and analysis methods, which will allow to reveal unexplored aspects of the complex kinematic phenomena of vascular tissue, the systematic application to clinical practice is not only feasible but also crucial for improving public health.

References

1. Martini FH, Nath JL, Bartholomew EF (2017) Fundamentals of anatomy and physiology, 11th edn. Pearson, USA
2. Wagenseil JE, Mecham RP (2009) Vascular extracellular matrix and arterial mechanics. Physiol Rev 89:957–989
3. Fung YC (1993) Biomechanics—mechanical properties of living tissues, 2nd edn. Springer, New York Inc
4. Nikita KS (2013) Atherosclerosis: the evolving role of vascular image analysis. Comput Med Imaging Graph 37(1):1–3
5. Greenwald SE (2007) Ageing of the conduit arteries. J Pathol 211(2):157–172
6. Mackenzie IS, Wilkinson IB, Cockroft JR (2002) Assessment of arterial stiffness in clinical practice. Q J Med 95:67–74
7. Sarvazyan A, Hall TJ, Urban MW, Fatemi M, Aglyamov SR, Garra BS (2011) An overview of elastography—an emerging branch of medical imaging. Curr Med Imaging Rev 7(4):255–282

8. Hoskins PR, Kenwright DA (2015) Recent developments in vascular ultrasound technology. Ultrasound 23(3):158–165
9. Gennisson JL, Deffieux T, Fink M, Tanter M (2013) Ultrasound elastography: principles and techniques. Diagn Interv Imaging 94(5):487–495
10. Tanter M, Fink M (2014) Ultrafast imaging in biomedical ultrasound. IEEE Trans Ultrason Ferroelectr Freq Contr 61(1):102–119
11. Golemati S, Gastounioti A, Nikita KS (2016) Ultrasound-image-based cardiovascular tissue motion estimation. IEEE Rev Biomed Eng 9:208–218
12. Wittek A, Karatolios K, Fritzen CP et al (2016) Cyclic three-dimensional wall motion of the human ascending and abdominal aorta characterized by time-resolved three-dimensional ultrasound speckle-tracking. Biomech Model Mechanobiol 15:1375–1388
13. Luo J, Konofagou EE (2011) Imaging of wall motion coupled with blood flow velocity in the heart and vessels *in vivo*: a feasibility study. Ultrasound Med Biol 37(6):980–995
14. van Disseldorp EM, Petterson NJ, Rutten MC, van de Vosse FN, van Sambeek MR, Lopata RG (2016) Patient specific wall stress analysis and mechanical characterization of abdominal aortic aneurysms using 4D ultrasound. Eur J Vasc Endovasc Surg 52(5):635–642
15. de Korte CL, Carlier SG, Mastik F, Doyley MM, van der Steen AF, Serruys PW, Bom N (2002) Morphological and mechanical information of coronary arteries obtained with intravascular elastography; feasibility study *in vivo*. Eur Heart J 23(5):405–413
16. Maurice RL, Fromageau J, Brusseau E, Finet G, Rioufol G, Cloutier G (2007) On the potential of the langrangian estimator for endovascular ultrasound elastography: *in vivo* human coronary artery study. Ultrasound Med Biol 33(8):1199–1205
17. Deleaval F, Bouvier A, Finet G, Cloutier G, Yazdani SK, Le Floc'h S, Clarysse P, Pettigrew RI, Ohayon J (2013) The intravascular ultrasound elasticity-palpography technique revisited: a reliable tool for the in vivo detection of vulnerable coronary atherosclerotic plaques. Ultrasound Med Biol 39(8):1469–1481
18. Tacheau A, Le Floc'h S, Finet G, Doyley MM, Pettigrew RI, Cloutier G, Ohayon J (2016) The imaging modulography technique revisited for high-definition intravascular ultrasound: theoretical framework. Ultrasound Med Biol 42(3):727–741
19. Golemati S, Nikita KS (2018) Carotid artery wall motion and strain analysis using tracking. In: Loizou CP, Pattichis CS, D'houge J (eds) Handbook of speckle filtering and tracking in cardiovascular ultrasound imaging and video. IET
20. Golemati S, Sassano A, Lever MJ, Bharath AA, Nicolaides AN (2003) Carotid artery wall motion estimated from B-mode ultrasound using region tracking and block matching. Ultrasound Med Biol 29(3):387–399
21. Cinthio M, Ahlgren AR, Bergkvist J, Jansson T, Persson HW, Lindström K (2006) Longitudinal movements and resulting shear strain of the arterial wall. Am J Physiol Heart Circ Physiol 291(1):H394–H402
22. Zahnd G, Boussel L, Marion A, Durand M, Moulin P, Sérusclat A, Vray D (2011) Measurement of two-dimensional movement parameters of the carotid artery wall for early detection of arteriosclerosis: a preliminary clinical study. Ultrasound Med Biol 37(9):1421–1429
23. Svedlund S, Eklund C, Robertsson P, Lomsky M, Gan LM (2011) Carotid artery longitudinal displacement predicts 1-year cardiovascular outcome in patients with suspected coronary artery disease. Arterioscler Thromb Vasc Biol 31(7):1668–1674
24. Gastounioti A, Golemati S, Stoitsis JS, Nikita KS (2013) Carotid artery wall motion analysis from B-mode ultrasound using adaptive block matching: in silico evaluation and *in vivo* application. Phys Med Biol 58(24):8647–8661
25. Tat J, Psaromiligkos IN, Daskalopoulou SS (2016) Carotid atherosclerotic plaque alters the direction of longitudinal motion in the artery wall. Ultrasound Med Biol 42(9):2114–2122
26. Dempsey RJ, Varghese T, Jackson DC, Wang X, Meshram NH, Mitchell CC, Hermann BP, Johnson SC, Berman SE, Wilbrand SM (2017) Carotid atherosclerotic plaque instability and cognition determined by ultrasound-measured plaque strain in asymptomatic patients with significant stenosis. J Neurosurg 10:1–9

27. Sisini F, Tessari M, Gadda G, DiDomenico G, Taibi A, Menegatti E, Gambaccini M, Zamboni P (2015) An ultrasonographic technique to assess the jugular venous pulse: a proof of concept. Ultrasound Med Biol 41(5):1334–1341
28. Herment A, Lefort M, Kachenoura N, DeCesare A, Taviani V, Graves MJ, Pellot-Barakat C, Frouin F, Mousseaux E (2011) Automated estimation of aortic strain from steady-state free-precession and phase contrast MR images. Magn Reson Med 65:986–993
29. Franquet A, Avril S, LeRiche R, Badel P, Schneider F, Li Z, Boissier C, Favre J (2013) A new method for the in vivo identification of mechanical properties in arteries from cine MRI images: theoretical framework and validation. IEEE Trans Med Imaging 6:1–16
30. Suever JD, Watson PJ, Eisner RL, Lerakis S, O'Donnell RE, Oshinski JN (2011) Time-resolved analysis of coronary vein motion and cross-sectional area. J Magn Reson Imaging 34(4):811–815
31. Ozturk C, Derbyshire JA, McVeigh ER (2003) Estimating motion from MRI data. Proc IEEE Inst Electr Electron Eng 9(10):1627–1648
32. Manduca A, Oliphant TE, Dresner MA, Mahowald JL, Kruse SA, Amromin E, Felmlee JP, Greenleaf JF, Ehman RL (2001) Magnetic resonance elastography: non-invasive mapping of tissue elasticity. Med Image Anal 5(4):237–254
33. Van der Geest RJ, Reiber JH (1999) Quantification in cardiac MRI. J Magn Reson Imaging 10(5):602–608
34. McVeigh ER (1996) MRI of myocardial function: motion tracking techniques. Magn Reson Imaging 14(2):137–150
35. Aletras AH, Ding S, Balaban RS, Wen H (1999) DENSE: displacement encoding with stimulated echoes in cardiac functional MRI. J Magn Reson 137:247–252
36. Abd-Elmoniem KZ, Sampath S, Osman NF, Prince JL (2007) Real-time monitoring of cardiac regional function using fastHARP MRI and region-of-interest reconstruction. IEEE Trans Biomed Eng 54(9):1650–1656
37. Wedding KL, Draney MT, Herfkens RJ, Zarins CK, Taylor CA, Pelc NJ (2002) Measurement of vessel wall strain using cine phase contrast MRI. J Magn Reson Imaging 15(4):418–428
38. Lin AP, Bennett E, Wisk LE, Gharib M, Fraser SE, Wen H (2008) Circumferential strain in the wall of the common carotid artery: comparing displacement-encoded and cine MRI in volunteers. Magn Reson Med 60(1):8–13
39. Krishnan K, Ge L, Haraldsson H, Hope MD, Saloner DA, Guccione JM, Tseng EE (2015) Ascending thoracic aortic aneurysm wall stress analysis using patient-specific finite element modeling of *in vivo* magnetic resonance imaging. Interact CardioVasc Thorac Surg 21(4):471–480
40. Xu L, Chen J, Glaser KJ, Yin M, Rossman PJ, Ehman RL (2013) MR elastography of the human abdominal aorta: a preliminary study. J Magn Reson Imaging 38:1549–1553
41. Kolipaka A, Woodrum D, Araoz PA, Ehman RL (2012) MR elastography of the *in vivo* abdominal aorta: a feasibility study for comparing aortic stiffness between hypertensives and normotensives. J Magn Reson Imaging 35(3):582–586
42. Litmanovich D, Bankier AA, Cantin L, Raptopoulos V, Boiselle PM (2009) CT and MRI in diseases of the aorta. Am J Roentgenol 193(4):928–940
43. Cesare E, Splendiani A, Barile A, Squillaci E, Cesare A, Brunese L, Masciocchi C (2016) CT and MR imaging of the thoracic aorta. Open Med (Wars) 11(1):143–151
44. Lin E, Alessio A (2009) What are the basic concepts of temporal, contrast, and spatial resolution in cardiac CT? J Cardiovasc Comput Tomogr 3(6):403–408
45. Morrison T, Choi G, Zarins CK, Taylor CA (2009) Circumferential and longitudinal cyclic strain of the human thoracic aorta: age-related changes. J Vasc Surg 49:1029–1036
46. Schlicht MS, Khanafer K, Duprey A, Cronin P, Berguer R (2013) Experimental foundation for *in vivo* measurement of the elasticity of the aorta in computed tomography angiography. Eur J Vasc Endovasc Surg 46:447–452
47. Martin C, Sun W, Primiano C, McKay R, Elefteriades J (2013) Age-dependent ascending aorta mechanics assessed through multiphase CT. Ann Biomed Eng 41:2565–2574

48. Weber TF, Müller T, Biesdorf A, Wörz S, Rengier F, Heye T, Holland-Letz T, Rohr K, Kauczor HU, von Tengg-Kobligk H (2014) True four-dimensional analysis of thoracic aortic displacement and distension using model-based segmentation of computed tomography angiography. Int J Cardiovasc Imaging 30:185–194
49. Lee MK, Holdsworth DW, Fenster A (2000) Dynamic 3D computed tomography: non-invasive method for determination of the aortic dynamic elastic modulus. In: Proceedings of the 22nd annual international conference of the IEEE engineering in medicine and biology society

Part IV
Mathematical and Computational Modelling

Modelling the Electrical Activity of the Heart

Sergio Alonso and Rodrigo Weber dos Santos

Abstract The electrocardiogram signal is a popular measurement of the electrical activity of the whole heart. It reflects the interaction and diversity of the electrical activity of cells from different parts of the heart. Rhythmically each cell changes the value of the transmembrane potential, and this change in the electrical properties of the cell propagates through the tissue producing the coordination of the electrical signal, which triggers the contraction of the whole heart. In this chapter we show the main ingredients for the description of the electrophysiology of a single cell and the different models for the propagation of the electrical signal along cardiac tissue. We discuss the main characteristics of certain arrhythmias and the corresponding patterns of electrical activity obtained in the numerical simulations.

1 Introduction

As excitable cells, cardiac myocytes are able to respond to an external stimulus with the generation of an Action Potential (AP), i.e. a specific signature of the transmembrane potential that varies along time for a certain characteristic duration, called Action Potential Duration (APD). The excitation appears only for stimulus over a certain threshold, resulting in an AP with always the same shape and leaving a refractory state which precludes a fast re-excitation of the cell [1, 2].

S. Alonso (✉)
Department of Physics, Universitat Politècnica de Catalunya, Barcelona, Spain
e-mail: s.alonso@upc.edu

R. W. dos Santos
Department of Computer Science, Universidade Federal de Juiz de Fora,
Juiz de Fora, Brazil
e-mail: rodrigo.weber@ufjf.edu.br

S. Golemati and K. S. Nikita (eds.), *Cardiovascular Computing—Methodologies and Clinical Applications*, Series in BioEngineering,
https://doi.org/10.1007/978-981-10-5092-3_10

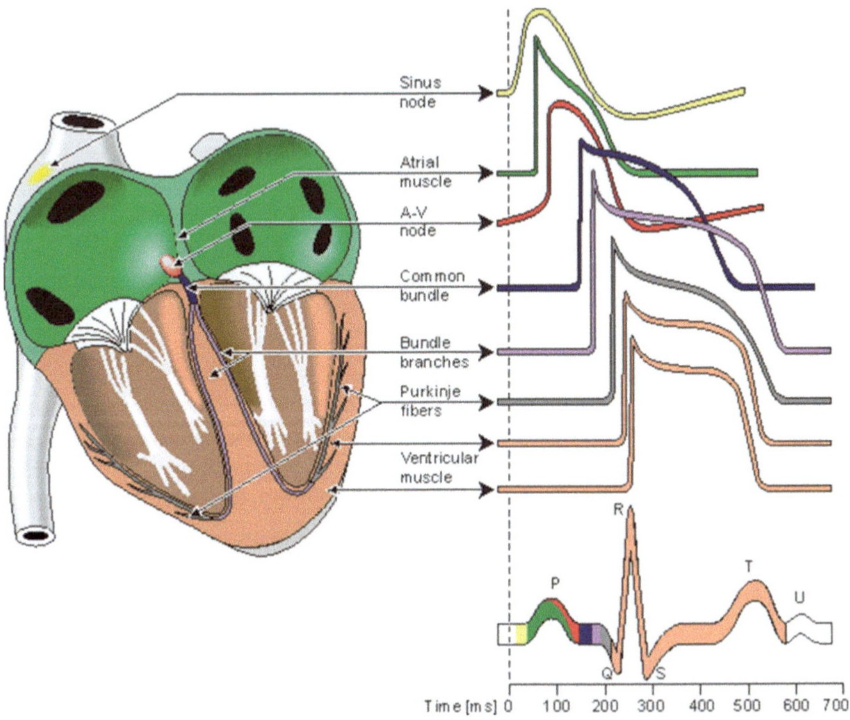

Fig. 1 Location of the different parts of the heart and relation of the electrocardiogram with the action potential curves in different types of myocytes. Reprinted from the free open access book [3]

In the heart, the AP has the important role of the synchronization of the whole cardiac tissue. To work as an efficient pump, the myocytes have to contract in a synchronized fashion. To this end, once an AP is initiated in a particular region (the sinoatrial node, SAN) it propagates from one cell to its neighbours, until all the cells of the heart are excited. The atria first pumps the blood to the ventricles, which later pumps blood out of the heart. The region that electrically connects the atria to the ventricles, called atrioventricular node (AVN), slows down the AP propagation so that the trigger for contraction arrives later in the ventricle than in the atria, see Fig. 1 [3]. A loss of synchronization of cardiac electrical impulses controlling the pumping of blood is associated with a number of arrhythmias including atrial (AF), ventricular (VF) fibrillation, and ventricular tachycardia (VT).

The electrical activity of the heart is visible in the electrocardiogram (ECG). A series of electrodes record the small voltage changes on the thorax of a person. With the ECG both the rhythm and the morphology of the electrical activity is recorded. The different phases of propagation along the heart leave different traces in the ECG, see Fig. 1. Thus, anomalies in propagation result in distinctive shape variations in the ECG.

Together with the ECG, there are other valuable experimental methods like optical imaging of the voltage and calcium content and electrophysiological studies, both at different scales ranging from individual cells to cardiac tissue, which permit the development of detailed cardiac models [4].

The modelling of the electrical properties of the cardiac tissue is the main purpose of this chapter. Computational models of the cardiac tissue are useful tools for the characterization of different mechanisms of arrhythmias; the definition of new effective defibrillation protocols; the effects of the different pathologies on cardiac tissue, like ischemia and fibrosis; the study of the effects of anti-arrhythmic drugs; and even the effects of genetic mutations on the behaviour of ion channels.

This chapter is organized as follows: in the next section, we present the basic ingredients to model the genesis of AP in cardiac myocytes. We show some simulation examples of myocytes located in different parts of the heart in Sect. 3. In Sect. 4, we discuss models for the propagation of AP in cardiac tissue. Such models of tissue are employed to describe wave propagation and different types of arrhythmias in Sect. 5. Finally, Sect. 6 provides a short discussion and outlook for future perspectives.

2 Celular Modelling

Cardiac myocytes are electrically active cells, or excitable cells, of the heart. They have a length of 100–120 μm and a diameter of 10–20 μm. Each myocyte is separated from the extracellular space by a phospholipid bilayer membrane. This cellular membrane permits the flow of some ions (Na^+, K^+, Ca^{2+}, Cl^-) between the extracellular and intracellular media through specific ion channels. The resulting different ionic concentrations between the interior and the exterior of the cell generates a transmembrane potential difference, i.e. a potential difference across the cell membrane. AP produces myocyte contraction because it triggers a pulse of intracellular Calcium concentration, $[Ca]_i$. The increase of $[Ca]_i$, enables the cellular contraction machinery to work, via crossbridge cycling tropomyosin slides over actin filaments and shortens the myocyte length. Figure 2 presents the typical waveforms of AP,

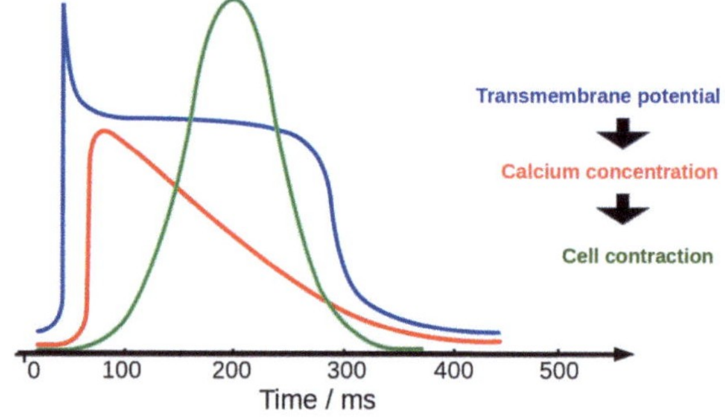

Fig. 2 Sequence of the processes inside a cardiac myocyte. First the transmembrane potential depolarizes, followed by an increase in Ca^{2+} concentration in the cytosol and the final contraction of the cell

$[Ca]_i$ pulse and corresponding cell contraction. Further details on cardiac contraction and electro-mechanical coupling can be found in [5].

2.1 Nernst Potential

Differences in the ionic concentrations between the interior and the exterior of the cell generates a potential difference across the membrane [2]. We may consider the intracellular space of the cell and the extracellular medium as two reservoirs that separates a certain ion S by a semipermeable membrane, i.e. let us for now consider that the membrane is only permeable to the ion S. The chemical potentials of S inside and outside of the cell are given by:

$$G_{S,i} = RT\ln([S]_i) + zFV_i, \qquad G_{S,e} = RT\ln([S]_e) + zFV_e, \tag{1}$$

where R, T, z and F are the gas constant, temperature, ion charge, and Faraday constant respectively. In a ideal case of equilibrium both chemical potentials are equal giving rise to transmembrane potential difference ($V_i - V_e$) which depends on the ion concentrations:

$$V_N^S = \frac{RT}{zF}\ln\left(\frac{[S]_e}{[S]_i}\right) \tag{2}$$

which is the definition of the Nernst potential for a given ion S.

For the case of a membrane that is permeable to multiple ion species [2] we have that the equilibrium potential, considering the most important ions inside myocytes, can be approximated by

$$V_r = \frac{g_{Na}V_N^{Na} + g_K V_N^K + g_{Ca}V_N^{Ca} + g_{Cl}V_N^{Cl}}{g_{Na} + g_K + g_{Ca} + g_{Cl}}, \tag{3}$$

where g_S is the permeability of ion S. The equilibrium potential depends on the permeabilities of the ions, which are controlled by the ion channels.

2.2 The Action Potential and Some Basic Properties

From the equilibrium equation presented above we can explain the different phases of the AP in terms of changes of the permeability values of some basic ions, such as K^+ and Na^+. At rest the largest permeability is because of potassium and therefore from Eq. (3): $V_r \sim V_N^K = -96$ mV. It is known that if the cell receives a stimulus above a given threshold the permeability of Na^+ rapidly increases and, again from Eq. (3), if g_{Na} is much larger than the other permeabilities, it results than $V_r \sim V_N^{Na} = +50$ mV and the potential depolarizes to positive values (phase 0). After the inactivation of sodium channels, dropping the permeability of Na^+, the potassium current produces a deflection of the membrane potential (phase 1) before the Ca^{2+} permeability increases to similar values than K^+ and $V_r \sim (V_N^K + V_N^{Ca})/2$ where $V_N^{Ca} = +134$ mV. The permeability of Ca^{2+} slowly decreases (phase 3) driving the membrane potential back to the $V_r \sim V_N^K$, typical for the rest state (phase 4).

2.3 Membrane Capacitance

Cell membrane separates charges between the interior and the exterior of the cell and therefore it can be interpreted as a capacitor with, $C_m V = q$, where C_m is the membrane capacitance, V is the transmembrane potential and q is the intracellular or extracellular charges. By taking the derivative with respect to time we have that $C_m dV/dt = dq/dt$ is the capacitive current that can be induced by the membrane. In the case a cell is isolated, and assuming a balance of charge, i.e. no charge is being created or destroyed, the sum of the currents from the ion channels, I_{ion} and the capacitive current $C_m dV/dt$ gives rise to a simple electric model presented in Fig. 3. This simple electric models is the basis for the electrophysiological models employed in cardiac modelling:

$$C_m \frac{dV}{dt} = -I_{ion}. \tag{4}$$

However, as we mentioned before, the permeability or conductance of each ion channels varies with time and is known to depend on the transmembrane potential (it may also depend on ion concentrations or other molecules or proteins). In the next section we present models for the so called gating of ion channels, where the

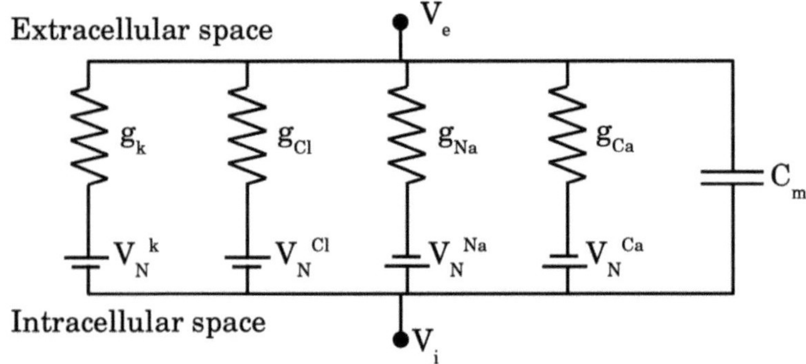

Fig. 3 Equivalent electric circuit model for the cellular membrane. The difference in the transmembrane potential between the extracellular and the intracellular spaces is maintained by the ion current of the different ions through the ion channels, the Nernst potential associated to each ion and the capacitance of the membrane

term gate is commonly used and refers to the fact that ion channels can be opened or closed to the flow of ions.

2.4 Ion Channels

The opening and close of the ion channels are complex processes. Assuming that a particular channel is ohmic the transmembrane potential depends on the Nernst potential of the particular ion V_N^{ion} plus the potential drop due to the current across the ion channel $\rho_{ion} I_{ion}$:

$$V = \rho_{ion} I_{ion} + V_N^{ion}, \tag{5}$$

where ρ_{ion} is the channel resistance, and the transmembrane potential V is the difference between the potentials in the intra- and extracellular media $V = V_i - V_e$. Then, from the previous equation one can obtain the current across the cell membrane for each ion as function of the membrane potential

$$I_{ion} = g_{ion}(V - V_N^{ion}), \tag{6}$$

where $g_{ion} = 1/\rho_{ion}$ is the membrane conductance for that ion, which is in general not constant. In general, the dependence with the potential may be non-linear and a generalization of Eq. (6) is

$$I_{ion} = g_{max} p_O \Phi(V), \tag{7}$$

where $\Phi(V)$ can be a non-linear function of the transmembrane potential, p_O is the proportion of open channels, and g_{max} is the maximum conductance when all the channels are open, i.e. when $p_O = 1$. The most common approach to model p_O is via the use of gating variables, as first proposed by Hodgkin and Huxley, in their pioneering model of AP [6]. For example, consider a K^+ channel that has a time rate $\alpha(V)$ to change from a closed state to an open state; and a time rate $\beta(V)$ to change from an opened state to a closed state. For the case we have many ion channels we can use a deterministic model based on Ordinary Differential Equation (ODE). Since the proportion of closed channels is $1 - p_O$ we have:

$$\frac{dp_O}{dt} = \alpha(V) p_O - \beta(V)(1 - p_O). \tag{8}$$

More complex behaviours, like the one we described for the Sodium channels, which first open and immediately after close (even for the same value of V), can not be described by a single gating variable. Two options are commonly used. The first is to assume that multiple independent gates have to be opened to let ions flow through the channel. For Sodium channel we could replace Eq. (7) by $I_{Na} = g_{NA}\, p_{Oa}\, p_{Oi} \Phi(V)$, where p_{Oa} is the gating variable associated to activation, p_{Oi} the one associated to inactivation, and both are controlled by equations similar to Eq. (8), but each one with different time rate functions. A more modern approach is to model p_O using a Markov Chain formulation [8].

3 Models of Myocytes

The sinoatrial node (SAN) is the natural pacemaker of the heart and initiates autonomously cardiac electrical activity. APs are produced periodically and propagate along the atria. The wave of AP arrives at the ventricular myocardium through the atrio-ventricular node (AVN) and the Purkinje fibres, depolarizing first the endocardium and proceeding transmurally to the epicardium.

The electrical properties of the heart tissue are very heterogeneous and each type of cells have particular features giving rise to a large diversity on the shape of the action potentials. Next, we present four models for human myocytes: SAN, atria, Purkinje fibres and ventricle. It is worth noting that there are still large differences on the AP shape even in the same region of the heart (e.g. APs are different in the ventricular endocardium and epicardium). In addition, substantial differences can also be found among species. Figure 4 presents a comparison of AP shapes of ventricular myocytes for different species. A small heart, like from a mouse, has higher heart rate and consequently a smaller APD than a human heart [9].

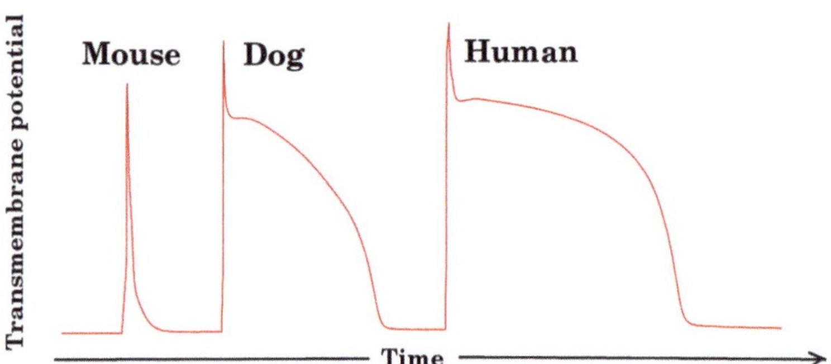

Fig. 4 Comparison of the action potential of a ventricular myocyte of three different animal species. All the action potentials have the same temporal and potential scales. Rest potential is however slightly modified for illustrative reasons. Action potential curves have been generated with program Myokit [7]

3.1 *Sinoatrial Node Myocyte*

In the right atrium there is a group of cells forming the sinoatrial node which spontaneously depolarize (60–90 min^{-1}). The property of continuous depolarization of such cells (automaticity) triggers repetitive electrical impulses, which defines the periodic contraction of the human heart. Contrary to the majority of the cardiac myocytes, these cells do not experience a rest state or phase 0. A continuous repolarization drives the cell to a hyperpolarization state, see Fig. 5a. At this phase, important ion currents, such as the funny current, I_f, is known to play an important role [10]. The term funny was coined because this current is activated at hyperpolarization and carries mainly Na^+ under physiological conditions. This flux of Na^+ into the pacemaker myocyte will eventually make the transmembrane potential to cross the threshold around −40 mV, where fast depolarization occurs and a new AP is generated.

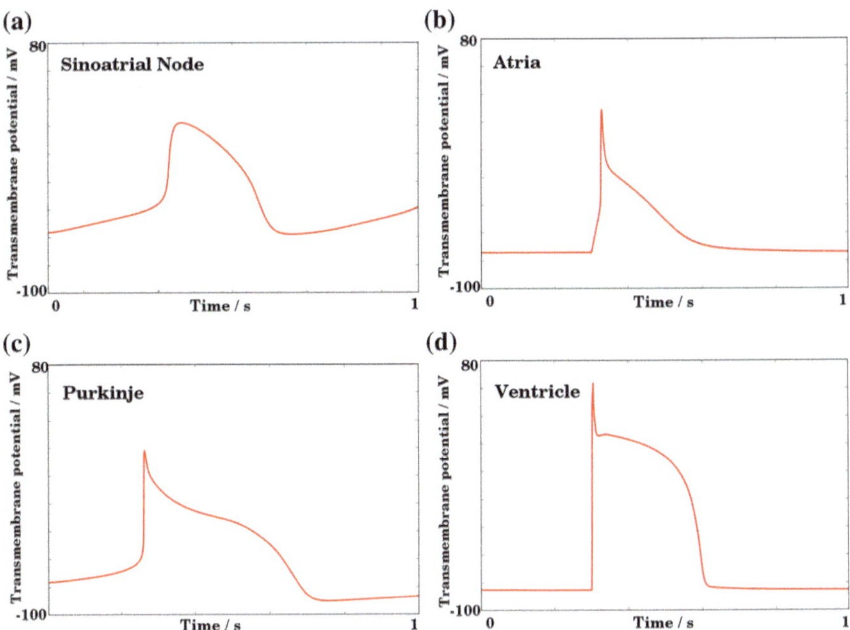

Fig. 5 Transmembrane potential obtained by four models of different cardiac myocytes: Simulated action potentials of a myocyte in the Sinoatrial node (**a**), a myocyte in a human atrium (**b**), a myocyte in human Purkinje fibres (**c**), and a myocyte in a human ventricle (**d**). Action potential curves have been generated with program Myokit [7]

3.2 *Atrial Myocyte*

Transmembrane potential of a cell in the atrium stays in a resting state of −74 mV when it not being stimulated. When the perturbation of the neighbouring cells and in particular from the sinoatrial node crosses a threshold a fast channel for sodium activates and induces the rapid entrance of sodium into the cell which suddenly depolarizes the cell to values around 20 mV. Phases 2 and 3 of the AP are mixed for atrial cells due to a continuous unbalanced of inward flow of Ca^{2+} and outward flow of K^+. This results in a gradual repolarization to the resting state, see an example in Fig. 5b.

3.3 *Purkinje Fiber Myocyte*

AP propagation slows down at the AVN node, but speeds up once entering the His bundle followed by the Purkinje fibres. The Purkinje fibres are AP highways that rapidly transport the electric signal to the ventricular myocytes. The myocytes forming the Purkinje fibres are the cells with the longest action potential duration, which arrives to 400 ms, see Fig. 5c to compare it with the other action potentials. In contrast with atrial and ventricular cells the myocytes forming the Purkinje fibres also have a certain automaticity. It means that cells in the Purkinje system are able to sustain low frequency oscillations (15–20 min^{-1}) in case the main pacemaker, the sinoatrial node, fails. Under normal conditions Purkinje fibres do not depolarize spontaneously because they are regularly stimulated at pacing rates higher than their own natural autonomous pacing activity.

3.4 *Ventricular Myocyte*

Ventricular cells present a stable resting state about −85 mV. Under suprathreshold perturbations the corresponding excitation is due to the opening of the fast Na^+ channels causing a rapid influx of Na^+ ions into the cell. The membrane potential is reversed from negative to positive and arrives to about +60 mV. The posterior deflection of the action potential is due to the movement of K^+ ion together with the inactivation of the fast Na^+ channels. In comparison with a atrial action potential, in ventricle cells the calcium influx is larger and balances the outward flux of K^+. This produces a plateau for about 200 ms, phase 3, which is the main difference between ventricular and atrial action potentials, see Fig. 5d for an example of AP from a model of the human ventricle.

4 Cardiac Tissue

Cardiac cells are electrically connected by special ion channels called gap junctions. These connections permit the propagation of the signal through the tissue and the synchronization of the whole heart. The models of transmembrane potential described in the previous section can be used to implement a model for AP propagation on cardiac tissue. Some particular dynamics observed in tissue models correspond to cardiac arrhythmias observed in the heart.

4.1 Bidomain Modelling

The bidomain model is based on the cable equation. Cardiac tissue is divided in two different regions which are interconnected, the intra- and extracellular regions, see Fig. 6a. The transmembrane potential is considered to vary along the tissue and, due to these variations, intra- and extracellular axial currents per unit length appear [2]:

$$I_i(x) = -g_i[V_i(x+dx) - V_i(x)]/dx, \qquad I_e(x) = -g_e[V_e(x+dx) - V_e(x)]/dx; \quad (9)$$

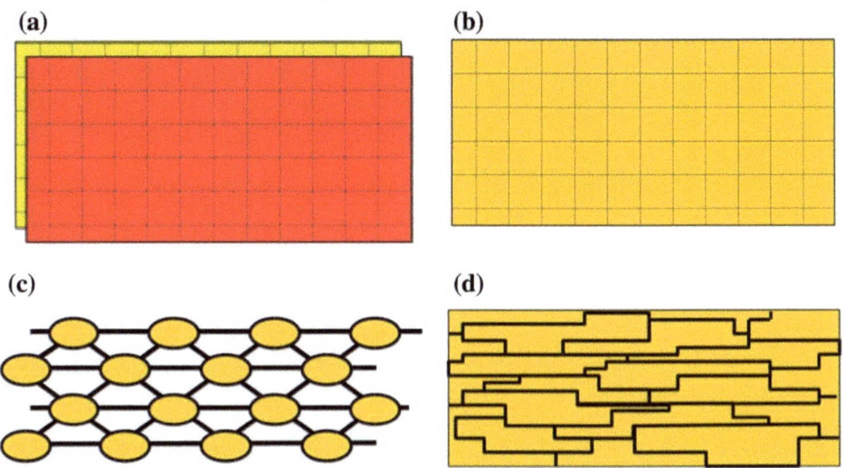

Fig. 6 Different modelling approaches to cardiac tissue: Bidomain model where intracellular (yellow) and extracellular (red) potentials are explicitly considered as two inteconnected continuous models (**a**). Monodomain model where the transmembrane voltage is considered in a continuous model (**b**). Discrete model where the myocyte is approached as an single element and electrically connected to the rest of cells in the tissue (**c**). Heterogeneous approach where single cells are discretized into smaller volume elements and effective and discrete gap junctions take into account cell to cell coupling

where g_i, g_e are the conductances per unit length of the intra- and extracellular media. The sum of the currents entering and leaving a given point of the tissue must be zero, and therefore:

$$I_i(x) - I_i(x+dx) = I_t dx = I_e(x+dx) - I_e(x), \tag{10}$$

where the transmembrane current, I_t is the sum of the ionic and capacitive currents:

$$I_t = p\left(C_m \frac{dV}{dt} + I_{ion}\right), \tag{11}$$

and p is the perimeter of the cell.

In the continuous limit $dx \to 0$, and assuming the 3D case, the previous Eq. (9) become:

$$I_i(x) = -\mathbf{g_i} \nabla V_i, \qquad I_e(x) = -\mathbf{g_e} \nabla V_e, \tag{12}$$

and Eq. (10):

$$I_t = -\nabla \cdot I_i = \nabla \cdot I_e, \tag{13}$$

where $\mathbf{g_i}$ and $\mathbf{g_e}$ are tensors that describe the anisotropy (cardiac fibre direction) of the intra- and extracellular domains, respectively, I_t satisfies:

$$I_t = \chi\left(C_m \frac{dV}{dt} + I_{ion}\right), \tag{14}$$

where χ is the surface to volume ratio of a cell, and I_{ion} is the sum of ion currents, where each one is modelled via equations similar to Eqs. (7–8).

Substituting Eq. (13) in Eq. (14) one obtains the three dimensional bidomain model. Using $V_i = V + V_e$ we have:

$$\chi(C_m \frac{\partial V}{\partial t} + I_{ion}) = \nabla \cdot (\mathbf{g_i} \nabla V) + \nabla \cdot (\mathbf{g_i} \nabla V_e). \tag{15}$$

In addition, from Eq. (13), we have:

$$\nabla \cdot (\mathbf{g_i} \nabla V_i + \mathbf{g_e} \nabla V_e) = \nabla \cdot \left[\mathbf{g_i} \nabla V + (\mathbf{g_i} + \mathbf{g_e}) \nabla V_e\right] = 0. \tag{16}$$

Equations (15–16) constitute the bidomain formulation of the cable equation written with the variables V and V_e, which solution depends on the choice of appropriate initial and boundary conditions. The numerical solution of the above system of equations is not a trivial task. In [11] the reader can find a review on sophisticated numerical methods for the solution of the cardiac bidomain equations.

The bidomain model is computationally demanding and it is usually reduced to a more tractable version, the monodomain approach, see next section. However, it is largely assumed that the full bidomain approach is necessary to properly model defibrillation [12] or to recover patient specific electrocardiogram (ECG) and magnetocardiogram (MCG) signals [13, 14].

4.2 Monodomain Modelling

In one dimension with homogeneous conductances it is always possible to reduce Eqs. (15–16) to a monodomain description. Note that, from Eq. (13), the divergence of the total axial current is zero, from which we obtain the monodomain cable equation.

In three-dimensions, if the anisotropy ratios are equal, i.e. $\mathbf{g_e} = \lambda \mathbf{g_i}$, the bidomain equations can be reduced to a monodomain model, see Fig. 6b. Under such conditions the resulting monodomain equation for the transmembrane potential is:

$$p\left(C_m \frac{\partial V}{\partial t} + I_{ion}\right) = \nabla \cdot (\mathbf{g_o} \nabla V), \tag{17}$$

where we define an effective conductance $\mathbf{g_o} = \lambda/(1+\lambda)\mathbf{g_i}$ [2]. In addition, for the case of plane wave propagation the bidomain equations also simplifies to the modomain equation with an expression for $\mathbf{g_o}$ that depends on the angle between the wave front and the cardiac fibre direction [15, 16].

However, cardiac tissue is known to have tensors with different anisotropy ratio and such equivalence does not hold for the general case. Nevertheless, in most applications of cardiac modelling both models produce similar dynamics [17].

4.3 Discrete Modelling

The previous models of cardiac tissue are based on the continuum and homogenized approach. For the numerical implementation such models are discretized into a grid or a mesh with spatial discretization that can arrive to small values as 100 μm. This is the characteristic size of a single myocyte. Such values may challenge the basis of the continuum and homogenized hypothesis. Therefore, for some applications the discrete nature of the tissue has to be taken into account. The resulting equation is

$$\left(C_m \frac{\partial V_i}{\partial t} + I_{ion}\right) = \sum_j \left(g_{ij}(V_j - V_i)\right), \tag{18}$$

where membrane potential is now a discrete variable V_i, the sum goes for all the neighbours of the cell i and conductivity may depend on the connected cells g_{ij}, see Fig. 6c.

Under slow conduction conditions, velocities are affected by the discreteness [18] and conduction block is observed in the numerical simulations [19]. However, conduction block is not capture by the continuum homogenized models.

Such discrete models have been shown to be convenient for the study of slow propagation, microfibrosis and the complex fractionated electrograms associated to it. A discrete distribution of cells into a square grid and the effects of reduced conductivity has been also analyzed and may induce the formation of ectopic beats [20, 21] or stabilize spiral breakup [22]. More realistic discrete meshes were also used for studies that associated microfibrosis and ectopic beats [23].

Another approach to capture discrete propagation in cardiac tissue is to include a corrector term in the discretization of the continuum homogenized monodomain model [24]. This approach allows the use of the classical continuum homogenized models (with spatial discretization larger than cell size) and yet capture the discrete features of the phenomenon.

4.4 Heterogeneous Modelling

A higher level of detail is obtained with microscopic models of the intracellular space of individual cells. Single cells are discretized at the subcellular level. It permits the description of the actual shape of the myocytes and consider different types of gap junctions depending on the direction of cell [25, 26]. Such models permit the direct simulations of two-dimensional processes at the intra-cellular level and are useful for the study of conduction block [27] and the effects of cardiac fibrosis [23, 28].

There are extensions to three-dimensions [29] and extensions that describe both extracellular and intracellular spaces [30].

5 Action Propagation Dynamics

The contraction of the heart is generated by a single wave of electrical excitation, see Fig. 7b, c for the propagation in a simple model of the ventricles. Tachycardia corresponds to a rotor that accelerates the rate of contraction, and typically is associated to a spiral wave, see Fig. 7d. Fibrillation occurs when the normal electrical activity is masked by higher frequency circulation waves which create small, out-of-phase localized contractions. One or more spiral waves break into multiple waves, see Fig. 7e–h, leading to fibrillation [31].

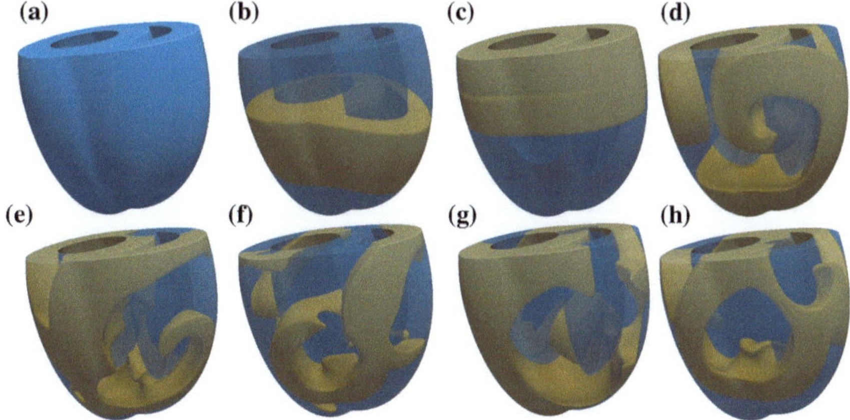

Fig. 7 Numerical simulation of the action potential wave (yellow) with a simple model in a regular domain (blue) with two cavities mimicking the geometrical properties of the ventricles (**a**) A wave is generated in the apex of the ventricles and propagates to the top (**b**, **c**). A secondary stimulus in the ventricles generates a spiral wave (**d**). Spiral wave is unstable (**e**, **f**) and gives rise to multiple spirals which desynchronize the ventricles (**g**, **h**)

5.1 Action Potential Pulse

Myocytes are connected through gap junctions, and action potential propagates along the tissue with roughly constant velocity, see such a wave in a simple model of the two ventricles in Fig. 7b, c.

The collision of two travelling waves in different directions produces their annihilation. However, interactions between consecutive waves travelling in the same direction are common due to the continuous forcing of the whole tissue by the sinoatrial node. The increase of the pacing frequency decreases the diastolic interval (DI) or distance between consecutive pulses. At low pacing frequencies, there is practically no interaction between waves and the wave-train propagates with the single travelling wave velocity, see Fig. 8. On the other hand, at fast pacing, a wave may not be able to propagate because it enters the refractory tail of the preceding wave and propagation is blocked. In between these two situations, waves tune their APD and CV to accommodate the propagation under the influence of the refractory tail of the previous wave, see the decrease of the APD and CV with the DI in Fig. 8, which is inversely proportional to the pacing frequency.

5.2 Tachycardia

Some cardiac arrhythmias appear when the regular synchronous propagation of the action potential along the tissue is disrupted. Tachycardia is a particular case of

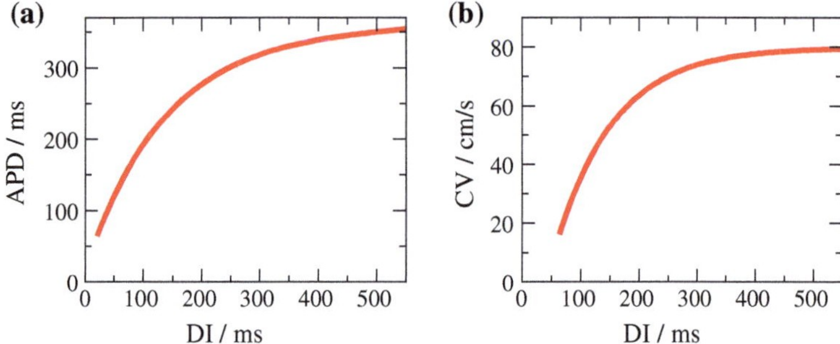

Fig. 8 Restitution curves or dependence of the action potential duration (**a**) and the conductions velocity (**b**) on the diastolic interval, which is related with the pacing frequency in models of the human ventricle

arrhythmia consisting in a fast but regular periodic contraction of the tissue. It has been associated to the appearance of a cardiac reentry around an inhomogeneity in the tissue, for example a vein (anatomical reentry), or it may appear and rotate without the existence of any particular heterogeneity (functional reentry). Reentry in cardiac tissue is often related with the appearance of a rotating spiral wave in the tissue as it has been observed in experiments. The generation of reentry in cardiac tissue is one of the main interests in the modelling of cardiac electrical activity. Next, we highlight two mechanisms of functional reentry observed in experiments and studied in numerical simulations.

The introduction of an extra excitation in the tail of travelling wave is known as ectopic beat. The new excitation cannot propagate in the direction of the refractory tail of the first wave. Hence, it slides along the refractory tail until the tissue becomes again excitable and then rotates giving rise to a spiral. The generation of the spiral wave after the second excitation only occurs during a particular window of time, known as the vulnerability window [32]. If the second perturbation comes too early, a new wave cannot be generated because that part of the tissue is still in the refractory state. If it comes too late, the perturbation generates a circular wave and no reentry is formed.

The alternation of the duration of the action potential at the single cell level results in the interchange of weak and strong contractions of the heart. It only happens when the dependence of the action potential duration on the pacing becomes very strong. An initially periodic wave-train may become unstable and evolve into alternans. In two or three dimensions when one of the pulses is locally too small, it may produce conduction block and initiate the formation of spiral waves due to the displacement of the broken end into the less dramatic region [33]. The probability for the conduction block depends on the pacing frequency of the tissue.

5.3 Fibrillation

One of the most relevant arrhythmias is fibrillation which corresponds to a state where the contraction of many cardiac myocytes are strongly desynchronized in the atria, i.e. atria fibrillation, or, with more dangerous consequences, in the ventricles, i.e. ventricular fibrillation. Electrical defibrillation, the only effective therapy when the ventricles fibrillate, resets the activity of the ventricle by delivering a strong electrical shock. Atrial fibrillation is typically treated by anti-arrhythmic drugs and, for severe cases, with catheter ablation of the most active regions of the atria.

Fibrillation is often attributed to a succession of multiple breakups and pairwise annihilations of spiral waves. Reentry is believed to be a necessary but not a sufficient condition for fibrillation. Computational modelling has shown different mechanisms to explain how the fibrillation can be triggered by a single reentry. For example, alternans can produce localized conduction blocks and break-up waves emitted by a spiral due to the alternation of waves with large and short action potentials. At fast rotation rates, the instability reaches the spiral core and produces a disordered state [34]. On the other hand, high meandering of the spiral waves, typically observed in models of cardiac tissue, may produce the interaction between consecutive waves and produce local conduction block, giving rise to spiral breakup.

Finally, there are other situations which may produce continuous breakup of waves, for example: when the tension of the filament of three-dimensional spirals, i.e. scroll waves, is negative [35]; or when the rotating anisotropy of cardiac fibres induces a scroll wave to breakup [36].

6 Conclusions and Final Remarks

We have described the main features of the computational electrophysiological modelling of the human heart. From the particular shapes of AP of the cardiac cells depending on their location in the heart to the modelling of diverse types of arrhythmias in cardiac tissue. We have also discussed the main methods to couple the electrophysiology of the individual cells to cardiac tissue.

Currently there are complex models of the geometry of the atria and the ventricles taking into account the anisotropy of the cardiac muscle fibres and the heterogeneous properties of the organ. The level of complexity and detail is arriving to permit patient-specific modelling of the electrical activity [37]. Furthermore, models have to couple the electrical part to the deformation of the muscle walls [38].

Therefore, the heart is a multiphysics problem [39] which has to consider the interplay among the electric wave propagation, the mechanics of the muscle contraction and the fluid dynamics inside the cardiac cavities to explain the correct performance of this electromechanical pump. It is also a multiscale problem [40], for example, the wrong operation of a ion channel at small spatial and temporal scales can definitely affect the behaviour on the whole organ. The complete computational modelling may permit the study of genetic mutations or the effects of drugs, processes, governing small spatial and temporal scales, in the function of the whole macroscopic organ.

Although many improvements on modelling of electrical activity of the heart have been done during the last decades, the complete description of the human heart is still a challenge for cardiac modellers.

Acknowledgements We acknowledge fruitful discussions with professors Blas Echebarria and Markus Bär. This work was partially supported by MINECO of Spain under the Ramon y Cajal program with the grant number RYC-2012-11265, and the Brazilian funding agencies FAPEMIG, CNPq, FINEP and CAPES.

References

1. Zipes D, Jalife J (2013) Cardiac electrophysiology: from cell to bedside. Elsevier, Amsterdam
2. Keener JP, Sneyd J (1998) Mathematical physiology. Springer, New York
3. Malmivuo J, Plonsey R (1995) Bioelectromagnetism: principles and applications of bioelectric and biomagnetic fields. Oxford University Press, Oxford
4. Clayton RH, Bernus O, Cherry EM, Dierckx H, Fenton FH, Mirabella L, Panfilov AV, Sachse FB, Seemann G, Zhang H (2011) Models of cardiac tissue electrophysiology: progress, challenges and open questions. Prog Biophys Mol Biol 104:22–48
5. Pfeiffer ER, Tangney JR, Omens JH, McCulloch AD (2014) Biomechanics of cardiac electromechanical coupling and mechanoelectric feedback. J Biomech Eng 136(2):021007
6. Hodgkin AL, Huxley AF (1952) A quantitative description of membrane current and its application to conduction and excitation in nerve. J Physiol 117(4):500
7. Clerx M, Collins P, de Lange E, Volders PGA (2016) Myokit: a simple interface to cardiac cellular electrophysiology. Prog Biophys Mol Biol 120(1–3):100–114
8. Qu Z, Hu G, Garfinkel A, Weiss JN (2014) Nonlinear and stochastic dynamics in the heart. Phys Rep 543(2):61–162
9. Kaese S, Verheule S (2013) Cardiac electrophysiology in mice: a matter of size. Transgenic models of cardiac arrhythmias and sudden death. 103
10. Campos FO, Davenport MH, dos Santos RW, Nygren A, Giles WR (2013) High heart rate in pregnancy is modulated by augmented expression of an ion channel, HCN-2, in pacemaker tissue. Circulation 20:127
11. Vigmond EJ, dos Santos RW, Prassl AJ, Deo M, Plank G (2008) Solvers for the cardiac bidomain equations. Prog Biophys Mol Biol 1:96
12. Trayanova N, Constantino J, Ashihara T, Plank G (2011) Modeling defibrillation of the heart: approaches and insights. IEEE Rev Biomed Eng 4:89–102
13. dos Santos RW, Kosch O, Steinhoff U, Bauer S, Trahms L, Koch H (2004) MCG to ECG source differences: measurements and a two-dimensional computer model study. J Electrocardiol 1:37
14. Mäntynen V, Konttila T, Stenroos M (2014) Investigations of sensitivity and resolution of ECG and MCG in a realistically shaped thorax model. Phys Med Biol 23:59
15. Roth BJ, Woods MC (1999) The magnetic field associated with a plane wave front propagating through cardiac tissue. IEEE Trans Biomed Eng 11:46
16. dos Santos RW, Koch H (2005) Interpreting biomagnetic fields of planar wave fronts in cardiac muscle. Biophys J 5:88
17. Potse M, Dubé B, Richer J, Vinet A, Gulrajani RM (2006) A comparison of monodomain and bidomain reaction-diffusion models for action potential propagation in the human heart. IEEE Trans Biomed Eng 53(12):2425–2435

18. Rudy Y, Quan W (1987) A model study of the effects of the discrete cellular structure on electrical propagation in cardiac tissue. Circ Res 61(6):815–823
19. Fast VG, Kléber AG (1995) Cardiac tissue geometry as a determinant of unidirectional conduction block: assessment of microscopic excitation spread by optical mapping in patterned cell cultures and in a computer model. Cardiovasc Res 29(5):697–707
20. Cherry EM, Ehrlich JR, Nattel S, Fenton FH (2007) Pulmonary vein reentry—properties and size matter: insights from a computational analysis. Heart Rhythm 4(12):1553–1562
21. Alonso S, Bär M (2013) Reentry near the percolation threshold in a heterogeneous discrete model for cardiac tissue. Phys Rev Lett 110(15):158101
22. Panfilov AV (2002) Spiral breakup in an array of coupled cells: the role of the intercellular conductance. Phys Rev Lett 88(11):118101
23. de Barros Gouvea B, Weber dos Santos R, Lobosco M, Alonso S (2015) Simulation of ectopic pacemakers in the heart: multiple ectopic beats generated by reentry inside fibrotic regions. BioMed Res Int 2015:713058
24. Costa CM, Silva PAA, dos Santos RW (2016) Mind the gap: a semicontinuum model for discrete electrical propagation in cardiac tissue. IEEE Trans Biomed Eng 4:63
25. Spach MS, Heidlage JF (1995) The stochastic nature of cardiac propagation at a microscopic level: electrical description of myocardial architecture and its application to conduction. Circ Res 76(3):366–380
26. de Barros Gouvea B, Sachetto Oliveira R, Meira W, Lobosco M, Weber dos Santos R (2012) Simulations of complex and microscopic models of cardiac electrophysiology powered by multi-GPU platforms. Comput Math Methods Med 2012:824569
27. Prudat Y, Kucera JP (2014) Nonlinear behaviour of conduction and block in cardiac tissue with heterogeneous expression of connexin 43. J Mol Cell Cardiol 76:46–54
28. Hubbard ML, Henriquez CS (2014) A microstructural model of reentry arising from focal breakthrough at sites of source-load mismatch in a central region of slow conduction. Am J Physiol Heart Circ Physiol 306(9):H1341–H1352
29. Spach MS, Barr RC (2000) Effects of cardiac microstructure on propagating electrical waveforms. Circ Res 86(2):e23–e28
30. Roberts SF, Stinstra JG, Henriquez CS (2008) Effect of nonuniform interstitial space properties on impulse propagation: a discrete multidomain model. Biophys J 95:3724–3737
31. Alonso S, Bär M, Echebarria B (2016) Nonlinear physics of electrical wave propagation in the heart: a review. Rep Prog Phys 79(9):096601
32. Qu Z, Garfinkel A, Weiss JN (2006) Vulnerable window for conduction block in a one-dimensional cable of cardiac cells, 1: single extrasystoles. Biophys J 91:793–804
33. Qu Z, Garfinkel A, Chen PS, Weiss JN (2000) Mechanisms of discordant alternans and induction of reentry in simulated cardiac tissue. Circulation 102:1664–1670
34. Karma A (1993) Spiral breakup in model equations of action potential propagation in cardiac tissue. Phys Rev Lett 71:1103
35. Alonso S, Bär M, Panfilov AV (2013) Negative tension of scroll wave filaments and turbulence in three-dimensional excitable media and application in cardiac dynamics. Bull Math Biol 75(8):1351–1376
36. Fenton F, Karma A (1998) Fiber-rotation-induced vortex turbulence in thick myocardium. Phys Rev Lett 81:481
37. Krishnamurthy A, Villongco CT, Chuang J, Frank LR, Nigam V, Belezzuoli E, Stark P, Krummen DE, Narayan S, Omens JH, McCulloch AD (2013) Patient-specific models of cardiac biomechanics. J Comput Phys 244:4–21
38. Oliveira BL, Rocha BM, Barra LPS, Toledo EM, Sundnes J, dos Santos Weber R (2013) Effects of deformation on transmural dispersion of repolarization using in silico models of human left ventricular wedge. Int J Numer Methods Biomed Eng 29:1323–1337

39. Nordsletten DA, Niederer SA, Nash MP, Hunter PJ, Smith NP (2011) Coupling multi-physics models to cardiac mechanics. Prog Biophys Mol Biol 104:77–88
40. Trayanova NA, Rice JJ (2011) Cardiac electromechanical models: from cell to organ. Front Physiol 2:43

Mathematical and Computational Modelling of Blood Pressure and Flow

Carole Leguy

Since William Harvey discovered in 1628 that blood circulates in a closed loop in the body, and that the contraction of the heart delivered the driving force to move the blood [1], cardiovascular mechanics has gained a lot of attention and is still subject to research. During the last decades, mathematical models have been developed to grasp the diversity of blood flow patterns and pressure propagation phenomena within the cardiovascular system [2]. The geometry of the arterial and venous system is difficult to describe; blood, a complex non-Newtonian fluid, circulates in vessels with non-linear viscoelastic walls. It is therefore very difficult to take into account the complexity of the cardiovascular system within mathematical or numerical models in a comprehensive manner. Thus, mathematical and numerical models generally focus on particular aspects of the cardiovascular circulation. Two approaches can be used to simulate blood flow: either a phenomenon is simulated locally (and in detail) using 3D Computational Fluid Dynamics (CFD) or fluid structure interaction (FSI) models, or with lumped or wave propagation models to simulate the entire systemic circulation considering a simplified geometry. These models have proven their value to understand normal physiology better [3], to simulate the effects of pathophysiological symptoms, or to predict the effect of medical interventions [4].

In the following sections, physiological considerations will be reviewed and the basic equations that govern blood flow and pressure dynamics within arteries and veins will be presented. Later, lumped, 1D and 3D models will be introduced and finally, clinical relevance and applications will be introduced.

C. Leguy (✉)
Department of Cardiovascular Engineering CVE, Institute of Applied Medical Engineering AME, RWTH Aachen University, Aachen, Germany
e-mail: leguy@ame.rwth-aachen.de

S. Golemati and K. S. Nikita (eds.), *Cardiovascular Computing—Methodologies and Clinical Applications*, Series in BioEngineering,
https://doi.org/10.1007/978-981-10-5092-3_11

1 Physiological Background

The cardiovascular system

The heart pumps roughly 5 l of blood every minute through 70 heart beats, for which the heart ejects on average 70 ml of blood into the resting body. Since the human circulation counts about 5 l of blood, on average a full circulation is obtained every minute [5]. In the systemic circulation, the blood is ejected from the left ventricle of the heart into the arterial tree composed of large arteries (diameter of 20–0.1 mm) that bifurcate into arterioles (diameter of 100–10 μm) and capillaries (diameter of 10–5 μm). The aorta is the most elastic artery of our cardiovascular system and is the buffer during the heart cycle. Its volume increases during systole (high blood pressure), whereas this extra-volume is sent to the peripheries during diastole. The compliance of systemic arteries decreases while decreasing in size down to the capillaries, which are mainly viscous vessels [6, 7]. In the capillaries, the blood exchanges oxygen, nutrients, and waste products with the tissues. The blood is then carried back to the right atrium of the heart via the venous system. The venous vessels are highly compliant and have the characteristic to collapse. Furthermore, veins are equipped with valves that avoid blood reflux and improve venous return to the heart. Then the blood is intermittently moved to the right ventricle and ejected into the pulmonary circulation. Afterwards the oxygenated blood returns back to the left atrium via the pulmonary veins, and, finally, it flows into the left ventricle and is forced again into the systemic circulation [5].

Vascular disorders

Cardiovascular diseases (CVD) are the major cause of death. Worldwide more people die annually from CVD than from any other cause. The World Health Organization has estimated that 17.5 million people died of CVD in 2012, representing 31% of all global deaths [8]. Of these deaths, an estimated 7.4 million were due to coronary heart disease and 6.7 million were due to stroke.

Heart failures are associated with insufficient pump function of the heart. The decrease in heart capacities mainly results from stenosis or leakage of one or more of the heart valves, or from a disturbed electrical activation of the heart muscle leading to systolic dysfunction. On of the other hand, a stiffening of the heart muscle, following chronic hypertension, can lead to diastolic dysfunction in which the heart ventricul does not fill adequately during diastole.

The pathological degradations of the arterial walls caused by CVD may also have dramatic consequences such as strokes or heart attacks. A rupture of atherosclerotic plaques located in large and medium-sized arteries is the major risk for CVD. Arteriosclerosis is associated with stiffening of the arterial wall, which is part of the aging process. Furthermore, high blood pressure, diabetes, high levels of cholesterol or smoking are risk factors that contribute to this development of atherosclerosis. The main associated symptom is the development of plaques on the inner walls of the blood vessels due to the build-up of fatty deposits. It has been shown that arterial stiffness is an independent predictor of cardiovascular risk at an early stage [9]. The elastin fibres that mediate the arterial compliance at low and normal blood pressures degrade with age, resulting in a stiffening of the arteries. Arterial stiffening may be both a cause and a consequence of hypertension. Consequently, pulsatile blood pressure rises [10] and the load on the heart increases. On the other hand, hemodynamics plays an important role in the development of these plaques. Plaques are prone to develop at low wall shear stress area such as bifurcations and curved vessels.

Arterial wall aging is also be associated with the growth of aneurysms. The vessel wall is locally weaker and does not fully sustain transmural arterial pressure anymore. The artery can then bulge out. The bulging aneurysms may leak or rupture. The rupture of aortic aneurysms often leads to fatal bleeding. Aneurysms may also occur in the arteries of the brain (intracranial aneurysms). Rupture of a cerebral aneurysm may cause bleeding into the brain tissue, resulting in a hemorrhagic stroke.

The venous circulation is also subject to insufficiencies. Varicose veins or thrombosis within the deep veins can cause venous insufficiency. The dysfunction of the venous valves can also impair venous return and cause blood to pool in your legs.

The relation between CVD and hemodynamics is multifaceted and associated with specific flow and pressure patterns.

2 Basics of Hemodynamics

2.1 Hemodynamics, Rheological Properties of Blood

Blood is a complex fluid mainly composed of plasma, which is the fluid medium of blood in which erythrocytes (red blood cells), leucocytes and platelets are suspended. Plasma is an aqueous saline solution with a density of 1.03 kg/m^3 that behaves like a Newtonian fluid with a viscosity of $3.5 \cdot 10^{-3}$ Pa $\cdot$ s. In suspension in plasma, red blood cells (erythrocytes) are the most abundant cells and account for 40–45% of blood volume. The density of erythrocytes is 1.08 kg/m^3. Each erythrocytes has a biconcave discoid form with a phospholipid bilayer membrane with a thickness of 80 nm. Red blood cells play an important role in the non-Newtonian behaviour of blood. At a low shear rate ($<100\,\text{s}^{-1}$) they aggregate and form rouleaux that increases the viscosity of blood. When the shear rate increases, these rouleaux disperse and will align with the flow direction while decreasing blood viscosity. Blood has a shear thinning behaviour and is therefore considered as a non-Newtonian fluid. Other components of blood are the leucocytes and platelets. However, they are present in very small quantities compared to erythrocytes and do not influence significantly blood hemodynamic properties.

Several mathematical models have been proposed to represent the non-Newtonian properties of blood. A power-law model can be used to depict the relationship between blood viscosity and the shear rate, where

$$\eta = \eta_0(\lambda\dot{\gamma})^{n-1} \tag{1}$$

with η the blood viscosity and η_0 the viscosity when the shear rate $\dot{\gamma}$ equals $1/\lambda$ with λ a time constant. The power law is defined by the index n and represents a shear thickening fluid if $n > 1$ or a shear thinning fluid if $n < 1$ [11]. The reference viscosity η_0 and the power-law index n depend on the constitution of the blood (e.g. hematocrit, fibrinogen, cholesterol). Although a power law can be acceptable for a defined shear rate range. At a very low shear rate, it goes to physically unrealistic values of 0 and to $+\infty$ for a very high shear rate.

A more realistic model has been proposed by Careau-Ysuda and is given by

$$\frac{\eta - \eta_\infty}{\eta_0 - \eta_\infty} = [1 + (\lambda\dot{\gamma})^a]^{(n-1)/a} \tag{2}$$

η_0 and η_∞ being the viscosity at low and high shear rate, respectively, λ is a time constant and n the power-law index [11–13]. The transition between the low shear rate region and the power law region is determined by the parameter a. Another model has been proposed by Casson. This model introduces a yield stress needed to "break" the red blood cell rouleaux.

The shear thinning behaviour of blood needs to be considered when shear stress at the vessel wall is investigated. However its influence is not significant on the blood flow in large arteries and veins, for which a Newtonian model suffices. Since the blood is mainly composed of water, it can be considered as an incompressible fluid.

2.2 *Mass and Momentum Balance Equations*

The blood flow velocity field and vessel wall deformation (distension waveform) are described by the laws of conservation of mass and momentum. Stress and velocity in function of space and time are the variables used for the blood (the fluid), whereas stress and displacement define the vessel wall state (the solid). The coupling between the fluid and solid domains is defined by specific constraints.

For a Newtonian and incompressible fluid, the momentum and conservation (or continuity) equations are described by the Navier-Stokes equations

$$\rho\frac{\partial v}{\partial t} + \rho(v \cdot \nabla)v = \rho f - \nabla p + \nu\nabla^2 v \tag{3}$$

$$\nabla \cdot v = 0, \tag{4}$$

wherein ρ is the blood density, v the blood velocity vector, p is the blood pressure and ν the blood viscosity. The left hand side of the momentum equation represents the inertial forces, with f the body forces (corresponding to earth gravity for the cardiovascular system), ∇p the pressure forces and $\nu\nabla^2 v$ the viscous forces. To obtain a close set of equation, the constitutive behaviour of the vessel wall has to be defined.

3 Vessel Wall Mechanical Properties

3.1 Arterial Wall Mechanics

The main component of the arterial wall are elastin, collagen fibres and smooth muscle cells that are arranged in a complex structure composed of mainly three layers. The first layer, called intima layer, is directly in contact with the blood and is composed of an endothelial cell layer, a laminal base layer. The intima layer plays an important role in vessel growth through blood wall shear stress and wall strain. This layer, due to its thickness of only 0.2–0.5 μm does not contribute to the overall elasticity of the vessel wall. The second layer is the tunica media and is composed of elastic lamina and smooth muscle cells. The structure of the tunica changes along the arterial tree. The proportion of smooth muscle cells versus elastic lamina increases towards the peripheries from large elastic arteries, as the aorta, to distal muscular arteries. The tunica is the component that mainly defines the mechanical properties of the arterial wall. The third layer is the adventitia that represents only 10% of the arterial wall and whose main function is to connect the blood vessel to its surrounding tissue. Due to this multilayer structure, the mechanical properties of the arterial wall is represented by an equivalent Young's modulus defined for the entire wall thickness.

For an healthy person, the arterial wall behaves linearly within the blood pressure range, where mainly elastin fibres contribute to the vessel elasticity. However, at high blood pressure (hypertensive patients) the collagen fibres become stretched and consequently contribute to an arterial stiffening at this high stretch. Because of the complex non-linear, and viscoelastic behaviour, the law of linear elasticity cannot be applied dirrectly. However, linearization at a specific equilibrium state, such as mean or diastolic pressure, results in a linearized or incremental effective Young's modulus. The effective Young's modulus can be obtained from a stress-strain relationship by local linearization of the strain/stress curve.

The wall stiffness can be derived from in-vivo ultrasound measurements of the vessel wall distension. The arterial wall distensibility coefficient D_0 is defined as the ratio between the linearized compliance coefficient C_0 and the time average cross-sectional area $\bar{A}$ [9, 14]

$$D_0 = \frac{C_0}{\bar{A}}, \; with \; C_0(p_{tr}) = \frac{\Delta A}{\Delta p_{tr}}, \tag{5}$$

with ΔA the maximum change in arterial cross-sectional area Δp the corresponding pressure difference within a heart cycle. The arterial stiffness S can then be defined from the distensibility by

$$S = Eh \approx \frac{2a(1-\nu^2)}{D_0}, \tag{6}$$

with E the linearized Young's modulus, h, the wall thickness, a the radius and ν the poisson ratio. The compliance C_0 can be be given in function of the Young's modulus

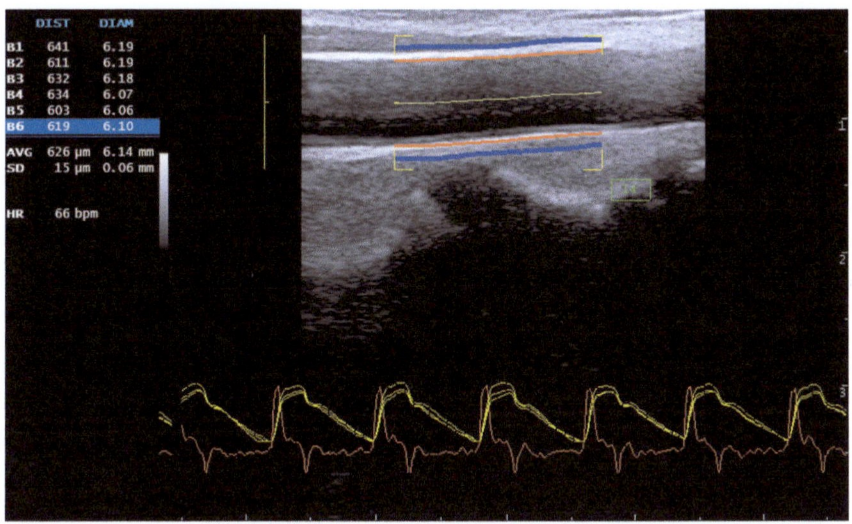

Fig. 1 Representative screenshot during an examination. Image of the CCA and detection of its vessel wall (orange lines) can be seen in the upper central part of the picture. Below vessel diameter (yellow) and the first derivative of the diameter (orange) are shown beat-to-beat. In the upper left corner numerical results of distension and diameter are given for each heartbeat. From Leguy et al. (2015) with permission

E:

$$C_0 = \frac{\partial A}{\partial p} = \frac{2\pi a^3}{h} \frac{(1-\nu^2)}{E}. \tag{7}$$

In clinical practice, arterial stiffness can be assessed from vascular ultrasound imaging with the assessment of arterial distensibility and intima media wall thickness (IMT), which is the vessel wall layers that mainly contribute to its elasticity [15], see Fig. 1. Magnetic resonance imaging (MRI) can also be used to assess the morphology of the vessel wall and atherosclerosis plaques as presented by Kwee et al. [16].

3.2 Poiseuille Flow

If the vessel wall elasticity is neglected, arteries can be compared to a stiff tube and assumed to be straight. The blood volume flow (Q) for a constant pressure drop over a tube section of length l is then given by the Poiseuille law [17] (Chap. 2)

$$Q = (\Delta P/l) \cdot (\pi/8\nu) \cdot r^4. \tag{8}$$

Such a flow is dependent on the vessel radius r to the fourth power, and corresponds to a flow dominated by friction forces. The velocity profile is parabolic (the maximum velocity at the centre equals 2 times the mean velocity). The wall shear stress at the vessel wall is giving by

$$\tau = 4\nu \cdot Q/(\pi r^3). \tag{9}$$

The resistance (relation between pressure difference and volume flow) can be defined as

$$R = \frac{\Delta p}{Q} = 8\nu l \pi r^4. \tag{10}$$

Even though the Poiseuille flow can be used as a first approximation for average blood flow over an heart cycle, the blood velocity profile will be influenced by blood pulsatility and is usually not parabolic as illustrated by Leguy et al., who compared blood volume flow estimates based on Poiseuille or Womersley profiles [18].

3.3 *Oscillatory Flow*

Womersley has derived an analytical solution of the Navier-Stokes equation, which describes flows through a straight tube for an oscillatory pressure drop [19]. The Womersley solution represents the pulsatility properties of blood flow in arteries with a blood flow profile that depends on the Womersley number α such as

$$\alpha = a\sqrt{\frac{\omega}{\nu}}, \tag{11}$$

where a is the vessel radius, ω the angular frequency of the flow ($\omega = 2\pi f$) and ν the dynamic viscosity.The dimensionless Womersley number denotes a ratio between viscous and inertial forces with a viscous-dominated flow that tends towards the Poiseuille profile for low Womersley numbers, and an inertia-dominated flow that tends towards a plug profile (uniform velocity) for high α numbers. For a sinusoidal flow, the axial velocity v is a function of the radial position r and time t is given by (Fig. 2)

$$v(r,t) = Real[(A * /i\omega\rho) \cdot \{1 - J_0(\alpha \cdot r/r_0 \cdot i^{3/2})/J_0(\alpha \cdot i^{3/2})\} \cdot e^{i\omega t}] \tag{12}$$

where r_0 is the vessel radius, J_i are the Bessel functions of order i. The velocity profiles can be obtained for different frequencies (Womersley number). A harmonic decomposition of the blood flow waveform will be used to reproduce the pulsatile blood flow profile [18].

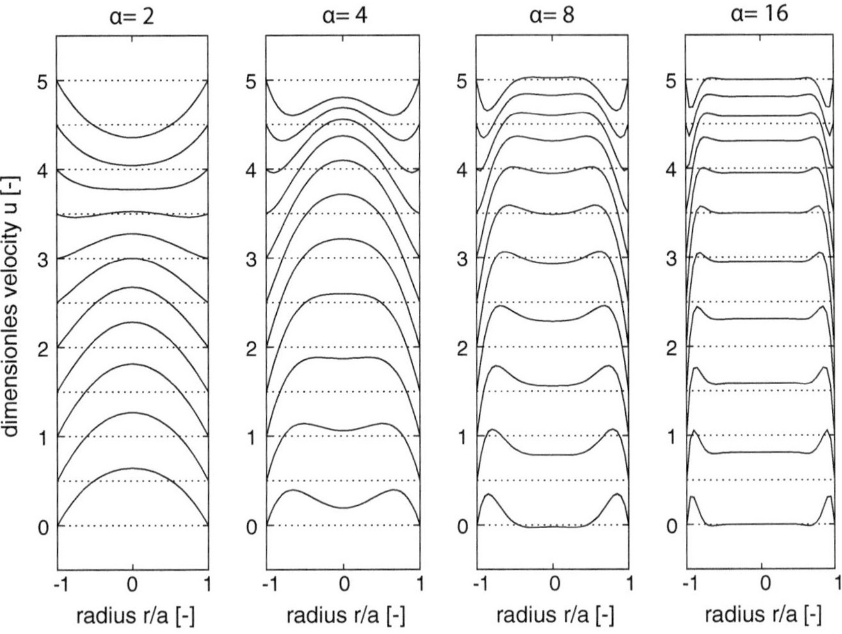

Fig. 2 Velocity profile for Womersley flow at different Womersley numbers α

3.4 Flow in Curved Tube and Bifurcation

Within the arterial tree, the velocity profiles are influenced by vessel curvatures and bifurcations. The curvature of the vessels induces an asymmetry of the velocity profile. A 3D CFD study performed by Leguy et al. reported velocity profiles in slightly curved tube that represent the brachial artery for physiological flow waveforms. One can notice that during the flow deceleration, the maximum velocity is shifted towards the outer wall due to the effect of curvature [20], see Fig. 3. This shifting induces a secondary flow that will transport the fluid along the upper and lower walls resulting in an helical movement of the fluid particles. The length needed for a flow be become axisymmetric within a straight part is called inlet length and depends on the Reynolds number. Schlichting has estimated that for laminar flow the inlet length can be estimated by $L_e/D = 0.056Re$, with D the vessel diameter and Re the Reynolds number [21]. With a Reynolds number of 300, the inlet length within the carotid artery corresponds to 40 times its radius. In general, one can consider that flow in arteries never fully develop.

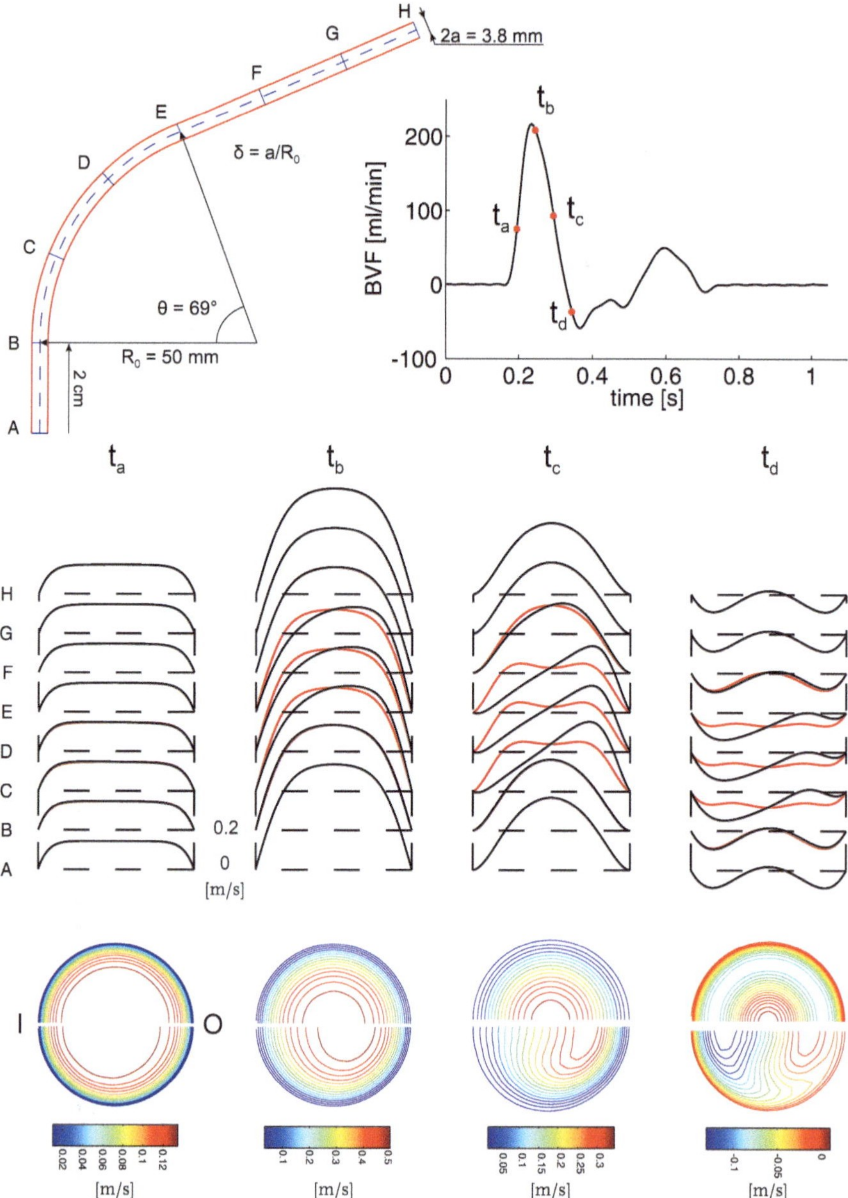

Fig. 3 Blood flow in curved artery, simulated for an in-vivo measured brachial artery flow and a radius of curvature of 50 mm. Topleft:geometry of the CFD model. Topright: blood volume flow. Center: axial-velocity profile in the plane of symmetry (in red) and of asymmetry (in black) at different cross-sections along the tube for 4 timesteps t_a to t_d; For each timestep,the top half disc depicts the axial-velocity profile at the inlet (cross-section A, whereas the bottom half disc depicts the velocity profile in the curve (cross-section D).The letters I and O represent the inner and outer wall positions, respectively. Adapted from Leguy et al. [20], used by permission

4 Reduced Numerical Models

4.1 0D Windkessel Model

To describe the relationship between blood pressure and blood volume flow in elastic arteries, a windkessel model was proposed by Frank [22]. The compliance of the systemic arterial tree is represented by an elastic chamber of compliance C and the distal blood vessels by a rigid tube of resistance (R). The blood volume flow, q, as a function of blood pressure, p, is then given by

$$q = C\frac{\partial p}{\partial t} + \frac{p}{R} \tag{13}$$

Later, a parallel resistance has been included to lead to a 3-element windkessel model. This extra resistance has been introduced to reflect more precisely the high-frequency behaviour of the input impedance [23] and thus minimize pressure reflection. Following this development, a 4-element model has been introduced with an additional inductance L that describes the total inertance of the arterial system [24–26]. Eventually, a frequency dependent lumped model with Womersley number dependant resistor and inductor and based on specific blood velocity profiles was developed [27]. Windkessel models are useful tools to study the pressure and flow relationships in large arteries. However, windkessel models provide a relation between pressure and flow at a specific arterial site but they ignore the pressure wave propagation phenomena along the arterial tree.

5 Lumped and Wave Propagation Models

5.1 Distributed Models

To study wave propagation phenomena in arteries, lumped parameter models have been used [23, 28, 29]. An (electrical) transmission line can be created with connecting segments of arteries, represented by windkessel models. Such distributed 0D models have been used to understand the propagation blood flow and pressure waves in the arterial system for normal physiological states [28, 30] or for pathophysiological states [31, 32]. The limitations of these models comes from the fact that only linear compliance is used for the mechanical behaviour of the arterial wall and that the transitions between segments are discrete and can generate non physiological reflections.

5.2 1D Wave Propagation Models

The 1D wave propagations models have been proposed to model blood pressure and flow along the vascular (arterial or venous) tree. One-dimentional wave propagation models are based on a 1D formulation of the Navier-Stokes equations. The momentum and conservation (or continuity) equations are integrated over the transverse cross-sections of the vessel and are completed by a constitutive relation between the local pressure and the cross-sectional area as used by Bessems et al. [33] or Alastruey et al. [34]. For a comprehensive overview of these models, see the review from van de Vosse and Stergiopulos [35].

When unidirectional flow along the vessel axis z is assumed, the momentum equation is then given by

$$\frac{\rho}{A}\frac{\partial q}{\partial t} + \frac{\rho}{A}\frac{\partial}{\partial z}\frac{q^2}{A} = \rho g - \frac{\partial p}{\partial z} + \frac{2}{a}\tau_\omega \tag{14}$$

with a the vessel radius, A the vessel cross-sectional area, q the blood flow over the cross-sectional area, p the pressure, and τ the shear stresses at the vessel wall. The continuity equation can be written as

$$C\frac{\partial p}{\partial t} + \frac{\partial q}{\partial z} + \Phi = 0 \tag{15}$$

with C the vessel compliance and Φ a blood leakage. When a linear-elastic model is used for the wall wall, the compliance C is defined so that

$$C = \frac{\partial A}{\partial p_{tr}} \tag{16}$$

with ∂p_{tr}, the transmural pressure. More complex arterial wall models that include non-linear or viscoelasticity properties of the wall can be included [36].

The venous system can also be represented by 1D wave propagation models with the inclusion of the collapsibility properties of the veins [37–39]. The venous system is a low pressure system that can be exposed to small or even negative transmural pressure due to increasing extravascular pressure and can thus collapse. This results in a non-linear pressure-area relationship that should be taken into account for the constitutive law of the vessel wall and that was approximated by Shapiro in 1977 for collapsible tubes [40].

The obtained set of equations can later be solved numerically using either finite-element or spectral-element methods for the arterial tree with gradual (smooth) changes in geometry. Lumped and wave propagation models are very time-efficient and are therefore appropriate for clinical applications. Pressure and flow within the entire arterial system can be provided within a few seconds. Many studies have demonstrated that such models have the capacity to describe blood pressure and blood volume flow wave propagation, not only quantitatively but also qualitatively if compared to physiological measurements [14, 41, 42]. However, these models present some limitations when discrete changes in geometries are considered since they do not take into account the perturbation of the velocity profiles due to complex geometries.

6 Three Dimensional Models

To study blood flow and pressure distribution within complex geometries as in curved vessels, at vessel bifurcations or in pathological cases of stenoses or aneurism (cerebral or aortic), 3-dimensional computational fluid dynamics (CFD) can be used. In such models, the full Navier-Stockes equations for non-compressible fluid are solved using finite-element methods. It is possible to include the non-Newtonian properties (shear-thinning) of the blood, which is relevant when accurate wall shear stress is assessed [13, 43]. A full 3D velocity profile and pressure distribution over the arterial cross-section is then obtained [44–46]. Pressure distribution, the flow pattern (that can be complex and turbulent at the ascending aorta or in case of stenosed arteries) and the local wall shear stress (important risk factor in the development of atherosclerosis) are derived.

The compliance of the vessel wall and the related vessel wall distension can decrease the maximum wall shear stresses since the arteries have a maximum diameter at systolic pressure around maximum flow. Imaging technics as 4D MRI can be used to assess the vessel wall movement and a deformable mesh can be used for the CFD model. The deformation of the wall can also be numerically calculated using fluid structure interaction (FSI) models, for which a solid model for the wall is coupled with the fluid problem [47, 48]. With such models, the flow around cardiac or venous valve can be obtained. The main limitation of either CDF or SFI models is that they are complex to solve and time consuming. Generally, only short arterial segments are considered.

Boundary conditions play an important role for such models and can either be given by patient-specific pressure and flow conditions obtained from medical imaging [49] or a reduced order model, such as 0D windkessel or 1D wave propagation, can be coupled to the 3D model to obtain more realistic conditions proximal ad distal to the considered section (Fig. 4).

7 Clinical Relevance

Mathematical and numerical models of blood flow and pressure in the cardiovascular system play an important role in the understanding of physical phenomena underlying specific flow or pressure patterns associated with physiological or pathophysiological states.

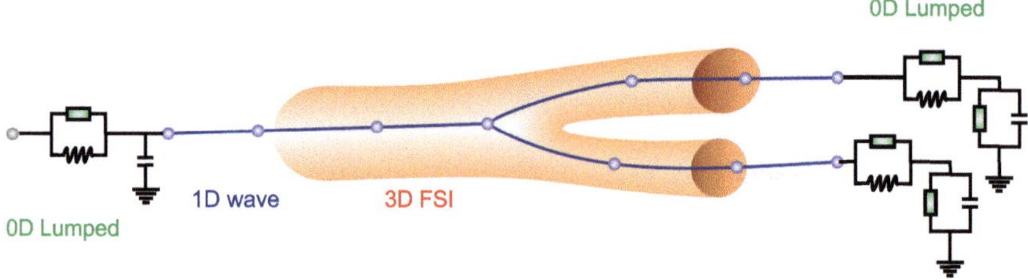

Fig. 4 Schematic view of 0D, 1D and 3D models

Lumped models such as 0D windkessel models have been used to determin total peripheral compliance and thus to analyze the load on the heart that comes from the systemic arterial system. 1D wave propagation models have be used to better understand the impact of arterial stiffening, which induces an augmentation of the pressure wave reflection and the load on the heart and which is an important factor in the evolution of pathological systolic hypertension. When geometrical details are relevant, 3D models have allowed to better associate low shear stress regions, e.g. at bifurcations or inner curvatures, where atherosclerosis plaques are more prone to develope [50]. Complex flows within cerebral or aortic aneurism were simulated by using arterial geometries provided by MRI or ultrasound. FSI models allow to design studies for cardiac valves replacement or left ventricular assisted devices [51] for which the interactions between the wall mechanics (or artificial valve) and blood flow pattern is extremely important.

Numerical models of the cardiovascular system are also relevant for the diagnosis and planning of treatment. 3D CFD models have been used by Speelman et al. in 2009 to localize high wall stress region within aortic aneurism from patient-specific geometries and flows obtained from MRI and ultrasound [52]. In the European Framework VPH (Virtual Physiological Human), Merkx et al. have used a 1D wave propagation model to predict the outcome of an arteriovenous fistula access for dialysis patients. The predictive value of such models have been demonstrated [53].

Considering the high number of input parameters which these models required and the uncertainty in the in vivo assessed data, global sensitivity analysis is used to determine which parameters are of main importance (parameter priorization). Inverse engineering approach has also been considered by Leguy et al. 2011 in order to find the best fit between simulated blood flow and pressure and in vivo assessed data [54]. These methods require relatively high computational power. However, such computational power is constantly increasing so it can be assumed that in the future these methods will be used to obtain patient-specific modelling [55] and be used as a supporting tools for clinicians and the biomedical industry.

References

1. Harvey W, Leake C (1928) Exercitatio anatomica de motu cordis et sanguinis in animalibus. Thomas, Springfield
2. van de Vosse F (2003) Mathematical modelling of the cardiovascular system. J Eng Math 47(3):175–183
3. Pedley TJ (2003) Mathematical modelling of arterial fluid dynamics. J Eng Math 47(3):419–444
4. Bode AS, Huberts W, Bosboom EMH, Kroon W, van der Linden WPM, Planken RN, van de Vosse FN, Tordoir JHM (2012) Patient-specific computational modeling of upper extremity arteriovenous fistula creation: its feasibility to support clinical decision-making. PloS one 7(4):e34491
5. Fung Y (1996) Biomechanics: circulation. Springer, Berlin
6. Nichols W, O'Rourke M (2005) Mc Donald's blood flow in arteries. Theoretic, experimental, and clinical principles, 5th edn. Oxford University Press, London
7. Segers P, Verdonck P (2000) Role of tapering in aortic wave reflection: hydraulic and mathematical model study. J Biomech 33(3):299–306
8. World Health Organization (2014) Global status report on noncommunicable diseases 2014
9. Laurent S, Cockcroft J, van Bortel L, Boutouyrie P, Giannattasio C, Hayoz D, Pannier B, Vlachopoulos C, Wilkinson I, Struijker-Boudier H (2006) Expert consensus document on arterial stiffness: methodological issues and clinical applications. Eur Heart J 27:2588–2605
10. Bussy C, Boutouyrie P, Lacolley P, Challande P, Laurent S (2000) Intrinsic stiffness of the carotid arterial wall material in essential hypertensives. Hypertension 35:1049–1054
11. Shibeshi SS, Collins WE (2005) The rheology of blood flow in a branched arterial system. Appl Rheol 15(6):398–405
12. Bessonov N, Sequeira A, Simakov S, Vassilevskii Y, Volpert V (2016) Methods of blood flow modelling. Math Model Nat Phenom 11(1):1–25
13. Gijsen F, Allanic E, van de Vosse F, Janssen J (1999) The influence of the non-newtonian properties of blood on the flow in large arteries: unsteady flow in a 90 degrees curved tube. J Biomech 32:705–713
14. Leguy CAD, Bosboom EMH, Gelderblom H, Hoeks APG, van de Vosse FN (2010) Estimation of distributed arterial mechanical properties using a wave propagation model in a reverse way. Med Eng Phys 32(9):957–67
15. Brands P, Hoeks A, Willigers J, Willekes C, Reneman R (1999) An integrated system for the non-invasive assessment of vessel wall and hemodynamic properties of large arteries by means of ultrasound. Eur J Ultrasound 9:257–266
16. Kwee RM, Truijman MTB, van Oostenbrugge RJ, Mess WH, Prins MH, Franke CL, Korten AGGC, Wildberger JE, Kooi ME (2012) Longitudinal MRI study on the natural history of carotid artery plaques in symptomatic patients. PLoS One 7(7)
17. Westerhof N (2010) Snapshots of hemodynamics: an aid for clinical research and graduate education
18. Leguy C, Bosboom E, Hoeks A, van de Vosse F (2009) Model-based assessment of dynamic arterial blood volume flow from ultrasound measurements. Med Biol Eng Comput 47:641–648
19. Womersley J (1955) Mathematical theory of oscillating flow in an elastic tube. J Physiol 127:37–8P
20. Leguy CAD, Bosboom EMH, Hoeks APG, van de Vosse FN (2009) Assessment of blood volume flow in slightly curved arteries from a single velocity profile. J Biomech 42(11):1664–72
21. Schlichting H (1960) Boundary layer theory, 1st edn. Mc Graw-Hill, New York
22. Frank O (1899) Die Grundform des arteriellen Pulses. Erste Abhandlung. Mathematische Analyse Z Biol 37:483–526
23. Westerhof N, Bosman F, de Vries C, Noordergraaf A (1969) Analog studies of the human systemic arterial tree. J Biomech 2:121–143

24. Stergiopulos N, Segers P, Westerhof N (1999) Use of pulse pressure method for estimating total arterial compliance in vivo. Am J Physiol 276:H424–H428
25. Stergiopulos N, Westerhof B, Westerhof N (1999) Total arterial inertance as the fourth element of the windkessel model. Am J Physiol 276:H81–H88
26. Westerhof N, Lankhaar J-W, Berend A, Westerhof E (2008) The arterial Windkessel
27. Huberts W, Bosboom E, van de Vosse F (2008) A lumped model for blood flow and pressure in the systemic arteries based on an approximate velocity profile function. Math Biosci Eng 6(1):27–40
28. Liang F, Liu H (2005) A closed-loop lumped parameter computational model for human cardiovascular system. JSME Int Ser C 48:84–493
29. Olufsen M, Peskin C, Kim W, Pedersen E, Nadim A, Larsen J (2000) Numerical simulation and experimental validation of blood flow in arteries with structured-tree outflow conditions. Ann Biomed Eng 28:1281–1299
30. Lanzarone E, Liani P, Baselli G, Costantino M (2007) Model of arterial tree and peripheral control for the study of physiological and assisted circulation. Med Eng Phys 29:542–555
31. Pietrabissa R, Mantero S, Marotta T, Menicanti L (1996) A lumped parameter model to evaluate the fluid dynamics of different coronary bypasses. Med Eng Phys 18:477–484
32. Wolters B, Emmer M, Rutten M, Schurink G, van de Vosse F (2007) Assessment of endoleak significance after endovascular repair of abdominal aortic aneurysms: a lumped parameter model. Med Eng Phys 29:1106–1118
33. Bessems D, Rutten M, van de Vosse F (2007) A wave propagation model of blood flow in large vessels using an approximate velocity profile function. J Fluid Mech 580:145–168
34. Alastruey J, Moore S, Parker K, David T, Peiro J, Sherwin S (2008) Reduced modelling of blood flow in the cerebral circulation: coupling 1-d, 0-d and cerebral auto-regulation models. Int J Numer Methods Fluids 56(8):1061–1067
35. van de Vosse FN, Stergiopulos N (2011) Pulse wave propagation in the arterial tree. Ann Rev Fluid Mech 43(1):467–499
36. Bessems D, Giannopapa CG, Rutten MCM, van de Vosse FN, Anliker M, Rockwell L, Anliker M, Moritz W, Ogden E, Bessems D, Cox R, Fung Y, Giannopapa C, Hughes T, Lubliner J, Learoyd B, Taylor M (2008) Experimental validation of a time-domain-based wave propagation model of blood flow in viscoelastic vessels. J Biomech 41(2):284–91
37. Fullana J-M, Zaleski S (2009) A branched one-dimensional model of vessel networks. J Fluid Mech 621:183
38. Keijsers JMT, Leguy CAD, Huberts W, Narracott AJ, Rittweger J, van de Vosse FN (2015) A 1D pulse wave propagation model of the hemodynamics of calf muscle pump function. Int J Numer Methods Biomed Eng 31(7):e02716
39. Marchandise E, Flaud P (2010) Accurate modelling of unsteady flows in collapsible tubes. Comput Methods Biomech Biomed Eng 13(2):279–290
40. Shapiro AH (1977) Steady flow in collapsible tubes. J Biomech Eng 99(3):126
41. Alastruey J, Khir AW, Matthys KS, Segers P, Sherwin SJ, Verdonck PR, Parker KH, Peiró J (2011) Pulse wave propagation in a model human arterial network: assessment of 1-D visco-elastic simulations against in vitro measurements. J Biomech 44(12):2250–2258
42. Reymond P, Merenda F, Perren F, Rüfenacht D, Stergiopulos N (2009) Validation of a one-dimensional model of the systemic arterial tree. Am J Physiol Heart Circ Physiol 297:H208–H222
43. Liu B, Tang D (2011) Influence of non-Newtonian properties of blood on the wall shear stress in human atherosclerotic right coronary arteries. Mol Cell Biomech MCB 8(1):3–90
44. Li M, Beech-Brandt J, John L, Hoskins P, Easson W (2007) Numerical analysis of pulsatile blood flow and vessel wall mechanics in different degrees of stenoses. J Biomech 40:715–3724
45. Morris PD, Narracott A, von Tengg-Kobligk H, Silva Soto DA, Hsiao S, Lungu A, Evans P, Bressloff NW, Lawford PV, Hose DR, Gunn JP (2016) Computational fluid dynamics modelling in cardiovascular medicine. Heart (Br Card Soc) 102(1):18–28
46. Steinman DA, Milner JS, Norley CJ, Lownie SP, Holdsworth DW (2003) Image-based computational simulation of flow dynamics in a giant intracranial aneurysm. AJNR. Am J Neuroradiol 24(4):559–66

47. Kayser-Herolda O, Matthies H (2007) A unified least-squares formulation for fluid-structure interaction problems. Comput Struct 85:998–1011
48. Moireau P, Xiao N, Astorino M, Figueroa CA, Chapelle D, Taylor CA, Gerbeau J-F (2012) External tissue support and fluid-structure simulation in blood flows. Biomech Model Mechanobiol 1(1–2):1–18
49. Taylor CA, Figueroa CA (2009) Patient-specific modeling of cardiovascular mechanics. Ann Rev Biomed Eng 11:109–34
50. Mynard JP, Wasserman BA, Steinman DA (2013) Errors in the estimation of wall shear stress by maximum Doppler velocity. Atherosclerosis 227(2):259–66
51. Neidlin M, Corsini C, Sonntag SJ, Schulte-Eistrup S, Schmitz-Rode T, Steinseifer U, Pennati G, Kaufmann TA (2016) Hemodynamic analysis of outflow grafting positions of a ventricular assist device using closed-loop multiscale CFD simulations: Preliminary results. J Biomech 49(13):2718–2725
52. Speelman L, Bosboom EMH, Schurink GWH, Buth J, Breeuwer M, Jacobs MJ, van de Vosse FN (2009) Initial stress and nonlinear material behavior in patient-specific AAA wall stress analysis. J Biomech 42(11):1713–9
53. Merkx MAG, Bode AS, Huberts W, Oliván Bescós J, Tordoir JHM, Breeuwer M, van de Vosse FN, Bosboom EMH (2013) Assisting vascular access surgery planning for hemodialysis by using MR, image segmentation techniques, and computer simulations. Med Biol Eng Comput 51(8):79–889
54. Leguy CAD, Bosboom EMH, Belloum ASZ, Hoeks APG, Van De Vosse FN (2011) Global sensitivity analysis of a wave propagation model for arm arteries. Med Eng Phys 33(8):1008–1016
55. Reymond P, Vardoulis O, Stergiopulos N (2012) Generic and patient-specific models of the arterial tree. J Clin Monit Comput 26(5):375–382

Artificial Organs

Theodore G. Papaioannou

Since antiquity humans develop and use technologies with the ultimate purpose to augment their ability to survive, to treat or eradicate diseases, to enhance quality of living, to better adjust to environmental changes and to prolong lifespan. From the ancient Theriac, an all-purpose cure for a wide range of illnesses [1], to the modern medical technologies, these purposes remain the same. The conceptualization, design, development, test, validation and clinical application of human-made artificial organs has been for centuries a great technological and clinical challenge that can serve these endless humans' objectives. In our days amazing achievements have occurred due to the rapid progress in technology and particularly in materials science, biotechnology, nanotechnology, tissue and genetic engineering, biomechanics, biosensors, robotics and information technologies. All these advances have been also translated into the design and developement of artificial organs.

1 Definition

The term "*artificial organ*" refers to any kind of material, device or machine that is used to replace the function of a missing or totally dysfunctional organ or part of human body, but also to support or enhance the function of a partially dysfunctional or diseased organ or part of the human body. The artificial organs can be implanted

T. G. Papaioannou (✉)
Biomedical Engineering and Cardiovascular Mechanics, Biomedical Engineering Unit,
First Department of Cardiology, Hippokration Hospital, Medical School,
National and Kapodistrian University of Athens, Athens, Greece
e-mail: thepap@med.uoa.gr

S. Golemati and K. S. Nikita (eds.), *Cardiovascular Computing—Methodologies and Clinical Applications*, Series in BioEngineering,
https://doi.org/10.1007/978-981-10-5092-3_12

or integrated into the body and their role can be either critical for life and survival or supportive for the improvement of quality of life.

The human circulatory system is a very attractive field for the application of various different types of artificial organs. Due to the electrical, mechanical, and "hydrodynamic" nature of the cardiovascular system numerous implantable devices are continuously developed aiming to treat, assist or rehabilitate various diseased cardiac, arterial and hemodynamic states. The most popular cardiovascular artificial organs include the artificial heart, the ventricular assist devices most commonly known as cardiac assist devices or blood pumps, the artificial valves, the pacemakers, the vascular prostheses such as stents and vascular grafts as well as implantable devices used for the treatment of structural heart diseases.

The design of an artificial organ is a highly complex procedure that requires a multidisciplinary methodological approach and research team. The first prerequisite for the optimal design of the device is the deep knowledge and understanding of the biological, physiological and pathophysiological parameters and mechanisms related to the structure and function of the original organ or part of the organ which is going to be replaced or assisted. Some of the most essential issues that will be dealt during the design of an artificial organ are briefly described below.

The structural and geometrical features of the artificial organ under design depend upon the respective features and properties of the native human organ but also of the surrounding tissues and organs. Anatomical, geometrical and structural data can be derived from anthropometry studies and databases. Anthropometry is the science and practice of measuring the size and shape of the human body and its parts and it plays a key role in the design of artificial organs. Although anthropometric data can provide valuable statistical information about human anatomy (i.e. organs' size and shape), recent developments in medical imaging with advanced computational tools, allow accurate and realistic 3D reconstruction of human organs. By current 3D imaging modalities it is possible to determine anatomical, geometrical and also functional information for the organ under examination thus allowing to personalize/individualize the design of the artificial organ.

The material(s) which will be used for the construction of the artificial organ is another critical issue of research and experimentation. The ideal materials should have properties that mimic the properties of the real tissues and organ that is going to be replaced or assisted. A key feature of a biomaterial is *biocompatibility*. Any biomaterial should ensure compatibility with living tissue or a living system and in particular it should not be toxic, injurious, or physiologically reactive and should not cause immunological rejection or other adverse effects such as hemolysis, thrombosis etc. Another essential feature of the biomaterial regards its *biomechanical* properties. The most critical biomechanical characteristics of the material(s) used for the development of cardiovascular artificial organs are the elasticity or stiffness, anisotropy, viscoelasticity and other properties such as stress-relaxation, creep, strain-rate sensitivity, hysteresis. Depending on the application other mechanical properties may be of interest as well. The complexity of the biological properties and biomechanical behavior of the real human tissues and organs renders the development of an artificial replicate of this organ or tissue a difficult task. For this reason many artificial prostheses and organs used in cardiovascular medicine still fail to successfully replace or assist the diseased organ without complications; i.e. artificial hearts are still accompanied by several technical and clinical limitations, vascular grafts and stents suffer from restenosis or thrombosis, artificial valves may present limited durability, thrombosis, hemolysis or mechanical deformations, pacemakers have power limitations or may induce infectious reactions and so on.

The biomechanical features of a prototype artificial organ, beyond the material properties, will determine its performance under real operating conditions and continuous functioning. Often several designs and different biomaterials are tested aiming to achieve optimal performance, safety and durability of the artificial organ. For this reason the device under development is first tested using models with many tests and re-tests performed in order to achieve an acceptable design of a prototype device.

Modeling of the anatomical, hemodynamic and biomechanical features of the cardiovascular system (or parts of it), is a typical methodological approach used for the understanding of pathophysiological phenomena as well as for the test of medical devices and artificial organs. There are three major categories of models of the cardiovascular system; (a) in silico models that use computational and mathematical principles and methods, (b) in vitro models mostly using tubes, pumps and other hydraulic elements and measurement/recording equipment and (c) in vivo models using animals and measurement/recording equipment. Obviously, the most cost effective and safe approach is the computational modeling that offers the ability to perform several tests, at different simulated conditions examining the performance of numerous different designs and biomechanical properties of the artificial organ under examination.

The computational models allow us to reach to the theoretically optimal design of the tested artificial organ before proceeding to in vitro and animal experiments and of course before the first clinical trials of the final product. Also these models are used to provide some initial proof of concept before conducting further detailed studies.

Different mathematical and computational approaches can be used for the development of an in silico model of the cardiovascular system [2, 3]. In the literature several one-dimensional (1-D), 2-D and 3-D models [4] or parts of it have been described. A typical 1-D mathematical model of the systemic arterial circulation is illustrated at the Fig. 1, which has been previously used for the evaluation of the hemodynamic impact of vascular grafts [5]. This model has been validated and it was found to be able to predict pressure and flow waves in good qualitative and quantitative agreement with in vivo measurements, especially with respect to the shape and wave details [6, 7]. A few examples of cardiovascular artificial organs

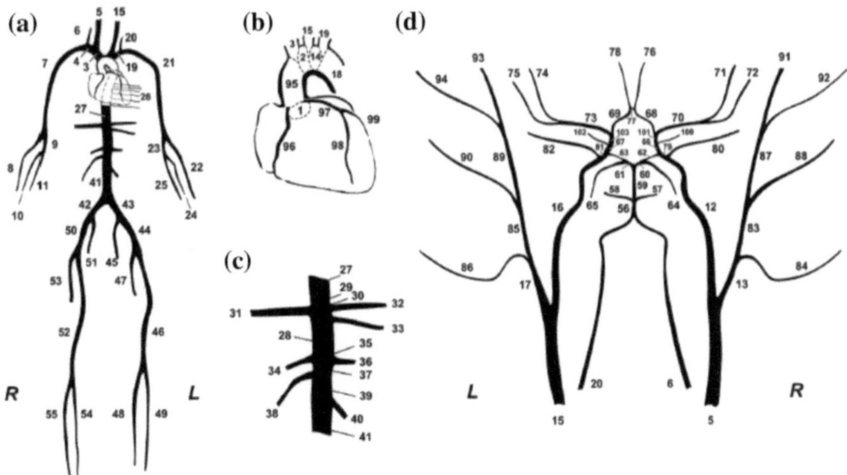

Fig. 1 Illustration of the main arterial segments used in an 1-D computational model [6, 7]. **a** Modelled segments of the main systemic arterial tree. **b** Braches of the aortic arch and coronary arteries, **c** braches of the abdominal aorta. **d** Segments of the cerebral arterial tree, which is connected via the carotids (segments 5 and 15) and the vertebrals (segments 6 and 20) to the main arterial tree. R, right; L, left

and the most critical features that determine their design and performance are briefly discussed below.

2 Stents

Vascular stents belong in the family of artificial organs as they can assist the vessel by holding up its lumen allowing blood to flow without the restrictions posed by arterial stenosis. However, stent structure, geometry and mechanical properties play a critical role on optimal blood flow conditions through stent as well as on the interaction of stent deployment with arterial lumen response. Other critical complications that depend on stent geometry and biomechanical properties are stent restenosis and thrombosis. Also, stent design and deployment are both related with plaque characteristics [8, 9]. Thus in order to estimate the optimal strut design, stent shape and deployment numerous mathematical and computational models have been developed in order to simulate and investigate blood flow conditions under different stent designs and at various hemodynamic scenario. Wall shear stress is an essential hemodynamic parameter which is related with the aforementioned complications and stent efficacy [10, 11], beyond other biological factors such as those related with the coating of the stent struts. Three-dimensional computational fluid dynamics models and finite element methods are widely used to investigate the hydrodynamic and biomechanical effects of various stent designs and deployment ratios [12, 13]. General

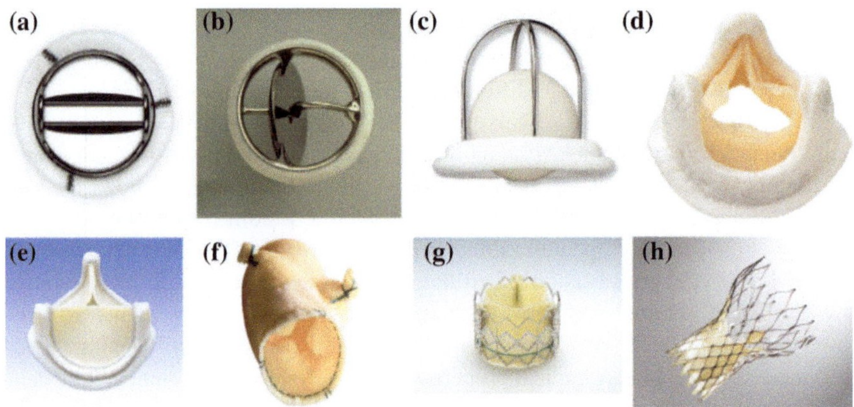

Fig. 2 Different types of prosthetic valves. **a** Bileaflet mechanical valve (St Jude), **b** monoleaflet mechanical valve (Medtronic Hall), **c** caged ball valve (Starr-Edwards), **d** stented porcine bioprosthesis (Medtronic Mosaic), **e** stented pericardial bioprosthesis (Carpentier-Edwards Magna), **f** stentless porcine bioprosthesis (Medtronic Freestyle), **g** percutaneous bioprosthesis expanded over a balloon (Edwards Sapien), **h** self-expandable percutaneous bioprosthesis (CoreValve). Reproduced with permission [14]

features pertaining to the "ideal" stent are: flexibility, biocompatibility, traceability, radio-opacity, resistance to thrombus formation, high radial strength, good expandability, hydrodynamic compatibility (i.e. uniform intra-stent shear stress profile). Other technical factors that determine stent performance are mechanisms related to the stent deployment (shelf-expandable or balloon expandable), the material used for stent construction (i.e. stainless steel, nitinol, cobalt-based alloy, coated materials, biodegradable materials), the geometrical configuration (i.e. coil, mesh, slotted tube, ring, or other costume designs).

3 Artificial Valves

The introduction of valve replacement surgery in the early 1960s has dramatically improved the outcome of patients with valvular heart disease. Despite the obvious improvements in artificial valve design and procedures/techniques of their implantation during the last decades, valve replacement is still accompanied by complications which are mainly due to prosthetic valve hemodynamics, durability, and thrombogenicity [14]. Nonetheless, many of these complications can be prevented or minimized through an optimal design and construction of the device, a personalized device selection, appropriate implantation and when needed proper re-positioning of the device. Several different types of artificial prosthetic heart valves (from first to latest generation) are illustrated in Fig. 2.

The ideal geometric, functional and biological features of an artificial valve and their design are based on data derived from the original human valves which have been thoroughly investigated at different methodological settings [15, 16].

Proper function of the heart valves is principally controlled by the surrounding hemodynamic environment. Although the four heart valves (tricuspid, pulmonary, mitral and aortic) present profoundly different anatomical and functional characteristics, their function basically aim to facilitate the unidirectional flow of blood while maximizing flow rate and minimizing flow resistance [16]. Furthermore, the proper design and construction of artificial valves should take into consideration how the valve material and function may impact hemodynamics, if the artificial valve will cause platelet aggregation or thrombosis, if the device will damage blood cells, and whether the mechanical properties of the device are sufficient to withstand the repeated cycles the valve will encounter in its lifetime. Numerous computational models and studies have been performed in order to understand, predict and optimize artificial valve design and function. As an example, the flow velocity distribution in bileaflet mechanical valves are depicted in Fig. 3 obtained by a previous numerical simulation study [14].

4 Artificial Heart and Cardiac Assist Devices

The most challenging engineering and clinical objective is the development of an artificial heart. The first steps in the development of devices for the mechanical support of the cardiovascular system were made in 1952 when temporary assistance of the circulation during cardiac repair operation was achieved by the development of the cardioplumonary bypass system [17]. Artificial hearts and cardiac assist devices are typically used as a bridge to heart transplantation or for permanent replacement of the heart in case transplantation is not possible.

The intra-aortic balloon pump (IABP), one of the most popular systems for the mechanical support of human circulation, was invented in early 60s based on the hemodynamic principle of counterpulsation [18]. The method was applicable only for temporary assistance of the failing heart and not for permanent or long-term use. However, the minimal invasive nature of the technique still remains an essential advantage. The hemodynamic performance of IABP depends on several technical parameters (i.e. balloon shape and size, timing and frequency of balloon inflation and deflation, balloon positioning, etc.) and clinical factors (i.e. arterial compliance, heart rate, severity of cardiac dysfunction, drug use, patient's position etc.) [19–24]. The primary objectives of IABP assistance is the reduction of left ventricular (LV) afterload (i.e. through a reduction in aortic end-diastolic blood pressure), the reduction in LV systolic work (i.e. via a decrease in aortic systolic pressure) and the increase in coronary artery perfusion and oxygen supply to the myocardium (i.e.

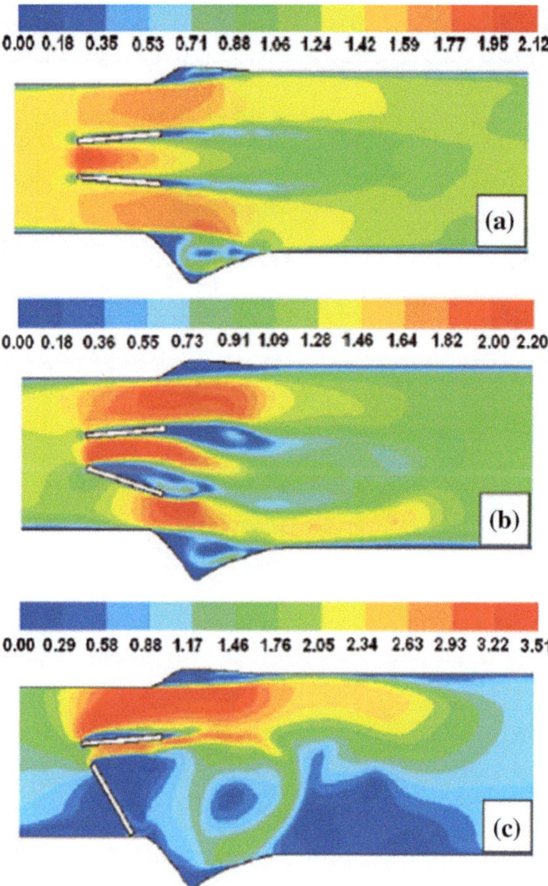

Fig. 3 **a** Normally functioning bileaflet prosthesis. The flow velocity within the central orifice is higher than that in the lateral orifices. **b** Mild prosthesis dysfunction with 25% restriction in the opening of 1 leaflet. **c** Severe prosthesis dysfunction with 1 leaflet blocked in the closed position. Courtesy of Drs Othman Smadi and Lyes Kadem, Concordia University, Montreal, Québec, Canada. Reproduced with permission from [14]

via the increase in mean diastolic aortic pressure and an increase in coronary blood flow). The understanding and the optimization of IABP function has been also based on computational studies which allow the multi-parametric modeling and analysis of IABP performance. Several mathematical models of various complexities have been developed in order to derive optimal conditions, hemodynamic states and operating parameters leading to maximum clinical efficacy of the IABP [25–27].

A few examples of cardiac assist devices for permanent or long-term use are illustrated in Fig. 4, with the total artificial heart being at the frontline of these technologies.

Computational models have been also used in order to examine a variety of design and functional configurations of assist devices. Computational fluid mechanics, in particular, allow the verification of experimental data derived by in vitro measurements. These models employ the development of digital grids that depict the physical

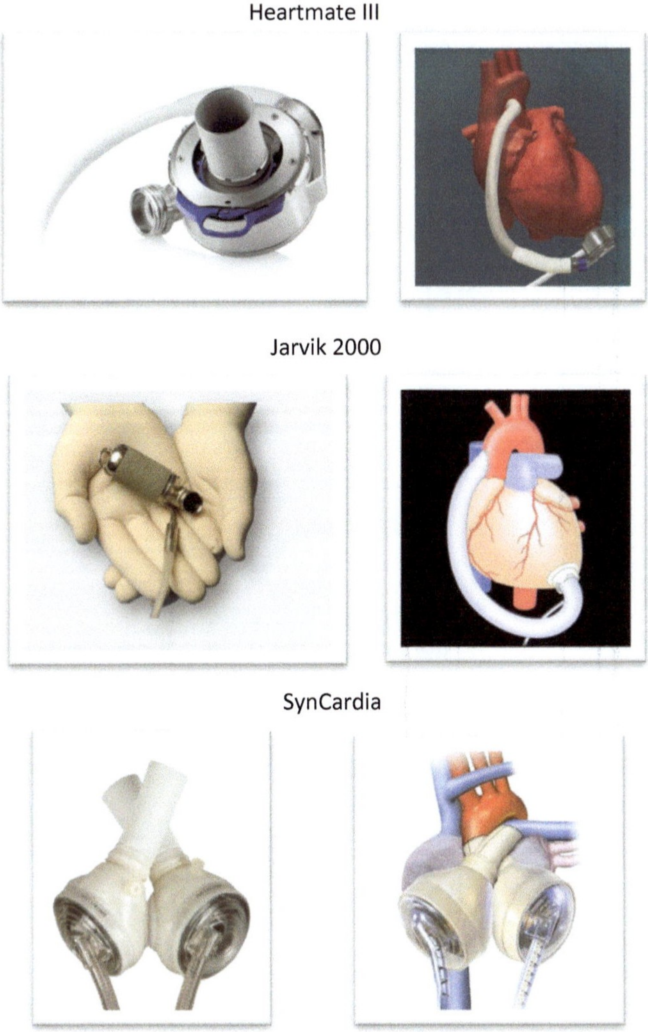

Fig. 4 Cardiac assist devices

boundaries of the flow field within which the pressure–flow relationships can be analyzed [28]. Another critical parameter that these models aim to examine is hemolysis which the pump may induce through the investigation of the generated flow fields and wall stresses. Several different types of cardiac assist devices have been developed; i.e. for the left ventricle's assistance (LVAD) or for bi-ventricular assistance (biVAD) as well as pneumatically or electrically driven systems. Blood pumps are also categorized based on their pressure flow relations and whether the produced flows are steady or pulsatile with a long-standing debate existing regarding the role of centrifugal and axial flow blood pumps generating steady flows [28].

5 Perspectives

The progress in biomaterials, biosensors, molecular biology, genetics, tissue engineering and nanotechnology promise future groundbreaking advances in the development of artificial organs. Scientists are already developing biological organs or part of them in the Lab [29, 30], transforming science fiction ideas into reality. Ethical issues arise, new philosophical movements are born, health policies and economics are reconsidered while the human species continuously abandon its biological limitations heading towards their complete transformation into a new trans-human or even post-human nature [31].

References

1. Karaberopoulos D, Karamanou M, Androutsos G (2012) The theriac in antiquity. Lancet 379:1942–1943
2. Morris PD, Narracott A, von Tengg-Kobligk H, Silva Soto DA, Hsiao S, Lungu A, Evans P, Bressloff NW, Lawford PV, Hose DR, Gunn JP (2016) Computational fluid dynamics modelling in cardiovascular medicine. Heart 102:18–28
3. Formaggia L, Quarteroni A, Veneziani A (2009) Cardiovascular mathematics: modeling and simulation of the circulatory system. Springer, Milan, New York, p xiii, 522
4. Lopez-Perez A, Sebastian R, Ferrero JM (2015) Three-dimensional cardiac computational modelling: methods, features and applications. Biomed Eng Online 14:35
5. Vardoulis O, Coppens E, Martin B, Reymond P, Tozzi P, Stergiopulos N (2011) Impact of aortic grafts on arterial pressure: a computational fluid dynamics study. Eur J Vasc Endovasc Surg 42:704–710
6. Reymond P, Bohraus Y, Perren F, Lazeyras F, Stergiopulos N (2011) Validation of a patient-specific one-dimensional model of the systemic arterial tree. Am J Physiol Heart Circ Physiol 301:H1173–H1182
7. Reymond P, Merenda F, Perren F, Rufenacht D, Stergiopulos N (2009) Validation of a one-dimensional model of the systemic arterial tree. Am J Physiol Heart Circ Physiol 297:H208–H222
8. Vavuranakis M, Papaioannou TG, Katsarou OA, Vrachatis DA, Sanidas EA, Siasos G, Kalogeras KI, Schizas D, Stefanadis CI, Tousoulis D (2016) Impact of atherosclerotic plaque components and their distribution on stent deployment: an intravascular-ultrasound virtual histology observational study. Minerva Cardioangiol 64:507–516
9. Lindsay AC, Paulo M, Kadriye K, Tejeiro R, Alegria-Barrero E, Chan PH, Foin N, Syrseloudis D, Di Mario C (2013) Predictors of stent strut malapposition in calcified vessels using frequency-domain optical coherence tomography. J Invasive Cardiol 25:429–434

10. Van der Heiden K, Gijsen FJ, Narracott A, Hsiao S, Halliday I, Gunn J, Wentzel JJ, Evans PC (2013) The effects of stenting on shear stress: relevance to endothelial injury and repair. Cardiovasc Res 99:269–275
11. Papaioannou TG, Karatzis EN, Vavuranakis M, Lekakis JP, Stefanadis C (2006) Assessment of vascular wall shear stress and implications for atherosclerotic disease. Int J Cardiol 113:12–18
12. LaDisa JF Jr, Olson LE, Guler I, Hettrick DA, Audi SH, Kersten JR, Warltier DC, Pagel PS (2004) Stent design properties and deployment ratio influence indexes of wall shear stress: a three-dimensional computational fluid dynamics investigation within a normal artery. J Appl Physiol 97:424–30. Discussion 416
13. Gervaso F, Capelli C, Petrini L, Lattanzio S, Di Virgilio L, Migliavacca F (2008) On the effects of different strategies in modelling balloon-expandable stenting by means of finite element method. J Biomech 41:1206–1212
14. Pibarot P, Dumesnil JG (2009) Prosthetic heart valves: selection of the optimal prosthesis and long-term management. Circulation 119:1034–1048
15. Hasan A, Ragaert K, Swieszkowski W, Selimovic S, Paul A, Camci-Unal G, Mofrad MR, Khademhosseini A (2014) Biomechanical properties of native and tissue engineered heart valve constructs. J Biomech 47:1949–1963
16. Sacks MS, David Merryman W, Schmidt DE (2009) On the biomechanics of heart valve function. J Biomech 42:1804–1824
17. Gibbon JH Jr (1954) Application of a mechanical heart and lung apparatus to cardiac surgery. Minn Med 37:171–185. Passim
18. Moulopoulos SD, Topaz S, Kolff WJ (1962) Diastolic balloon pumping (with carbon dioxide) in the aorta–a mechanical assistance to the failing circulation. Am Heart J 63:669–675
19. Papaioannou TG, Stefanadis C (2005) Basic principles of the intraaortic balloon pump and mechanisms affecting its performance. ASAIO J 51:296–300
20. Nanas JN, Moulopoulos SD (1994) Counterpulsation: historical background, technical improvements, hemodynamic and metabolic effects. Cardiology 84:156–167
21. Papaioannou TG, Mathioulakis DS, Stamatelopoulos KS, Gialafos EJ, Lekakis JP, Nanas J, Stamatelopoulos SF, Tsangaris SG (2004) New aspects on the role of blood pressure and arterial stiffness in mechanical assistance by intra-aortic balloon pump: in-vitro data and their application in clinical practice. Artif Organs 28:717–727
22. Papaioannou TG, Terrovitis J, Kanakakis J, Stamatelopoulos KS, Protogerou AD, Lekakis JP, Nanas JN, Stamatelopoulos SF (2002) Heart rate effect on hemodynamics during mechanical assistance by the intra-aortic balloon pump. Int J Artif Organs 25:1160–1165
23. Kolyva C, Pepper JR, Khir AW (2016) Newly shaped intra-aortic balloons improve the performance of counterpulsation at the semirecumbent position: an in vitro study. Artif Organs 40:E146–E157
24. Khir AW (2013) The balancing act of timing the intra-aortic balloon pump. Artif Organs 37:848–850
25. Aye TP, Htet ZL, Singhavilai T, Naiyanetr P (2015) Effect of intra-aortic balloon pump on coronary blood flow during different balloon cycles support: a computer study. Conf Proc IEEE Eng Med Biol Soc 2015:3303–3306
26. Giridharan GA, Koenig SC, Mitchell M, Gartner M, Pantalos GM (2007) A computer model of the pediatric circulatory system for testing pediatric assist devices. ASAIO J 53:74–81
27. Schampaert S, Rutten MC, van TVM, van Nunen LX, Tonino PA, Pijls NH, van de Vosse FN (2013) Modeling the interaction between the intra-aortic balloon pump and the cardiovascular system: the effect of timing. ASAIO J 59:30–36
28. Miller GE (2006) Artificial heart and cardiac assist devices. In: Miller GE (ed) Artificial Organs, 1st edn. Morgan & Claypool, USA, pp 11–19
29. Marx V (2015) Tissue engineering: organs from the lab. Nature 522:373–377

30. Murphy SV, Atala A (2014) 3D bioprinting of tissues and organs. Nat Biotechnol 32:773–785
31. Deretic I, Lorenz Sorgner S (2015) From humanism to meta-, post- and transhumanism? Peter Lang AG

Part V
Cardiovascular Informatics

Tele-, Mobile- and Web-Based Technologies in Cardiovascular Medicine

Ioannis I. Andreadis and Konstantina S. Nikita

Abstract The rapid growth of information and communications technology (ICT) and the recent advances of sensors enable the acquisition, transmission, and interpretation of different vital biosigns leading to the development of two emerging scientific fields, the electronic health (e-Health) and the mobile health (m-Health). Innovative services in healthcare have been developed, including timely collection of clinical information from different points, fixed or mobile, and remote analysis by physicians that aims in better prevention, well being and efficient management through prompt diagnostic tools. These services go beyond medical professionals to the general public, healthy individuals, patients and their families, who probably lack any medical training. They may have in particular a potential broad application to the management of chronic diseases, where the patients are in the need of continuous assistance, wishing to live independently. Cardiovascular diseases (CVDs) consist one of the most serious chronic conditions and a leading cause of deaths globally. They have already attracted the attention of many researchers towards developing novel approaches for their management, providing a wide variety of applications ranging from clinical setting to individual's daily environment. This chapter presents current advances on the management of CVDs, focusing on the acquisition of the related biosigns and the use of both telemedicine and mobile technologies for their transmission and remote analysis. The potential and perspectives on e-Health and m-Health applications for the health management of patients and healthy individuals are discussed.

I. I. Andreadis (✉) · K. S. Nikita
Athens, Greece
e-mail: iandr@biosim.ntua.gr

K. S. Nikita
e-mail: knikita@ece.ntua.gr

S. Golemati and K. S. Nikita (eds.), *Cardiovascular Computing—Methodologies and Clinical Applications*, Series in BioEngineering,
https://doi.org/10.1007/978-981-10-5092-3_13

1 Introduction

Cardiovascular diseases (CVDs) consist the primary cause of deaths globally and it is expected to remain the leading cause of mortality during next years, particularly in low- and middle-income countries, where over three quarters of CVDs deaths take place [56]. CVDs include mainly acute events (heart attacks and strokes) originated from disorders of the heart and blood vessels, such as coronary heart disease (CHD), heart failure (HF), hypertension (HTN) and carotid atherosclerosis (CA-a degenerative disease leading to lesions that narrow carotid arteries) [59]. The main cause of these conditions may be attributed to a combination of risk factors, including unhealthy diet and obesity, hypertension, physical inactivity and harmful use of alcohol [104]. Despite the substantial improvements in health care delivery for cardiac care, one in three deaths is still attributed to CVDs. Additionally, concerning the spending costs for the healthcare delivery, it is estimated that health care costs in the United States will grow by 5.8% per year for the period 2010–2020 and are projected to reach $4.64 trillion by 2020, representing almost 20% of the gross domestic product [40]. Heart conditions are ranked first in the relative ranking of chronic illnesses for the medical expenses in the United States [101]. Therefore, the accompanying rising costs, along with the disease burden from CVDs, provoke the struggling of global healthcare systems, making thus the improvement of interventions to ameliorate CVDs prevention an urgent need [60].

In response to these challenges, scientific community envisages a fundamental redesign of the healthcare processes that should be based on the integration of Information and Communication Technologies (ICT) at all levels, leading to a preventive, personalized, precise and pervasive health care system [87]. The exponential growth of communication technology in the past years has opened up new possibilities towards improving health management. The rapid exchange of medical information may be exploited to substantially improve patient's health status allowing better transmission of health care delivery. Therefore, health care may be shifted away from the medical institutions, promoting the proliferation of innovative modalities, including telemedicine, tele-health, mobile health applications and web-based strategies.

Telemedicine mainly refers to the use and transmittance of medical information in cases where the distance consists a critical factor. Telemedicine has been introduced four decades ago towards the delivery of health care services to patients in remote areas. Currently, it is being used as a common tool in healthcare and it is considered synonymous to tele-health and electronic health (e-Health), which implies the use of digital technologies in the healthcare domain [26]. Among the wide range of applications associated to tele-health services, we may mention remote meetings for patient consultation, prevention and treatment of diseases and injuries, telemonitoring of patient's biosigns, websites for patients, as well as continuing medical education of healthcare providers and remote training for healthcare professionals [46]. It is estimated that the beneficiaries of telemedicine services are set to grow tenfold between 2013 and 2018 [35].

As in the case of telemedicine, the revolution in the field of wireless communications and the rapid adoption of mobile smart devices during the last decade offer new chances in health care delivery, in an attempt to overcome barriers and limitations coming from traditional services. Along with the rapid advancements in sensors, a pervasive wireless environment is currently created that may address a wide range of major health-related challenges, including chronic and non-communicable diseases (NCDs), support for well-being and healthier lifestyle, infectious diseases and aging population. This emerging field of mobile health (m-Health) has the potential to reshape the future of healthcare, promoting disease management and wellness.

Specifically considering CVDs, the use of technology has been initially limited to the development of devices able to measure physiological signs and image anatomical structures. However, the continuous exploitation of technological advancements in the context of tele-health and m-Health has significantly enhanced all aspects of healthcare delivery and is even more promising for further improving them. Telemedicine in CVDs has already been applied since 1970 when the trans-telephonic transmission of electrocardiographic data has been introduced. Since then, much work has been done towards CVDs management via electronic health, leading to revolutionary ways of tele-monitoring cardiac signs and providing tele-consultation by health experts [33]. Additionally, thanks to innovative unobtrusive and wearable sensors, the measurement of physiological parameters is completely transformed, enabling the continuous monitoring of vital signs during the daily life of a subject and permitting therefore the detection of acute events, such as heart attacks and strokes, in real-time [110, 111].

The objectives of this chapter are to provide an overview of the state-of-the-art technologies in the context of e-Health and m-Health and update the reader on the role of these technologies in the management of CVDs. The rest of the chapter is organized as follows: Sect. 2 presents e-health applications, while Sect. 3 outlines the recent advances in the area of m-Health for CVDs management.

2 e-Health in the Management of CVDs

The World Health Organization has adopted the following description of telemedicine: "The delivery of health care services, where distance is a critical factor, by all health care professionals using information and communication technologies for the exchange of valid information for diagnosis, treatment and prevention of disease and injuries, research and evaluation, and for the continuing education of health care providers, all in the interests of advancing the health of individuals and their communities" [89]. Hereafter, we focus on the abovementioned aspects of telemedicine targeted to the diagnosis, treatment and prevention of CVDs.

As stated previously, the scientific field of telehealth has met revolutionary growth during the last decades, thanks to the combination of Information and Communication Technologies (ICT) and modern infrastructure (Fig. 1). CVDs management has been beneficiated by this growth in several ways, including the real-time collection

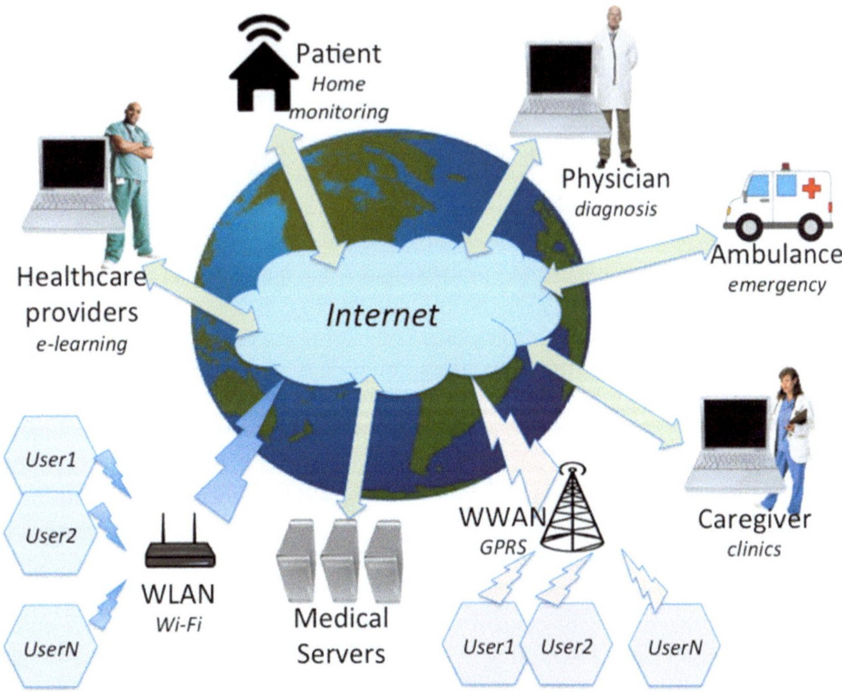

Fig. 1 Schematic representation for e-Health network and services

of crucial data (medical, physiological, behavioural) and their remote analysis and evaluation by physicians, enabling direct precautionary actions. Several studies have investigated the contribution of telemedicine technologies on the telecardiology field, including primary and secondary prevention of CVDs, cardiac rehabilitation, monitoring of chronic HF and diagnosis of acute coronary syndrome.

Primary preventions are considered the interventions aiming to the delay of the onset of the disease, while secondary prevention include the actions followed for the delay of the progression of the disease. Both areas have been significantly beneficiated by the use of telemedicine technologies [69]. The transmission of ECG via telephone lines and the remote consulting by expert cardiologists have shown promising results for the assessment of chest pain [79, 80], the detection of atrial fibrillation [8] and the support of frail elderly patients [79, 80]. The results of related studies [54, 55] focusing on the effect of telecardiology in the number of hospital admissions of patients with suspected cardiac events (following trans-telephonic electrocardiography and tele-consultation) have indicated that both reduction of unnecessary admissions and promotion of home-care may be achieved.

Based on the same main principles, telemedicine technologies may serve also in the case of rehabilitation after cardiac events. Preliminary studies [19, 77, 90, 96, 113] have investigated the effect of telemonitoring patients with diagnosed CVDs on the progress of the cardiac rehabilitation program. In the majority of cases the reported observations are quite encouraging, since the patients participating in the examination group presented higher adherence to the program, improved physical activity, weight loss, as well as reduced hospital readmissions, fewer major events and thus higher survival rates.

As in the case of monitoring cardiac rehabilitation, patients suffering from chronic HF are in the need of constant monitoring. Exploiting the advantages of telemedicine technologies, various methods, mainly based on telephone transactions, have evolved for enabling telemonitoring of the HF population from their home environment. In the majority of the studies conducted, significant positive effects on the healthcare delivery are reported. In particular, the main contribution appears to be the reduction of hospital stays and re-hospitalizations [9]. This conclusion has been extracted from several studies that proposed telemanagement of chronic HF patients [20, 27, 36, 49, 88]. Additional beneficial effects reported include better quality of life and reduced mortality [88], improved family function during the post-hospital period [15] and significant reduction in costs [47]. Furthermore, since HF consists a chronic disease, the proper and complete education of the patients plays a significant role towards the management of the healthcare delivery. As a result, many studies have focused on the factor of patient's education by nurses through telephone calls or specific web-based software, to improve self-care and emphasize in adherence to diet, drug treatment and symptoms monitoring [18, 21, 76]. The outcomes of these studies indicate also both reduced hospital costs and re-admissions for a 6-month period after the discharge from the hospital.

In contrast to the practices followed for chronic situations, as those described above, there are certain cases where the timely analysis of biosigns is of enormous importance for patient's health. Such circumstances mainly occur in pre-hospital applications, where precaution measures have to be followed before the arrival of the patient to the hospital. Early diagnosis of acute coronary syndrome consists probably the most representative example of this type of applications, since the efficient use of telemedicine technologies may prove to be catalytic for patient's life. The record of pre-hospital ECG, along with its transmission by the ambulance to the medical institution, has been investigated during the last twenty years [28] and consists nowadays a quite common practice warmly recommended given the achieved advantages. Specifically, lower rates of false negative diagnosis [7], reduction of infarct size [78] and drop in mortality rates [11, 100] have been reported in studies investigating the contribution of pre-hospital triage of ECG following telemedicine technologies.

3 m-Health in the Management of CVDs

After the initial evolution of the e-Health domain, the combined integration of mobile devices and medical sensors has led to the development of the m-Health scientific field. m-Health consists a multidimensional scientific field combining mainly mobile

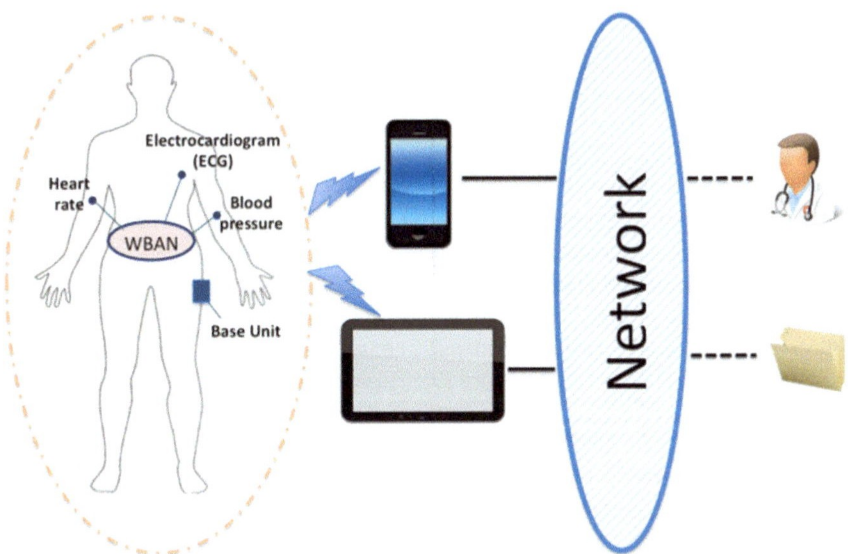

Fig. 2 Illustration of a typical architecture of m-Health services for the management of CVDs including a wireless body area network (WBAN)

technologies, mobile computing, data analysis, data storage and electronics in health practice, targeting to improved patient monitoring and communication. The extended use of mobile phones and other smart devices broadens the capacities of these devices in intervention of human-health related activities, as opportunities for continuous and accurate monitoring of human lifestyle are opened up. In brief, m-Health concerns mainly the analysis and transmission of health information through mobile devices (Fig. 2). Its ultimate goal is to improve disease management and to play a key role in the prevention of non-communicable or chronic diseases.

CVDs consist one of the "big four NCDs" that has already attracted the attention of many research teams in the context of developing novel m-Health technologies for their management. Typical examples of the innovative solutions in the area of CVD management that research on m-Health aspires to offer include: ensure collection of vital parameters (electrocardiogram, cardiac pressures, blood pressure) by analyzing context information (physical activity, stress), encourage adherence to physical activity plan or adherence to treatment to prevent heart disease, promote home- and self-care and detect the onset or provide warnings in case of acute events. Such applications address different audiences, not only the patients themselves but also their families, professionals (physicians, nurses) and any other group involved in the delivery of healthcare services.

In the context of the current study, we focus on the analysis of two main axes, including the process of data collection of vital signs associated to CVDs and the exploit of mobile phone functions towards vital events tracking and electronic decision support.

3.1 Collection of Related Biosigns

Among the most common vital signs associated to CVDs, electrocardiogram (ECG), blood pressure (BP) and heart rate (HR) are included. Towards the first axis considered, the record and collection of these signs, a variety of smart devices have been presented in the literature [1, 110, 111]. Such devices are mainly wearable, in the form of clothing or accessories, and their objective consists on measuring, through unobtrusive sensing, physiological parameters during the daily life of a subject to enable continuous monitoring. Apart from wearable devices, sensors embedded in smart objects in the living environment of the subject have also been proposed, that measure unobtrusively the corresponding signs through the interaction with the subject. A few examples of both wearable devices and smart objects are presented hereafter.

For the measurement of ECG using sensors embedded in the clothing of the subject, several approaches have been proposed where the electrodes are integrated into a cotton T-shirt [57], into the garment [4, 24, 107] or embedded within the fabric [14]. Park et al. [63] have proposed the adoption of their monitoring system on the belt of the subject. Furthermore, ECG necklaces for reliable cardiac activity monitoring have been presented [66, 108].

Regarding the measurement of HR, the photoplethysmographic (PPG) sensing has been widely used. Since the direct contact with the skin is prerequisite for the accurate measurement of the pressure pulse, many approaches introducing the use of sensors in daily gadgets and accessories have been proposed. Such studies include the application of ear-worn sensors [10, 50, 51, 65, 71, 72, 86, 85, 97], glove and hat sensors [91], ring-type devices [106, 3] and eyeglasses [112].

As far as the measurement of BP is concerned, unobtrusive application has showed significant advance during the last years, introducing approaches deviating from the traditional ones that are mainly based on the use of cuff. One of the first studies reported for the unobtrusive measurement of BP was based on the integration of e-textile materials in a T-shirt [109]. Many mobile systems have been presented since then, including clothing [30, 31], watches [73, 94], rings [84], systems mounted on ears [103] or arms [110, 111] and eyeglasses [112].

Regarding the use of smart objects, several approaches have been reported in the literature, such as sleeping bed [17, 30, 31], weighing scale [86, 85], steering wheel [29], toilet seat [43], smart chairs [5, 13, 99, 105] or even directly mobile smartphones [12, 67], and cameras [38] for the measurement of the vital signs related to CVDs.

In all the abovementioned cases, data can be gathered wirelessly by a smart device and possibly transmitted to another workstation for storage or further analysis.

3.2 m-Health Applications

Apart from the use of sensors, discussed in the previous section, to monitor signs and transmit feedback to healthcare providers, the ubiquity of mobile phones and smart devices has extended disease management from clinical setting to individual's daily environment. More simple mobile functionalities have been exploited during the past decade in the area of m-Health. These technologies include simple strategies, such as text messaging and short message services (SMS), or more complex functionalities including Bluetooth technologies and smart phone applications. We provide typical examples of m-Health systems incorporating such technologies, in an attempt to provide insights on the framework followed by current research studies towards the introduction of mobile technologies in today's healthcare. This list is by no means exhaustive.

One of the initial mobile technologies that consists basic feature of almost all mobile phones is text messaging. The usage of SMS text services in the healthcare domain is in general an intervention effort aiming mainly to medication adherence, intrinsic motivation and appointment reminders. This technology has already been widely used for various applications, such as diabetes management [32, 75], smoking cessation [23], adherence to physical activity [34] and weight loss [64].

Towards the use of text messaging for CVD management, TEXTME is a randomized trial clinical study conducted in Australia, considering as study population adults with coronary (CHD), established either angiographically or by a prior myocardial infraction [16]. The subjects included in the study population were provided with advices, support and motivation through four text messages per week for a period of six month. The messages aimed to promote healthy eating, adherence to physical activity and tobacco abstinence. After the end of the 6-month period, the authors indicated that the use of text messaging has contributed to reduction in systolic blood pressure, LDL-cholesterol, body mass index and smoking. Frederix et al. [22] performed also a clinical trial study using a population consisted of 140 patients with CHD. Through the provision of SMS coaching, along with conventional cardiac rehabilitation, they demonstrated that, after a 24-weeks period, self reported physical activity and health-related quality of life were significantly improved, after proper comparisons between the experimental and the control group. Corresponding conclusions have been extracted from a similar trial [2], where physical activity was higher in the experimental group (69 patients with CHD) than in control after a period of 3 months providing SMS and e-mail messages to complete intervention tasks. Kamal et al. [39] investigated the potential of reminder SMS messages to improve medication adherence, studying a group of 200 patients having a cerebrovascular accident. The authors verified the improved adherence to medication in the experimental group, after a period of two months. The significance of SMS reminders for medical and medication adherence has been investigated through various clinical trials [41, 45, 61, 62, 68, 74] studying groups of patients suffering from CVDs. In the majority of the considered studies, medical adherence was better in the experimental than in the control group.

Advancing the potential of text messaging, the development of smartphone applications may have enormous benefit in healthcare delivery, as both technologies may transform smartphone devices to a platform providing both health tracking and monitoring. Many mobile applications have been proposed targeting weight loss [25], dietary intake [98], physical activity [6], blood glucose tracking [42] and diabetes management in general [44].

As far as the management of the CVDs through mobile applications is concerned, various approaches have been proposed during the last years to identify the potential of smartphones features to be used as profitable interventions. Initial studies have investigated the potential of mobile devices to transmit data, either answers to questionnaires or fragments and values of physiological signs (ECG, BP, body weight), to telemedical centres and physicians to enable telemonitoring and further analysis [48, 52, 70]. Seto et al. [82] conducted a randomized clinical trial study, using mobile phones for daily transmission of the values of BP and weight and weekly transmission of ECG signs. The comparison between the control and experimental group revealed significant differences that lead to improved quality of life, self-care maintenance and management for the experimental population.

Furthermore, more recent studies have also included the development of smart applications based on certain specifications for handling the issue of telemonitoring CVDs. Feasibility studies have been conducted where mobile applications enabled both the daily risk acquisition of risk factor parameters and the manual entry of data by the subject itself, as well as the efficient transmission of these information to healthcare providers [81, 93]. In a randomized clinical trial, Varnfield et al. [95], using an experimental group of 120 patients with a recent myocardial infraction, demonstrated that the use of a mobile application, along with phone coaching, resulted in better quality of life and improved adherence to the completion of cardiac rehabilitation programs. More recently, Widmer et al. [102] proposed the use of a mobile application prior to or after traditional cardiac rehabilitation, indicating that both lower rates of re-hospitalization and improvements in systolic BP, weight and exercise capacity were achieved. Similarly, Steventon et al. [92], using a great number (3230) of adults with chronic diseases (including HF), investigated the contribution of telehealth devices in the management of chronic diseases, which proved to be quite significant as both lower risk of hospital admissions and death were observed.

Concluding, the major advances in the field of smartphone technologies and wireless communications have ended in a great variety of mobile applications (apps) oriented for issues related to the management of CVDs [26, 53, 58]. Many opportunities exist for the use of apps in helping to prevent CVD throughout life, from childhood where behavioral, environmental and social actions may be promoted to late adulthood where significant risk-factor reduction and primary and secondary CVD management are needed. Given the high use of mobile devices in childhood and adolescence, apps targeted to behavior change and promotion of healthier lifestyle may facilitate the prevention of developing CVD risk factors. Towards this direction, apps have been developed that encourage individuals to make healthy food choices (e.g. Eatery, FoodSwitch) or enable daily step count/running distances tracking and duration of activity (e.g. MyFitnessPal). Apart from childhood and adolescence, mobile apps may also be suitable both for primary prevention, in order to limit disease progression, and secondary prevention, in order to reduce CVD risk factors. Applications (such as Blood Pressure Monitor, HeartWise) have been recently introduced for the measurement of vital physiological signs, while a number of different applications (e.g. Heart Risk Calculator, MyHeart-MyLife) have been proposed towards risk evaluation. Such tools enable patients to manage different aspects of CVD from tracking medication and collecting personal health statistics, to helping them being educated regarding signs of heart attack.

Finally, there exists a great number of alternative applications that have been proposed for both the prevention and the management of diabetes, a condition that is partly related to the majority of CVDs [32]. Towards the prevention of diabetes, the available applications target mainly weight loss, physical activity and dietary intake. Regarding the management of the disease, several aspects (including adherence to physical activity and medication, healthy eating) have been recognized as essential steps towards the specific direction. The most prominent however feature of such applications is related to the blood glucose monitoring, through either manual entry or connection with related devices (e.g. glucometers) [37]. Finally, an additional category of smartphone applications contains educational tools that aim in delivering lessons on diabetes care and self-management [83].

4 Conclusions

This chapter provides a review of the published literature on the effectiveness of e-Health and m-Health technologies for the management of CVDs. Many solutions today use communication technology-based tools aiming in prevention, diagnosis, treatment, lifestyle monitoring and in general disease management. Typical examples include telemedicine services, wearable and portable systems and electronic health records.

Concerning the issue of telemedicine and web-based services in the management of CVDs, we have initially presented an extended overview of studies evaluating the contribution of telemedicine technologies for the management of CVDs, including both post-hospital (primary preventions, monitoring cardiac rehabilitation after acute events, management of chronic heart failure) and pre-hospital applications (acute coronary syndrome). Regarding the post-hospital settings, it seems that the role of telemedicine is of enormous importance, since its implementation in rehabilitation programs may significantly reduce both the re-hospitalization rates and the corresponding costs. As a result, promotion of home care is achieved. Considering pre-hospital cases, it has been shown that the timely analysis of pre-hospital biosigns may lead to lower mortality rates.

As far as the application of m-Health technologies in CVD management is concerned, various smart ubiquitous health care systems have been proposed following the advances in sensor technology. These innovative developments have lead to novel biomedical devices, such as health-related smart clothes, wearable gadgets or smart objects embedded in the living environment of the subject and health-oriented smart home platforms, offering the potential to acquire, transmit and store data and clinical information from the recording of vital biosigns. Despite the significant progress achieved in the development of sensing equipment, various issues related to miniaturization, security, personalization, user acceptance and energy efficiency have to be addressed in order to improve the usability of such devices for practical use. It is believed that future developments of sensing equipment would reform the monitoring and measuring activity of patients, revolutionizing therefore the way healthcare is provided. Preliminary studies investigating the potential of applying m-Health technologies in the management of CVDs have indicated a number of positive outcomes, including promotion of healthy eating, adherence to physical activity and medication, and improved health monitoring through smart phone applications. It appears therefore that m-Health solutions can improve the efficiency of health services, promote home care, remote disease management and wellness and become, thus, the cornerstone for supporting continuity of care for elderly citizens or patients suffering from a chronic disease.

Concluding, there is emerging evidence that internet-based interventions targeting CVD may be beneficial to health management and well being, acting efficiently towards the reduction of risk factors. Both e-Health and m-Health technologies could play an important role in the delivery of effective health care for patients suffering from cardiovascular diseases, especially for those with limited access to health services.

References

1. Ajami S, Teimouri F (2015) Features and application of wearable biosensors in medical care. J Res Med Sci: Off J Isfahan Univ Med Sci 20(12):1208–1215
2. Antypas K, Wangberg SC (2014) An Internet- and mobile-based tailored intervention to enhance maintenance of physical activity after cardiac rehabilitation: short-term results of a randomized controlled trial. J Med Internet Res. 16(3):e77
3. Asada HH, Shaltis P, Reisner A, Rhee S, Hutchinson RC (2003) Mobile monitoring with wearable photoplethysmographic biosensors. IEEE Eng Med Biol 22(3):28–40
4. Atallah L, Serteyn A, Meftah M, Schellekens M, Vullings R, Bergmans JW, Osagiator A, Oetomo SB (2014) Unobtrusive ECG monitoring in the NICU using a capacitive sensing array. Physiol Meas 35(5):895–913
5. Baek H, Chung G, Kim K, Park K (2012) A smart health monitoring chair for nonintrusive measurement of biological signals. IEEE Trans Inf Technol Biomed 16(1):150–158
6. Bort-Roig J, Gilson ND, Puig-Ribera A, Contreras RS, Trost SG (2014) Measuring and influencing physical activity with smartphone technology: a systematic review. Sports Med 44(5):671–686
7. Brunetti ND, De Gennaro L, Amodio G, Dellegrottaglie G, Pellegrino PL, Di Biase M et al (2010) Telecardiology improves quality of diagnosis and reduces delay to treatment in elderly patients with acute myocardial infarction and atypical presentation. Eur J Cardiovasc Prev Rehabil 17:615–620
8. Brunetti ND, De Gennaro L, Pellegrino PL, Dellegrottaglie G, Antonelli G, Di Biase M (2012) Atrial fibrillation with symptoms other than palpitations: incremental diagnostic sensitivity

with at-home telecardiology assessment for emergency medical service. Eur J Cardiovasc Prev Rehabil 19:306–313

9. Brunetti ND, Scalvini S, Acquistapace F, Parati G, Volteranni M, Fedele F et al (2015) Telemedicine for cardiovascular disease continuum: a position paper from the Italian Society of Cardiology Working Group on Telecardiology and Informatics. Int J Cardiol 184:452–458
10. Celka P, Verjus C, Vetter R, Renevey P, Neuman V (2004) Motion resistant earphone located infrared based heart rate measurement device. Paper presented at the 2nd IASTED international conference of biomedical engineering, Innsbruck, Austria, 16–18 Feb 2004
11. Chan AW, Kornder J, Elliott H, Brown RI, Dorval JF, Charania J et al (2012) Improved survival associated with pre-hospital triage strategy in a large regional ST-segment elevation myocardial infarction program. JACC Cardiovasc Interv 5:1239–1246
12. Chandrasekaran V, Dantu R, Jonnada S, Thiyagaraja S, Subbu KP (2013) Cuffless differential blood pressure estimation using smart phones. IEEE Trans Biomed Eng 60(4):1080–1089
13. Cheng J, Sundholm M, Zhou B, Hirsch M, Lukowicz P (2016) Smart-surface: large scale textile pressure sensors arrays for activity recognition. Pervasive Mob Comput 30:97–112
14. Chi YM, Cauwenberghs G (2010) Wireless non-contact EEG/ECG electrodes for body sensor networks. Paper presented at the international conference body sensor networks, Singapore, 7–9 June 2010
15. Chiang LC, Chen WC, Dai YT, Ho YL (2012) The effectiveness of telehealth care on caregiverburden, mastery of stress, and family function among family caregivers of heart failure patients: a quasi-experimental study. Int J Nurs Stud 49:1230–1242
16. Chow CK, Redfern J, Hillis GS, Thakkar J, Santo K, Hackett ML et al (2015) Effect of lifestyle-focused text messaging on risk factor modification in patients with coronary heart disease: a randomized clinical trial. JAMA 314(12):1255–1263
17. Cikajlo I, Sprager S, Erjavec T, Zazula D (2015) Cardiac arrhythmia alarm from optical interferometric signals during resting or sleeping for early intervention. Biocybern Biomed Eng 36(1):267–275
18. Conway A, Inglis SC, Clark RA (2014) Effective technologies for noninvasive remote monitoring in heart failure. Telemed J E Health 20:531–538
19. Dalleck LC, Schmidt LK, Lueker R (2011) Cardiac rehabilitation outcomes in a conventional versus telemedicine-based programme. J. Telemed. Telecare 17(5):217–221
20. Dendale P, De Keulenaer G, Troisfontaines P, Weytjens C, Mullens W, Elegeert I et al (2012) Effect of a telemonitoring-facilitated collaboration between general practitioner and heart failure clinic on mortality and rehospitalization rates in severe heart failure: the TEMA-HF 1 (TElemonitoring in the MAnagement of Heart Failure) study. Eur J Heart Fail 14:333–340
21. Dunagan WC, Littenberg B, Ewald GA, Jones CA, Emery VB, Waterman BM et al (2005) Randomized trial of a nurse administered, telephone-based disease management for patients with heart failure. J Card Fail 11:358–365
22. Frederix I, Hansen D, Coninx K, Vandervoort P, Vandijck D, Hens N et al (2015) Medium-term effectiveness of a comprehensive internet-based and patient-specific telerehabilitation program with text messaging support for cardiac patients: randomized control trial. J Med Internet Res 17(7):e185
23. Free C, Knight R, Robertson S, Whittaker R, Edwards P, Zhou W et al (2011) Smoking cessation support delivered via mobile phone text messaging (txt2stop): a single-blind, randomised trial. Lancet 378(9785):49–55
24. Fuhrhop S, Lamparth S, Heuer S (2009) A textile integrated longterm ECG monitor with capacitively coupled electrodes. Paper presented at the IEEE biomedical circuits and systems conference, Beijing, China, 26–28 Nov 2009
25. Fukuoka Y, Gay CL, Joiner KL, Vittinghoff E (2015) A novel diabetes prevention intervention using a mobile app: a randomized controlled trial with overweight adults at risk. Am J Prev Med 49(2):223–237
26. Gastounioti A, Golemati S, Andreadis I, Kolias VD, Nikita KS (2015) Cardiovascular disease management via electronic health. In: Eren H, Webster J (eds) Telehealth and mobile health. CRC Press Taylor & Francis Group, pp 187–202

27. Giordano A, Scalvini S, Paganoni AM, Baraldo S, Frigerio M, Vittori C et al (2013) Home-based telesurveillance program in chronic heart failure: effects on clinical status and implications for 1-year prognosis. Telemed J E Health 19:605–612
28. Giovas P, Papadoyannis D, Thomakos D, Papazachos G, Rallidis M, Soulis D et al (1998) Transmission of electrocardiograms from a moving ambulance. J Telemed Telecare 4:5–7
29. Gomez-Clapers J, Casanella R (2012) A fast and easy-to-use ECG acquisition and heart rate monitoring system using a wireless steering wheel. IEEE Sens J 12(3):610–616
30. Gu WB, Poon CCH, Leung HK, Sy MY, Wong MYM, Zhang YT (2009) A novel method for the contactless and continuous measurement of arterial blood pressure on a sleeping bed. Paper presented at the 31th annual international conference of the IEEE in engineering in medicine and biology society, 3–6 Sept 2009
31. Gu WB, Poon CCY, Sy MY, Leung HK, Liang YP, Zhang YT (2009) A h-shirt-based body sensor network for cuffless calibration and estimation of arterial blood pressure. Paper presented at the 6th international workshop on wearable and implantable body sensor networks, Berkeley, CA, 3–5 June 2009
32. Hartz J, Yingling L, Powell-Wiley TM (2016) Use of mobile health technology in the prevention and management of diabetes mellitus. Curr Cardiol Rep 18(12):130–141
33. Hsieh JC, Li AH, Yang CC (2013) Mobile, cloud, and big data computing: contributions, challenges, and new directions in telecardiology. Int J Environ Res Public Health 10(11):6131–6153
34. Hurling R, Catt M, Boni MD, Fairley BW, Hurst T, Murray P et al (2007) Using internet and mobile phone technology to deliver an automated physical activity program: randomized controlled trial. J Med Internet Res 9(2):e7
35. IHS (2014) Telehealth report. https://www.ihs.com/index.html. Accessed 12 Dec 2016
36. Inglis SC, Clark RA, McAlister FA, Stewart S, Cleland JG (2011) Which components of heart failure programmes are effective? A systematic review and meta-analysis of the outcomes of structured telephone support or telemonitoring as the primary component of chronic heart failure management in 8323 patients: Abridged Cochrane Review. Eur J Heart Fail 13:1028–1040
37. Issom DZ, Woldaregay AZ, Chomutare T et al (2015) Mobile applications for people with diabetes published between 2010 and 2015. Diabetes Manag 5(6):539–550
38. Jeong IC, Finkelstein J (2016) Introducing contactless blood pressure assessment using a high speed video camera. J Med Syst 40(4):77
39. Kamal AK, Shaikh Q, Pasha O, Azam I, Islam M, Memon AA et al (2015) A randomized controlled behavioral intervention trial to improve medication adherence in adult stroke patients with prescription tailored short messaging service (SMS)-SMS4Stroke study. BMC Neurol 15:212
40. Keehan SP, Sisco AM, Truffer CJ, Poisal JA, Cuckler JA, Madison AJ et al (2011) National health spending projections through 2020: economic recovery and reform drive faster spending growth. Health Aff 30(8):1594–1605
41. Khonsari S, Subramanian P, Chinna K, Latif LA, Ling LW, Gholami O (2015) Effect of a reminder system using an automated short message service on medication adherence following acute coronary syndrome. Eur J Cardiovasc Nurs 14(2):170–179
42. Kim HS, Choi W, Baek EK, Kim YA, Yang SJ, Choi IY et al (2014) Efficacy of the smartphone-based glucose management application stratified by user satisfaction. Diabetes Metab J 38(3):204–210
43. Kim KK, Lim YK, Park KS (2004) The electrically noncontacting ECG measurement on the toilet seat using the capacitively coupled insulated electrodes. Paper presented at the 26th annual international conference of the IEEE engineering in medicine and biology society, San Francisco, CA, USA, 1–5 Sept 2004
44. Kirwan M, Vandelanotte C, Fenning A, Duncan MJ (2013) Diabetes self-management smartphone application for adults with type 1 diabetes: randomized controlled trial. J Med Internet Res 15(11):e235
45. Kiselev OM, Gridnev VI, Shvartz VA, Posnenkova OM, Dovgalevsky PY (2012) Active ambulatory care management supported by short message services and mobile phone technology in patients with arterial hypertension. J Am Soc Hypertens 6(5):346–355

46. Klaassen B, van Beijnum BJF, Hermens HJ (2016) Usability in telemedicine systems—a literature survey. Int J Med Inform. 93:57–69
47. Klersy C, De Silvestri A, Gabutti G, Raisaro A, Curti M, Regoli F et al (2011) Economic impact of remote patient monitoring: an integrated economic model derived from a meta-analysis of randomized controlled trials in heart failure. Eur J Heart Fail 13:450–459
48. Koehler F, Winkler S, Schieber M, Sechtem U, Stangl K, Bohm M et al (2011) Impact of remote telemedical management on mortality and hospitalizations in ambulatory patients with chronic heart failure: The telemedical interventional monitoring in heart failure study. Circulation 123(17):1873–1880
49. Kurtz B, Lemercier M, Pouchin SC, Benmokhtar E, Vallet C, Cribier A et al (2011) Automated home telephone self-monitoring reduces hospitalization in patients with advanced heart failure. J Telemed Telecare 17:298–302
50. Lei W, Lo B, Yang GZ (2007) Multichannel reflective PPG earpiece sensor with passive motion cancellation. IEEE Trans Biomed Circuits Syst 1(4):235–241
51. Lin YH, Lin CF, You HZ (2011) A driver's physiological monitoring system based on a wearable PPG sensor and a smartphone. In: Chang RS, Kim T, Peng SL (eds) Security-enriched urban computing and smart grid. Communications in computer and information science, vol 223. Springer, Berlin, Heidelberg
52. Logan AG, McIsaac WJ, Tisler A, Irvine MJ, Saunders A, Dunai A et al (2007) Mobile phone-based remote patient monitoring system for management of hypertension in diabetic patients. AJH. 20(9):942–948
53. Martínez-Pérez B, de la Torre-Díez I, López-Coronado M, Herreros-González J (2013) Mobile apps in cardiology: review. JMIR Mhealth Uhealth 1(2):e15
54. Molinari G, Reboa G, Frascio M, Leoncini M, Rolandi A, Balzan C, Barsotti A (2002) The role of telecardiology in supporting the decision-making process of general practitioners during the management of patients with suspected cardiac events. J Telemed Telecare 8:97–101
55. Molinari G, Valbusa A, Terrizzano M, Bazzano M, Torelli L, Girardi N, Barsotti A (2004) Nine years' experience of telecardiology in primary care. J Telemed Telecare 10:249–253
56. Mozaffarian D, Benjamin EJ, Go AS, Arnett DK, Blaha MJ, Cushman M et al (2016) Heart disease and stroke statistics-2016 update a report from the American Heart Association. Circulation. https://doi.org/10.1161/CIR.0000000000000350
57. Nemati E, Deen MJ, Mondal T (2012) A wireless wearable ECG sensor for long-term applications. IEEE Commun Mag 50:36–43
58. Neubeck L, Lowres N, Benjamin EJ, Freedman SB, Coorey G, Redfern J (2015) The mobile revolution—using smartphone apps to prevent cardiovascular disease. Nat Rev Cardiol 12(6):350–360
59. Nikita KS (2013) Atherosclerosis: the evolving role of vascular image analysis. Comput Med Imaging Graph 37:1–3
60. Nikita KS (2014) Handbook of biomedical telemetry. Wiley, Wiley-IEEE Press
61. Nundy S, Razi RR, Dick JJ, Smith B, Mayo A, O'Connor A et al (2013) A text messaging intervention to improve heart failure self-management after hospital discharge in a largely African-American population: before-after study. J Med Internet Res. 15(3):e53
62. Park LG, Howie-Esquivel J, Chung ML, Dracup K (2014) A text messaging intervention to promote medication adherence for patients with coronary heart disease: a randomized controlled trial. Patient Educ Couns 94(2):261–268
63. Park C, Chou PH, Bai Y, Matthews R, Hibbs A (2006) An ultrawearable, wireless, low power ECG monitoring system. Paper presented at the IEEE biomedical circuits and systems conference, London, U.K., 29 Nov–1 Dec 2006
64. Patrick K, Raab F, Adams MA, Dillon L, Zabinski M, Rock CL et al (2009) A text message-based intervention for weight loss: randomized controlled trial. J Med Internet Res. 11(1):e1
65. Patterson JAC, McIlwraith DC, Yang GZ (2009) A flexible, low noise reflective PPG sensor platform for ear-worn heart rate monitoring. Paper presented at the 6th international workshop on wearable and implantable body sensor networks, Berkeley, 3–5 June 2009

66. Penders J, van de Molengraft J, Altini M, Yazicioglu F, Van Hoof C (2011) A low-power wireless ECG necklace for reliable cardiac activity monitoring on-the-move. Paper presented at the 33rd international conference of the IEEE engineering in medicine and biology society, Boston, USA, 30 Aug–3 Sept 2011
67. Peng RC, Yan WR, Zhang NL, Lin WH, Zhou XL, Zhang YT (2015) Cuffless and continuous blood pressure estimation from the heart sound signals. Sensors 15(9):23653–23666
68. Pfaeffli Dale L, Whittaker R, Jiang Y, Stewart R, Rolleston A, Maddison R (2015) Text message and internet support for coronary heart disease self-management: results from the Text4Heart randomized controlled trial. J Med Internet Res 17:e237
69. Pietrzak E, Cotea C, Pullman S (2014) Primary and secondary prevention of cardiovascular disease: is there a place for internet-based interventions? J Cardiopulm Rehabil Prev 34:303–317
70. Piotrowicz E, Jasionowska A, Banaszak-Bednarczyk M, Gwilkowska J, Piotrowicz R (2012) ECG telemonitoring during home-based cardiac rehabilitation in heart failure patients. J Telemed Telecare 18(4):193–197
71. Poh MZ, Kim K, Goessling A, Swenson S, Picard R (2012) Cardiovascular monitoring using earphones and a mobile device. IEEE Pervasive Comput 11:18–26
72. Poh MZ, Swenson NC, Picard RW (2010) Motion-tolerant magnetic earring sensor and wireless earpiece for wearable photoplethysmography. IEEE Trans Inf Technol Biomed 14:786–794
73. Poon CCY, Wong YM, Zhang YT (2006) M-health: the development of cuff-less and wearable blood pressure meters for use in body sensor networks. Paper presented at the IEEE/NLM life science systems and applications workshop, 13–14 July 2006
74. Quilici J, Fugon L, Beguin S, Morange PE, Bonnet JL, Alessi MC et al (2013) Effect of motivational mobile phone short message service on aspirin adherence after coronary stenting for acute coronary syndrome. Int J Cardiol 168(1):568–569
75. Ramachandran A, Snehalatha C, Ram J, Selvam S, Simon M, Nanditha A, Shetty AS, Godsland IF, Chaturvedi N, Majeed A, Oliver N, Toumazou C, Alberti KG, Johnston DG (2013) Effectiveness of mobile phone messaging in prevention of type 2 diabetes by lifestyle modification in men in India: a prospective, parallel-group, randomised controlled trial. Lancet Diab Endocrinol 1(3):191–198
76. Riegel B, Carlson B, Kopp Z, LePetri B, Glaser D, Unger A (2002) Effect of a standardized nurse case management telephone intervention on resource use in patients with chronic heart failure. Arch Intern Med 162:705–712
77. Roth A, Malov N, Steinberg DM, Yanay Y, Elizur M, Tamari M et al (2009) Telemedicine for post-myocardial infarction patients: an observational study. Telemed J E Health 15(1):24–30
78. Sanchez-Ross M, Oghlakian G, Maher J, Patel B, Mazza V, Hom D et al (2011) The STAT-MI (ST-segment analysis using wireless technology in acute myocardial infarction) trial improves outcomes. JACC Cardiovasc. Interv. 4:222–227
79. Scalvini S, Zanelli E (2002) Telecardiology: a new support for general practitioners in the management of elderly patients. Age Ageing 31:153
80. Scalvini S, Zanelli E, Conti C, Volterrani M, Pollina R, Giordano A et al (2002) Assessment of prehospital chest pain using telecardiology. J Telemed Telecare 8:231–236
81. Seo WK, Kang J, Jeon M, Lee K, Lee S, Kim JH et al (2015) Feasibility of using a mobile application for the monitoring and management of stroke-associated risk factors. J Clin Neurol 11(2):142–148
82. Seto E, Leonard KJ, Cafazzo JA, Barnsley J, Masino R, Ross HJ (2012) Mobile phone-based telemonitoring for heart failure management: a randomized controlled trial. J Med Internet Res 14(1):e31
83. Shah VN, Garg SK (2015) Managing diabetes in the digital age. ClinDiabetes Endocrinol 1(1):1–7
84. Shaltis PA, Reisner AT, Asada HH (2008) Cuffless blood pressure monitoring using hydrostatic pressure changes. IEEE Trans Biomed Eng 55(6):1775–1777

85. Shin JH, Lee KM, Park KS (2009) Non-constrained monitoring of systolic blood pressure on a weighing scale. Physiol Meas 30(7):679–693
86. Shin K, Kim Y, Bae S, Park K, Kim S (2009) A novel headset with a transmissive PPG sensor for heart rate measurement. In: Lim CT, Goh JCH (eds) 13th International conference on biomedical engineering. IFMBE Proceedings, vol 23. Springer, Berlin, Heidelberg
87. Silva BM, Rodrigues JJ, de la Torre Díez I, López-Coronado M, Saleem K (2015) Mobile-health: a review of current state in 2015. J Biomed Inform 56:265–272
88. Sohn S, Helms TM, Pelleter JT, Müller A, Kröttinger AI, Schöffski O (2012) Costs and benefits of personalized healthcare for patients with chronic heart failure in the care and education program "Telemedicine for the Heart". Telemed J E Health 18:198–204
89. Sood S, Mbarika V, Jugoo S, Dookhy R, Doarn CR, Prakash N et al (2007) What is telemedicine? A collection of 104 peer-reviewed perspectives and theoretical underpinnings. Telemed J E Health 13:573–590
90. Southard BH, Southard DR, Nuckolls J (2003) Clinical trial of an Internet-based case management system for secondary prevention of heart disease. J Cardiopulm Rehabil 23:341–348
91. Spigulis J, Erts R, Nikiforovs V, Kviesis-Kipge E (2008) Wearable wireless photoplethysmography sensors. Proc. SPIE, vol. 6991 (Photonics Europe, Strasbourg, FR), 6991120
92. Steventon A, Bardsley M, Billings J, Dixon J, Doll H, Hirani S, et al (2012) Effect of telehealth on use of secondary care and mortality: findings from the Whole System Demonstrator cluster randomised trial. BMJ 344:e3874
93. Stuckey M, Fulkerson R, Read E, Rusell-Minda E, Munoz C, Kleinstiver P et al (2011) Remote monitoring technologies for the prevention of metabolic syndrome: the diabetes and technology for increased activity (DaTA) study. J Diabetes Sci Technol 5(4):936–944
94. Thomas SS, Nathan V, Zong C, Soundarapandian K, Shi X, Jafari R (2016) BioWatch: a non-invasive wrist-based blood pressure monitor that incorporates training techniques for posture and subject variability. IEEE J Biomed Health Inform. 20(5):1291–1300
95. Varnfield M, Karunanithi M, Lee CK, Honeyman E, Arnold D, Ding H et al (2014) Smartphone-based home care model improved use of cardiac rehabilitation in postmyocardial infarction patients: results from a randomised controlled trial. Heart 100(22):1770–1779
96. Vernooij JW, Kaasjager HA, van der Graaf Y, Wierdsma J, Grandjean HM, Hovens MM et al (2012) Internet based vascular risk factor management for patients with clinically manifest vascular disease: randomised controlled trial. BMJ 344:1–13
97. Vogel S, Hulsbusch M, Hennig T, Blazek V, Leonhardt S (2009) In-ear vital signs monitoring using a novel microoptic reflective sensor. IEEE Trans Inf Technol Biomed 13:882–889
98. Waki K, Fujita H, Uchimura Y, Aramaki E, Omae K, Kadowaki K et al (2013) Dialbetics: smart phone-based self-management for type 2 diabetes patients. J Diabetes Sci Technol 6(4):983–985
99. Walter M, Eilebrecht B, Wartzek T, Leonhardt S (2011) The smart car seat: Personalized monitoring of vital signs in automotive applications. Pers Ubiquit Comput 15(7):707–715
100. de Waure C, Cadeddu C, Gualano MR, Ricciardi W (2012) Telemedicine for the reduction of myocardial infarction mortality: a systematic review and a meta-analysis of published studies. Telemed J E Health 18:323–328
101. WebMD (2012) Slideshow: top 11 medical expenses. http://www.webmd.com/healthy-aging/medical-cost-disability-11/slideshow. Accessed 12 Dec 2016
102. Widmer RJ, Allison TG, Lerman LO, Lerman A (2015) Digital health intervention as an adjunct to cardiac rehabilitation reduces cardiovascular risk factors and rehospitalizations. J Cardiovasc Transl Res 8(5):283–292
103. Winokur ES, Da He D, Sodini CG (2012) A wearable vital signs monitor at the ear for continuous heart rate and pulse transit time measurements. Paper presented at the 34th annual international conference of the IEEE engineering in medicine and biology society, San Diego, CA, 28 Aug–1 Sept 2012
104. World Health Organization (2016) Cardiovascular diseases. http://www.who.int/topics/cardiovascular_diseases/en/. Accessed 12 Dec 2016

105. Wu KF, Chan CH, Zhang YT (2006) Contactless and cuffless monitoring of blood pressure on a chair using e-textile materials. Paper presented at the 3rd IEEE/EMBS international summer school on medical devices and biosensors, Cambridge, MA, 4–6 Sept 2006
106. Wu Y-C, Chang C-S, Sawaguchi Y, Yu W-C, Chen M-J, Lin J-Y, et al (2011) A Mobile-Phone-Based Health Management System. https://doi.org/10.5772/20044
107. Yama Y, Ueno A, Uchikawa Y (2007) Development of a wireless capacitive sensor for ambulatory ECG monitoring over clothes. Paper presented at the 29th annual international conference of the IEEE engineering in medicine and biology society, Lyon, France, 22–26 Aug 2007
108. Yu J, Chen X (2017) Integrated application research about the necklace type wearable health sensing system under the internet of things. In: Yang C, Virk G, Yang H (eds) Wearable sensors and robots. Lecture notes in electrical engineering, vol 399. Springer, Singapore
109. Zhang YT, Poon CCH, Chan CH, Tsang MW, Wu KF (2006) A health-shirt using e-textile materials for the continuous and cuffless monitoring of arterial blood pressure. Paper presented at the 3rd IEEE/EMBS international summer school on medical devices and biosensors, 4–6 Sept 2006
110. Zheng YL, Ding XR, Poon CCY, Lo BPL, Zhang H, Zhou XL et al (2014) Unobtrusive sensing and wearable devices for health informatics. IEEE Trans Biomed Eng 61(5):1538–1584
111. Zheng YL, Yan BP, Zhang YT, Poon CCY (2014) An armband wearable device for overnight and cuff-less blood pressure measurement. IEEE Trans Biomed Eng 61(7):2179–2186
112. Zheng YL, Leung B, Sy S, Zhang YT, Poon CCY (2012) A clipfree eyeglasses-based wearable monitoring device for measuring photoplethysmographic signals. Paper presented at the 34th annual international conference of the IEEE engineering in medicine and biology society, San Diego, CA, 28 Aug–1 Sept 2012
113. Zutz A, Ignaszewski A, Bates J, Lear SA (2007) Utilization of the Internet to deliver cardiac rehabilitation at a distance: a pilot study. Telemed J E-Health 13:323–330

Artificial Intelligence and Data Mining Methods for Cardiovascular Risk Prediction

Eleni I. Georga, Nikolaos S. Tachos, Antonis I. Sakellarios, Vassiliki I. Kigka, Themis P. Exarchos, Gualtiero Pelosi, Oberdan Parodi, Lampros K. Michalis and Dimitrios I. Fotiadis

Abstract This chapter describes the state-of-the-art in artificial intelligence and machine learning methods for cardiovascular disease diagnosis and prognosis, focusing on Coronary Artery Disease (CAD). We aim at providing a cohesive overview of the existing methodologies in the topic and the most exploitable predictors for CAD staging and evolution. Thus, the relevant literature is analysed and contrasted with respect to the acquired dataset, the examined feature space, the employed predictive modelling schemes and their discriminative or predictive capacity. Moreover, important challenges stemming from the increasing ubiquity of electronic health records, personal health records and big data are discussed and, given the limitations of current approaches, future directions are delineated.

Keywords Machine learning · Artificial intelligence · Cardiovascular disease
Coronary artery disease · Atherosclerosis · Diagnosis · Prediction

---

E. I. Georga · V. I. Kigka · T. P. Exarchos · D. I. Fotiadis (✉)
Unit of Medical Technology and Intelligent Information Systems, Materials Science and Engineering Department, University of Ioannina, Ioannina 45110, Greece
e-mail: fotiadis@cc.uoi.gr

N. S. Tachos · A. I. Sakellarios · V. I. Kigka · D. I. Fotiadis
Biomedical Research Department, FORTH, Institute of Molecular Biology and Biotechnology, Ioannina 45110, Greece

G. Pelosi · O. Parodi
Institute of Clinical Physiology, National Research Council, Pisa 56124, Italy

L. K. Michalis
Department of Cardiology, Medical School, University of Ioannina, Ioannina 45110, Greece

S. Golemati and K. S. Nikita (eds.), *Cardiovascular Computing—Methodologies and Clinical Applications*, Series in BioEngineering,
https://doi.org/10.1007/978-981-10-5092-3_14

List of Abbreviations

ATS	Atherosclerosis
AUC	Area Under the ROC Curve
BMI	Body Mass Index
CA	Coronary Angiography
CAD	Coronary Artery Disease
CART	Classification and Regression Trees
CFS	Correlation-based Feature Selection
CTA	Computed Tomography Angiography
CVD	Cardiovascular Disease
DBN	Dynamic Bayesian Network
EHR	Electronic Health Record
FFNN	Feed-forward Neural Network
FRS	Framingham Risk Score
FURIA	Fuzzy Unordered Rule Induction Algorithm
GAM	Generalized Additive Model
GBT	Gradient Boosted Trees
HDL	High-density Lipoprotein
IVUS	Intravascular Ultrasound
LAD	Left Anterior Descending
LCX	Left Circumflex
LDL	Low-density Lipoprotein
LR	Logistic Regression
MRI	Magnetic Resonance Imaging
NPV	Negative Predictive Value
OCT	Optical Coherence Tomography
PHR	Personal Health Record
PPV	Positive Predictive Value
RBF	Radial Basis Function Network
RCA	Right Coronary Artery
RF	Random Forest
ROC	Receiver Operating Curve
RTF	Rotation Forest
SMOTE	Synthetic Minority Oversampling Technique
SOFM	Self-organizing Feature Map
SVM	Support Vector Machine
TA	Temporal Abstraction

1 Introduction

According to the World Health Organisation approximately 45% of total deaths in Europe are caused by cardiovascular disease (CVD), while 20% of total deaths occur in coronary artery disease (CAD) patients. CAD diagnosis is validated through invasive coronary angiography (CA); however, different invasive (e.g. intravascular ultrasound [IVUS], optical coherence tomography [OCT]) and non-invasive imaging modalities (e.g. computed tomography angiography [CTA], magnetic resonance imaging [MRI]) are nowadays available to visualize the vessel wall, quantify the plaque burden and characterize the type of the atherosclerotic plaque. CAD is a multi-factorial disease characterized by the accumulation of lipids into the arterial wall and the subsequent inflammatory response [1, 2]. The phenotype of disease progression is affected by several factors, including clinical risk factors (gender, smoking, hyperlipidaemia, hypertension, diabetes), but also molecular, biohumoral and biomechanical factors, such as the low endothelial shear stress. According to the guidelines of the European Society of Cardiology and the American Heart Association, the early prevention, diagnosis and prediction of disease stage may have a potential influence to the patient health status, but also may reduce the healthcare costs for the management and treatment of CAD patients [3, 4].

Predicting the risk of CVD constitutes a widely-studied problem from the perspective of statistical modelling. The majority of existing risk models, such as the Framingham risk score (FRS) [5], the Systematic COronary Risk Evaluation (SCORE) [6] and the QRISK [7], postulate a Cox proportional hazard regression or logistic regression (LR) model of relatively few traditional predictors of the disease, focusing on CAD or CVD. Most frequently applied predictor variables describe information on family history, lifestyle, comorbidities, blood pressure, physical examinations and blood lipids; whereas, other blood variables, treatment and genetics are less frequently exploited. In spite of the reported good discrimination ability of such parametric regression models, a recent systematic review demonstrated the paucity of external validation and head-to-head comparisons, the poor reporting of their technical characteristics as well as the variability in outcome variables, predictors and prediction horizons, which limits their applicability in evidence-based decision making in healthcare [8]. More importantly: (i) precision medicine suggests more dynamic individualized nonlinear predictive modelling approaches not being hypotheses-driven, and (ii) the increasing availability of electronic health records (EHRs), personal health records (PHRs) and omics big data give rise to multiscale multi parametric predictive big data analytics. In this context, artificial intelligence and machine learning naturally arise as favourable solutions to CVD risk prediction.

A case study addressing the prediction of in hospital mortality after diagnosis of acute myocardial infarction illustrated the main shortcomings of statistical methods, including non-linearity and homogeneity of interactions, as well as the challenges introduced to machine learning by CVD risk prediction models [9]. Classical machine learning and data mining techniques can be certainly employed to solve a variety of classification, regression, clustering and rule mining problems related to personalized medicine in cardiovascular research and clinical practice [10–23]. Moreover, the potential for utilizing big data analytics to improve cardiovascular health care and the emerging literature on CVD risk predictive modelling has been discussed in [24, 25].

In this chapter, we provide an overview of the state of the art on data-driven solutions to CAD diagnosis and prognosis focusing on studies employing non-imaging data. Methodological and technical issues pertaining to the development and evaluation of such models are described in detail, whereas special emphasis is placed on the predictive value of the examined feature sets and on how complex input-output interactions can be captured by the different algorithms. Our aim is to provide a clear picture of the existing methodologies to CAD diagnosis or prediction contributing to synthesizing innovative predictive schemes.

2 Non-imaging CAD Diagnosis Based on Machine Learning Methods

The diagnosis of clinically significant (obstructive) CAD is typically formulated as a binary classification problem on the basis of a confined set of features (e.g. imaging, clinical, laboratory and demographic data), with a $\geq$50% diameter stenosis in at least one main coronary artery vessel, as assessed by CA or other imaging modality, characterizing patients with CAD. Herein, we provide an overview of the literature studies approaching the CAD diagnosis problem through artificial intelligence and non-imaging procedures of data acquisition (Table 1).

Machine learning algorithms, ranging from parametric (e.g. neural networks, dynamic Bayesian networks [DBN], decision trees) to non-parametric (e.g. kernel methods) ones, have been examined towards discriminating subjects with respect to CAD existence. Feature evaluation techniques, such as filter to wrapper approaches are used, in conjunction with classification or regression algorithms, to identify the most informative features with respect to the CAD diagnosis or prediction. Kurt et al. demonstrated that a feature set comprised of traditional heart disease risk factors (i.e. age, sex, body mass index [BMI], smoking status, diabetes, hypertension, hypercholesterolemia, family history of CAD) yields predictions of low specificity, though a high sensitivity is obtained, irrespective of the employed classification algorithm [15]. More specifically, the overall accuracy of LR, classification and regression trees (CART), and feed-forward neural networks (FFNN) was comparable (~80%), whereas radial basis function network (RBF) exhibited a slightly lower performance; on the other hand, self-organizing feature maps (SOFM) behaved inaccurately regarding the identification of negative samples resulting in 7.4% specificity.

More comprehensive datasets, exploited by purely nonlinear classifiers, can improve substantially the accuracy of predictions. In that case, feature subset selection becomes a prerequisite for avoiding overfitting stemming from the increased input size. Correlation-based feature selection (CFS) using particle swarm optimization identified Duke Treadmill Score and post exercise recovery period with

Table 1 Characteristic non-imaging CAD diagnosis methods based on machine learning methods

Study	Dataset	Outcome	Methods	Feature set	Performance		
Kurt et al. [15]	n = 1245 subjects with angina associated with evidence for myocardial ischemia **Exclusion criteria**: Non-atherosclerotic CAD	**Class I—CAD (n = 865)**: ≥50% stenosis in at least one coronary artery vessel in CA **Class II—Normal (n = 380)**: Otherwise	**Classification**: LR, CART, FFNN, RBF, SOFM **Evaluation**: Training, test, validation sets (60%–20%–20%)	Age, sex, BMI, smoking status, diabetes mellitus, systemic hypertension, hypercholesterolemia, family history of CAD	**LR** Acc. (%) 79.5 Se. (%) 92.3 Sp. (%) 45.6	**CART** Acc. (%) 79.9 Se. (%) 92.3 Sp. (%) 47.1	**FFNN** Acc. (%) 79.1 Se. (%) 91.7 Sp. (%) 45.6
					RBF Acc. (%) 76.7 Se. (%) 89.5 Sp. (%) 42.6	**SOFM** Acc. (%) 73.9 Se. (%) 98.9 Sp. (%) 7.4	
Tsipouras et al. [26]	n = 199 subjects who were suspected for CAD **Exclusion Criteria**: Acute coronary syndrome, known CAD, or more than mild valvular heart disease	**Class I—Significant CAD** (**n = 110**):≥ 50% diameter stenosis in at least one coronary artery vessel. **Class II—Absence of CAD** (**n = 89**): Completely smooth epicardial coronary arteries without any narrowing visible in CA	**Optimized fuzzy model** 1. Decision tree (C4.5) induction 2. Extraction of the rule base from the tree 3. Development of a fuzzy model 4. Optimization of the fuzzy model's parameters **Evaluation**: ten-fold stratified cross-validation	Age, sex, family history, smoking, diabetes mellitus, hypertension, hyperlipidaemia, creatinine, glucose, total cholesterol, HDL, Triglycerides, BMI, waist, heart rate, systolic blood pressure, diastolic blood pressure, carotid femoral pulse wave velocity, augmentation index	Acc. (%) 73.4 Se. (%) 80.0 Sp. (%) 65.2		

(continued)

Table 1 (continued)

Study	Dataset	Outcome	Methods	Feature set	Performance
Anooj 2012 [27]	The UCI heart disease dataset ($n = 303$)—Cleveland data Hungarian data Switzerland data	**Class I—Existence of heart disease**:$\geq$ 50% diameter stenosis in at least one coronary artery vessel Cleveland data: 46% positive cases Hungarian data: 37.5% positive cases Switzerland data: 93.5% positive cases **Class II—Absence of heart disease**: otherwise Cleveland data: 54% positive cases Hungarian data: 62.5% positive cases Switzerland data: 6.5% positive cases	**Automated generation of weighted fuzzy rules**: Mamdani fuzzy inference system **Evaluation**: Training-Test sets	**Cleeveland data** Age, resting blood pressure, serum cholesterol, maximum heart rate achieved (Thalach), ST depression induced by exercise relative to rest, Thal (Categorical variable, normal: 3; fixed defect: 6; reversible defect:7)	**Cleeveland data** Acc. (%) 62.4 Se. (%) 44.7 Sp. (%) 76.6
				Hungarian data Age, resting blood pressure, serum cholesterol, resting electrocardiographic results, maximum heart rate achieved (Thalach), exercise induced angina, ST depression induced by exercise relative to rest, slope of the peak exercise ST segment	**Hungarian data** Acc. (%) 46.9 Se. (%) 74.3 Sp. (%) 31.7

(continued)

Table 1 (continued)

Study	Dataset	Outcome	Methods	Feature set	Performance
				Switzerland data Age, sex, chest pain type, resting blood pressure, fasting blood glucose, resting electrocardiographic results, maximum heart rate achieved (Thalach), ST depression induced by exercise relative to rest, slope of the peak exercise ST segment, number of major vessels, Thal (Categorical variable, normal: 3; fixed defect: 6; reversible defect:7)	**Switzerland data** Acc. (%) 51.2 Se. (%) 52.6 Sp. (%) 33.3
Karabulut and Ibrikci [28]	The UCI heart disease dataset ($n = 303$)	**Class I—Existence of heart disease (*n* = 165)** :≥ 50% diameter stenosis **Class II—Absence of heart disease (*n* = 138)**: otherwise	**Classification**: RTF with FFNNs as the base classifier **Evaluation**: ten-fold cross-validation	Age, sex, chest pain type, resting systolic blood pressure, serum cholesterol, fasting blood glucose, resting electrocardiographic results, maximum heart rate achieved, exercise induced angina, ST depression induced by exercise relative to rest, slope of the peak exercise ST segment, number of major vessels coloured by fluoroscopy, exercise thallium scintigraphic defects	Acc. (%) 91.2 Se. (%) 95.6 Sp. (%) 86.7 AUC 0.915
Nahar et al. [29]	The UCI heart disease dataset ($n = 303$)	**Class I—Existence of heart disease**:≥ 50% diameter stenosis **Class II—Absence of heart disease**: otherwise	**Feature Selection**: CFS, knowledge-based feature selection (MFS) **Classification**: SMO **Evaluation**: Approach I ten-fold cross-validation Approach II training—test sets (66–33%) combined with internal ten-fold cross-validation for hyper-parameter optimization	**CFS** Old peak, number of vessels coloured, Thal (categorical variable, normal: 3; fixed defect: 6; reversible defect: 7)	Approach II - MFS: Acc. (%) 77.95 Se. (%) 81.1

(continued)

Table 1 (continued)

Study	Dataset	Outcome	Methods	Feature set	Performance	
				Knowledge-based feature selection (MFS) Age, chest pain type, resting blood pressure, cholesterol, fasting blood glucose, resting heart rate, maximum heart rate, and exercise induced angina	Approach II - MFS combined with CFS: Acc. (%) 83.83 Se. (%) 91.9	
Alizadehsani et al. [30]	$n = 303$ subjects	**Class I—CAD (*n* = 865)**:≥ 50% stenosis in at least one coronary artery vessel in CA **Class II—Normal (*n* = 380)**: Otherwise	**Feature selection**: Embedded in SVM weights **Classification**: SVM, Naïve Bayes, bagging of SVMs, FFNN **Association rule mining**: Apriori **Evaluation**: ten-fold cross-validation	Typical chest pain, region with regional wall motion abnormality*, age, ejection fraction*, hypertension, diabetes, T inversion, erythrocyte sedimentation rate, Q wave, ST elevation, pulse rate, BMI, lymph, blood pressure*, dyspnoea, HDL, creatinine*, white blood cell*, weight, valvular heart disease, function class, airway disease, haemoglobin, triglycerides*, bundle branch block, Na*, sex, Left ventricular hypertrophy, haemoglobin*, family history	**SVM** Acc. (%) 93.39 ± 5.14 Se. (%) 95.37 Sp. (%) 88.51	**Bagging SVM** Acc. (%) 92.74 ± 6.43 Se. (%) 95.37 Sp. (%) 86.21
					FFNN Acc. (%) 87.13 ± 5.84 Se. (%) 90.28 Sp. (%) 79.31	**Naïve Bayes** Acc. (%) 55.37 ± 9.62 Se. (%) 38.89 Sp. (%) 96.55

(continued)

Table 1 (continued)

Study	Dataset	Outcome	Methods	Feature set	Performance	
Alizadehsani et al. [30]	$n = 303$ subjects	**Class I—CAD ($n = 865$):**$\geq 50\%$ stenosis in at least one coronary artery vessel in CA **Class II—Normal ($n = 380$):** Otherwise	**Feature selection**: Embedded in SVM weights **Classification**: SVM, Naïve Bayes, bagging of SVMs, FFNN **Association rule mining**: Apriori **Evaluation**: ten-fold cross-validation	Typical chest pain, region with regional wall motion abnormality*, age, ejection fraction*, hypertension, diabetes, T inversion, erythrocyte sedimentation rate, Q wave, ST elevation, pulse rate, BMI, lymph, blood pressure*, dyspnoea, HDL, creatinine*, white blood cell*, weight, valvular heart disease, function class, airway disease, haemoglobin, triglycerides*, bundle branch block, Na*, sex, Left ventricular hypertrophy, haemoglobin*, family history		
Alizadehsani et al. [31]	$n = 303$	**Problem I** Class I—LAD stenotic: $\geq 50\%$ stenosis in LAD artery Class II—LAD normal: Otherwise **Problem II** Class I—LCX stenotic: $\geq 50\%$ stenosis in LCX artery Class II—LCX normal: Otherwise **Problem III** Class I—RCA stenotic: $\geq 50\%$ diameter stenosis in RCA artery Class II—RCA normal: Otherwise	**Feature selection** Approach I Different feature set for each artery: SVM weights Approach II Common feature set for all arteries: Information Gain **Classification**: SVM with kernel fusion **Association rule mining**: Apriori **Evaluation**: ten-fold cross-validation	**Feature selection approach II** Typical chest pain, atypical chest pain, ejection fraction, region with regional wall motion abnormality, age, valvular heart disease, diabetes, hypertension, T inversion, lymphocyte, fasting blood glucose*, neutrophil, blood pressure, Nonanginal chest pain, fasting blood glucose, erythrocyte sedimentation rate, Na, K, creatinine, creatinine*, blood urea nitrogen, ST elevation, white blood cell count, neutrophil*, Q wave, white blood cell*, weight	**Feature selection approach I**	**Feature selection approach II**

(continued)

Table 1 (continued)

Study	Dataset	Outcome	Methods	Feature set	Performance	
					LAD Acc. (%) 85.81 ± 1.7 Se. (%) 92.66 ± 1.9 Sp. (%) 76.19 ± 1.2	LAD Acc. (%) 86.14 ± 1.1 Se. (%) 90.96 ± 0.9 Sp. (%) 79.37 ± 1.4
					LCX Acc. (%) 77.23 ± 1.6 Se. (%) 69.75 ± 1.9 Sp. (%) 82.07 ± 1.9	LCX Acc. (%) 83.17 ± 0.4 Se. (%) 90.96 ± 0.3 Sp. (%) 72.22 ± 0.6
					RCA Acc. (%) 81.85 ± 0.4 Se. (%) 68.42 ± 0.6 Sp. (%) 89.95 ± 0.1	RCA Acc. (%) 83.50 ± 0.8 Se. (%) 87.01 ± 1.2 Sp. (%) 78.57 ± 0.7
Verma et al. [32]	$n = 335$ subjects who were suspected for CAD	**Class I—CAD (48.9%)** **Class II—No CAD (51.1%)**	**Feature Selection**: CFS with particle swarm optimization **Clustering**: k-means **Classification**: FFNN, LR, Fuzzy unordered rule induction algorithm (FURIA), Decision tree (C4.5) **Evaluation**: ten-fold cross-validation	Smoking, diabetes, HDL, duke treadmill score, duration of recovery with persistent ST changes	**FFNN** Acc. (%) 88.40	**FURIA** Acc. (%) 82.80
					LR Acc. (%) 84.11	**C4.5** Acc. (%) 80.68

Acc accuracy, *Se* sensitivity, *Sp* specificity
* Discretized according to “Braunwald’s heart disease: a textbook of cardiovascular medicine”

persistent electrocardiographic ST-segment changes, following a treadmill stress testing, amongst the most informative features with respect to CAD diagnosis [32]. In particular, a FFNN fed additionally with information on smoking, diabetes, and high-density lipoprotein (HDL) attains 88.4% accuracy. Besides filter-based feature selection methods, feature selection embedded in learning algorithms have been applied to reduce the dimensionality of the feature space. The two-stage methodology by Alizadehsani et al. encompassed: (i) an evaluation of the discriminative capability of 54 features concerning demographic, clinical, electrocardiographic, echocardiographic, and laboratory data based on the support vector machine (SVM) weight vector, and (ii) a comparative study of the performance of four algorithms including naïve Bayes, SVM, bagging SVM, and FFNN [30]. The kernel-based methods (i.e. SVM and bagging SVM) outperformed both FFNN and naïve Bayes, exhibiting 93.4 and 92.7% accuracy as well as high sensitivity and specificity rates. In a subsequent study, Alizadehsani et al. examined the diagnostic accuracy of the same feature set with respect to the level of stenosis of each coronary artery [i.e. left anterior descending (LAD) artery, left circumflex (LCX) artery and right coronary artery (RCA)] separately, formulating a 2-class problem where a $\geq$50% diameter stenosis characterizes a stenotic artery [31]. In particular, (i) a common feature set was used for the diagnosis of the stenosis of each coronary artery, encompassing the 24 top ranked features according to a combined info-gain index, and (ii) a new multiple kernel learning algorithm was proposed to define the most appropriate hyperplane which may classify the dataset. The stenosis of LAD, LCX and RCA is diagnosed with 86.14%, 83.17% and 83.5% accuracy, respectively. On the other hand, Nahar et al. [29], using the UCI Cleveland heart disease dataset, showed that knowledge-based feature selection is an asset for the diagnosis of heart disease [33]. Nahar et al. decomposed the 5-class problem into 5 binary classification problems, which were solved employing well-known classification algorithms, i.e. naïve Bayes, SVM, k-nearest neighbour algorithm, Adaboost.M1, J48 decision tree, and PART rule-based classifier. The results indicated that: (i) the best performing algorithm in the case where the whole feature set is considered was SVM, and (ii) feature selection enhances the accuracy for the majority of algorithms and for all binary problems.

Ensemble learning of the UCI Cleveland heart disease dataset, when focusing on the heart disease diagnosis problem (Class 0 vs. Class1–4), has been shown to improve the accuracy of FFNN [29, 34]; an ensemble of three FFNNs yielded 89.01% accuracy, 80.95% sensitivity and 95.91% specificity, whereas rotation forest (RTF) using FFNN as the base classifier improved its accuracy by 7% reaching 91.2%.

Unlike most machine learning techniques, fuzzy rule-based classifiers provide interpretable decision making. To that end, Tsipouras et al. proposed an optimized fuzzy model for the diagnosis of CAD considering traditional cardiovascular risk factors as well as two non-invasive indices of pulse wave velocity, namely carotid–femoral and augmentation index. A four-stage methodology was developed including: (i) induction of a decision tree, (ii) extraction of the rule base from the decision tree, in disjunctive normal form and formulation of a crisp model, (iii) transformation of the crisp set of rules into a fuzzy model, and (iv) optimization of the parameters of the fuzzy model [26]. The optimized fuzzy model resulted in 73.4% accuracy, 80.0% sensitivity and 65.2% specificity, exhibiting comparable performance with a FFNN (73.9% accuracy) and significantly better results than an adaptive neuro-fuzzy inference system (56.8% accuracy), both applied to the same task.

3 Non-imaging CAD Prediction Based on Machine Learning Methods

Prediction of CAD development or CAD progression can be also viewed as a classification problem which involves a temporal dimension. The existing machine learning predictive modelling approaches of CAD, which are based on non-imaging data, utilize information obtained either at a specific time instance t (at baseline) or up to a specific time instance t in order to predict one patient's status at time $t+h$ (at follow-up), where h is the prediction horizon, typically, expressed in years. Well-designed prospective clinical studies constitute the standard data source of CAD prediction machine learning methods. Nevertheless, the consolidation of EHRs have inspired researchers to explore longitudinal patient health information from EHRs towards constructing data-driven CAD risk prediction models. The studies presented in this section are representative of the spectrum of methodologies which are employed in the related literature (Table 2).

Exarchos et al. assembled and analyzed a multivariate dataset aiming at: (i) identifying the most significant features towards the progression of atherosclerosis (ATS), and (ii) developing a decision support system inferencing the prognosis of the disease [35]. Patients underwent angiographic assessment by CTA or CA both at the baseline visit as well as during the follow-up, whereas demographic data, clinical data, standard biohumoral analytes, adhesion molecules, markers of monocyte activation, and therapy, were measured at the same time-slices. To this end, Exarchos et al. defined two binary outcome variables capturing the severity and progression of ATS: (i) number of stenoses: Binary variable indicating whether any coronary vessels exhibit stenosis >50%, (ii) ATS progression: Binary variable indicating whether the number or percentage of stenosis in any vessel increased from the baseline to the follow-up visit. A hybrid score is also utilized according to which each patient is assigned a severity level in the range [0, ..., 17], with 17 denoting the most severe condition. In addition, two analysis axes were defined. The first one concerns the solution of the binary classification problem employing baseline data and encompasses: (i) class imbalance handling through the synthetic minority oversampling technique (SMOTE), (ii) feature selection by the CFS, gain ratio and wrapper algorithms, and (iii) evaluation and comparison of a multitude of classification algorithms (i.e. Bayesian network, naïve Bayes, FFNN, SVM, decision tree, and random forest [RF]). The second axis of analysis considers temporal modelling of the information obtained both at baseline and follow-up visits by DBN. The results pertaining to the first analysis axis indicated that naïve Bayes yields the highest performance, 91.7%

Table 2 Characteristic non-imaging CAD prediction methods based on machine learning methods

Study	Dataset	Outcome	Methods	Feature Set	Performance
Exarchos et al. [35]	$n = 39$ subjects **Average follow-up time**: 31.4 ± 17.2 months	**Problem I—Number of stenoses**: Binary variable indicating whether one or more coronary vessels exhibit stenosis >50% **Problem II—ATS progression**: Binary variable indicating whether the number or percentage of stenosis in any vessel increased from the baseline to the follow-up visit **Problem III—Hybrid score**: Each patient is assigned a severity level in the range [0,…17], with 17 denoting the most severe condition	**Axis I—Baseline analysis**: Baseline information is used to predict the progression of ATS **Resampling**: SMOTE algorithm **Feature selection**: CFS, gain ratio algorithm, wrapper algorithm **Classification**: Bayesian network, Naïve Bayes, FFNN, SVM, Decision tree, RF **Evaluation**: ten-fold cross-validation, leave 1 patient out	**Axis I**: **Problem I** Age, sex, weight, diabetes, family history, left ventricular ejection fraction, cholesterol, HDL, creatinine clearance, glucose. E-selectin, vascular cell adhesion molecule 1 (VCAM-1), beta-blockers, statins **Problem II** Weight, diabetes, hypertension, smoke, FRS, infarct site, cholesterol, statins **Problem III** Hypercholesterolemia, hypertension, monocytes, ca antagonists	**Axis I**: **Problem I** Wrapper and Naïve Bayes Acc. (%) 91.7 Se. (%) 93.3 Sp. (%) 90% PPV(%) 90.3 AUC 0.944 **Problem II** CFS and Naïve Bayes Acc. (%) 93.3 Se. (%) 96.7 Sp. (%) 90% PPV (%) 90.6 AUC 0.937

(continued)

Table 2 (continued)

Study	Dataset	Outcome	Methods	Feature Set		Performance	
			Axis II—Temporal analysis: Snapshots of the patient's status over the follow-up period are analyzed to model ATS evolvement **Resampling**: SMOTE algorithm Statistical testing: Chi-square test, Fischer's test **Temporal analysis**: DBN	**Axis II**: **Problem I** Diabetes, hypercholesterolemia, total cholesterol to HDL ratio, triglycerides, Glucose **Problem II** Diabetes, low-density lipoprotein (LDL), infarct site, creatinine, creatinine clearance, monocytes, Total cholesterol to HDL ratio, white blood cell, Smoke		**Axis II**: **Problem I** Acc. (%) 79 **Problem II** Acc. (%) 83	
Weng et al. [19]	$n = 378256$ subjects free from cardiovascular disease at outset	The first recorded diagnosis of a fatal or non-fatal cardio-vascular event over 10 years ($n = 24970$)	**Feature selection**: Ranking mechanism embedded into machine learning classification algorithms **Classification**: RF, LR, gradient boosting machines, FFNN **Evaluation**: Training-Test sets	**RF** Age, gender, ethnicity, smoking, HDL, glycated haemoglobin (HbA1c), triglycerides, townsend deprivation index, BMI, total cholesterol	**LR** Ethnicity, age, townsend deprivation index, gender, smoking, atrial fibrillation, chronic kidney disease, rheumatoid arthritis, family history of premature CAD, chronic obstructive pulmonary disease	**RF** Se. (%) 65.3% Sp. (%) 70.5% PPV(%) 17.8% NPV(%) 95.4% AUC 0.745	**Gradient boosting machines** Se. (%) 67.5% Sp. (%) 70.7% PPV(%) 18.4% NPV(%) 95.7% AUC 0.761

(continued)

Table 2 (continued)

Study	Dataset	Outcome	Methods	Feature Set		Performance		
				Gradient boosting machines Age, gender, ethnicity, smoking, HDL, triglycerides, total cholesterol, glycated haemoglobin (HbA1c), systolic blood pressure, townsend deprivation index	**FFNN** Atrial fibrillation, ethnicity, oral corticosteroid prescribed, age, severe mental illness, townsend deprivation index, chronic kidney disease, bmi, smoking, gender	**LR** Se. (%) 67.1% Sp. (%) 70.7% PPV(%) 18.3% NPV(%) 95.6% AUC 0.760	**FFNN** Se. (%) 67.5% Sp. (%) 70.7% PPV(%) 18.4% NPV(%) 95.7% AUC 0.764	
Kennedy et al. [36]	$n = 113973$ subjects **Exclusion criteria**: Cerebrovascular disease or CVD diagnosis or event during the baseline year	Occurrence of a fatal cerebrovascular or CVD event over a 5-year period ($n = 4995$)	**Feature selection**: Three feature sets were explored: 1. Feature set 1: Traditional risk predictors 2. Feature set 2: Traditional risk predictors and Medication 3. Feature set 3: Traditional risk predictors, medication, and labs/vital signs/diagnoses/other **Classification**: FRS, LR, GAM, GBT **Evaluation**: ten-fold cross-validation	**Traditional risk predictors**: Age, male, Systolic BP, Total cholesterol to HDL ratio, Diabetes **Medication**: Hypertension, Lipids, Diabetes, Narcotics or opiates, Benzodiazepines, Levothyroxines, Anticoagulants **Labs/vital signs/diagnoses/other**: Albumin, blood urea nitrogen, LDL, serum creatinine, pulse, pulse pressure, baseline diagnoses: chronic obstructive pulmonary disease, periodontitis, inflammatory arthritis, sleep apnea, body mass index, number of visits		**Feature set 1**	**Feature set 2**	**Feature set 3**

(continued)

Table 2 (continued)

Study	Dataset	Outcome	Methods	Feature Set	Performance		
					FRS AUC(%) 71.3 ± 1.0 ***LR*** AUC(%) 72.6 ± 1.0 ***GAM*** AUC(%) 73.1 ± 0.9 ***GBT*** AUC(%) 73.1 ± 0.9	***FRS*** AUC(%) - ***LR*** AUC(%) 74.3 ± 0.8 ***GAM*** AUC(%) 74.8 ± 0.7 ***GBT*** AUC(%) 74.9 ± 0.7	***FRS*** AUC(%) - ***LR*** AUC(%) 76.3 ± 1.0 ***GAM*** AUC(%) 77.5 ± 0.9 ***GBT*** AUC(%) 77.8 ± 0.9
Orphanou et al. [37]	STULONG dataset—849 men monitored from 2 to 21 years	Occurence of CAD event in the last 3 years of the total observation period (21 years)	Prediction of the risk of a patient suffering a CAD event during a particular time period t, based on the patient's medical history up to time t-1 **Resampling**: SMOTE-N oversampling with clustering undersampling **Feature selection**: Knowledge-based **Temporal abstractions derivation** (State, trend and persistence TAs) **Classification**: Extended DBN **Evaluation**: k-fold cross-validation	Age, blood pressure, dyslipidemia levels, obesity history, diabetes history, cholesterol and hypertension medication, smoking, diet, exercise	Precision: 0.7207 Recall: 0.75 F1 score: 0.7351 AUC: 0.778		

Acc accuracy, *Se* sensitivity, *Sp* specificity

and 93.3%, for the prediction of both the number of stenoses and ATS progression, respectively. With regard to the temporal analysis, DBN provided a satisfactory accuracy of 87 and 84% for the two aforementioned outcome variables. Nevertheless, Exarchos et al. note that the application of the SMOTE algorithm might have introduced an overestimation of the performance metrics.

Identifying patients at high risk of a CVD event in the follow-up period constitutes a different endpoint than estimating asymptomatic CAD progression. Recently, Weng et al. evaluated four machine-learning algorithms (i.e. RF, LR, gradient boosting machines and FFNNs) with respect to the prediction of first CVD event over a 10-year follow-up period on EHR data of a cohort of patients ($n = 378256$), who were free from cardiovascular disease at outset [19]. In total, 30 variables, concerning patient's characteristics, clinical and laboratory data, CVD risk factors, history, lifestyle and medications, with potential to be associated with CVD were examined. Their importance was determined by the embedded in each algorithm mechanisms of feature ranking, and the overall ranking was consistent with the standard risk factors included in the American College of Cardiology/American Heart Association (ACC/AHA) model. Compared with the established recommendations on the assessment of cardiovascular risk by the ACC/AHA [38], a considerable improvement in the area under the receiver operating curve (AUC) measure was obtained: RF +1.7% (AUC 0.745), LR +3.2% (AUC 0.760), gradient boosting +3.3% (AUC 0.761), FFNN +3.6% (AUC 0.764). More specifically, the highest achieving algorithm, i.e. FFNN, featured 67.5% sensitivity, 70.7% specificity, 18.4% positive predictive value (PPV) and 95.7% negative predictive value (NPV), resulting in a net increase of 355 true positive CVD cases (4,998 out of 7,404 total CVD cases) as compared with ACC/AHA model (sensitivity 62.7%, specificity 70.3%, PPV 17.1%, NPV 95.1%).

Similarly, a systematic comparative study of modelling approaches for predicting the risk of a fatal cardiovascular event over a 5-year period based on comprehensive EHR data demonstrated the predominance of gradient boosted trees over the FRS; the AUC increased from 71 to 78% [36]. In particular, the predictive capacity of traditional risk factors (i.e. age, gender, systolic blood pressure, total cholesterol to HDL ratio, diabetes) along with medication information, laboratory and clinical data, was examined, with non-parametric algorithms (i.e. generalized additive model [GAM], gradient boosted trees [GBT]) capturing better the relationships in the feature set as its size increases. Nevertheless, we should note that in the two aforementioned studies the values of all features were recorded during the baseline year, without exploring the longitudinal nature of EHR data.

From a different perspective, Orphanou et al. proposed a dynamic approach to CAD prognosis integrating DBN and temporal abstractions (TAs) and which has been applied to a longitudinal benchmark dataset [37]. In particular, the STULONG dataset comprises from 1 to 20 examinations for each patient, which corresponds to 1–24 years of clinical monitoring. Essentially, the proposed approach consisted of the following steps: (i) data pre-processing and knowledge-based feature selection, (ii) derivation of basic TAs (state, trend, and persistence TAs), and (iii) deployment and evaluation of the extended DBN. The selected feature set, which was incorporated into the extended DBN, contained information on well-established CAD risk factors; namely, hypertension, smoking status, dyslipidaemia level, obesity, diabetes, patient's and family history, age, hypertension and high-cholesterol medication, diet, and exercise. The maximum observation period was set equal to 21 years, whereas the outcome variable describes the occurrence of CAD event in the last 3 years of the total observation period (19–21 years). Therefore, the examined problem is postulated as follows: prediction of the risk of a patient suffering a CAD event during a particular time period $\Delta t = [t, t + 2]$, based on the patient's medical history up to time t. Orphanou et al. applied two oversampling methods (SMOTE, random oversampling of the minority class) as well as a combination of oversampling with undersampling (SMOTE combined with k = 2-means clustering undersampling, random oversampling combined with k = 2-means clustering undersampling), aiming at addressing the class imbalance problem. A 72% precision accompanied with a 75% recall and 74% F1 score were obtained for the combination of random oversampling with k = 2-means clustering undersampling. Moreover, the extended DBN model outperformed a DBN model without TAs applied to the same task.

4 Discussion and Future Trends

CAD diagnosis is currently performed according to well-known screening strategies (i.e. CA, IVUS, OCT, CTA, MRI), whereas CVD risk can be assessed by linear regression models of baseline clinical, laboratory and anthropometric features, assuming linearity as well as time-invariance of the underlying input-output relationships. Nonlinearity is addressed by black-box parameterizations (neural networks and kernel-based models) or more transparent architectures (decision trees, DBN) or ensembles of classification models (RF, RTF), which feature space, however, resembles that of linear approaches (i.e. established risk factors). The generalization capability of the existing machine learning models for the diagnosis of CAD or the estimation of eventful or asymptomatic CAD progression is promising; however, no consensus has been reached on feature learning and model identification and validation.

New research approaches to CVD risk prediction can be enhanced as follows:

i. First, the input space can be partitioned into coherent and well-separated clusters which portray the innate data similarities or structures. Unsupervised learning (k-means, expectation maximization clustering, hierarchical agglomerative clustering) can be investigated towards identifying groups of patients with similar characteristics, especially for omics data, or organize patients into a hierarchy of clusters. Profile analysis can also rely on pattern mining aiming at identifying dynamic dependencies into genomics, clinical, biohumoral, molecular/cellular, and environmental/lifestyle information, which may have a prognostic relevance in CAD. Especially longitudinal data trajectories (PHRs, EHRs) has to be explored for co-occurrence relationships (static data analytics) as well as sequences of events (dynamic data analytics) aiming at inferring high-level context describing a patient or a group of individuals [39]. For this purpose, innovative temporal pattern mining algorithms have been proposed that consider the temporal dimension of the data [40–45] as well as deep-learning approaches to EHRs representation [46].

ii. Second, special emphasis should be placed to the identification of a minimum subset of the most informative features, aiming at, eventually, refining the existing stratification scores and, in parallel, increasing their accuracy. Modality and feature learning should be addressed such that conditional dependencies between input and output variables are effectively detected in the quantized space even in the presence of groups of highly-correlated features. To this end, sequential (backward or forward) feature selection, evaluating the incremental predictive value of the input space, would allow the adoption of only those parameters that contribute to the improvement in accuracy of CAD stratification.
iii. Third, the core of predictive modelling ought to be built upon adaptive non-linear regression or classification solutions on the basis of the results of patient's profiling analysis, feature learning and dynamic pattern analysis. In this direction, contemporary powerful learning methods (e.g. deep-learning, DBN and continuous time Bayesian networks) and big data solutions can be employed to identify novel correlations and causal relationships, strongly related with the onset of CAD. In addition, the discriminative/predictive capacity of the extracted clusters or temporal patterns (grouping of patients), can be studied, resulting to a hybrid prediction scheme. On top of these, a comprehensive pre-processing procedure has to be applied in order to resolve issues related with data heterogeneities, missing data unbalanced classes and sampling times, and assure a high-quality adequately-synchronized dataset.
iv. Finally, the expected generalization performance of the computational model should be evaluated on large-scale multivariate datasets using well-established statistical measures and approaches aiming at balancing the trade-off among accuracy, interpretability and time and space complexity. The efficient integration of personalized behavioural and psychosocial data with health data can provide a better understanding of the effect of patient's daily context on clinical health outcomes.

Concluding, predictive modelling of CAD diagnosis or CAD progression should aim to develop hybrid multi-level multi-scale schemes, combining unsupervised and supervised adaptive learning systems and being built upon novel multi-sensor, multi-source and multi-process information fusion schemes. Intelligent data mining and machine learning algorithms integrating previous clinical risk stratification models and refining novel ones using new knowledge coming from big data sources (e.g. molecular, cellular, inflammatory and omics data) could advance existing modelling methods in terms of accuracy, precision and interpretability. New paradigms should emphasize on both architecture and algorithms of the predictive model aiming at promoting the synergism among different information analysis levels.

Acknowledgements This work is partially funded by the European Commission: Project SMARTOOL, "Simulation Modeling of coronary ARTery disease: a tool for clinical decision support—SMARTool" GA number: 689068.

References

1. Stone PH, Saito S, Takahashi S, Makita Y, Nakamura S, Kawasaki T, Takahashi A, Katsuki T, Nakamura S, Namiki A, Hirohata A, Matsumura T, Yamazaki S, Yokoi H, Tanaka S, Otsuji S, Yoshimachi F, Honye J, Harwood D, Reitman M, Coskun AU, Papafaklis MI, Feldman CL (2012) Prediction of progression of coronary artery disease and clinical outcomes using vascular profiling of endothelial shear stress and arterial plaque characteristics: the PREDICTION study. Circulation 126(2):172–181. https://doi.org/10.1161/circulationaha.112.096438
2. Sakellarios A, Bourantas CV, Papadopoulou S-L, Tsirka Z, de Vries T, Kitslaar PH, Girasis C, Naka KK, Fotiadis DI, Veldhof S, Stone GW, Reiber JHC, Michalis LK, Serruys PW, de Feyter PJ, Garcia-Garcia HM (2017) Prediction of atherosclerotic disease progression using LDL transport modelling: a serial computed tomographic coronary angiographic study. Eur Heart J Cardiovasc Imaging 18(1):11–18. https://doi.org/10.1093/ehjci/jew035
3. Piepoli MF, Hoes AW, Agewall S, Albus C, Brotons C, Catapano AL, Cooney MT, Corra U, Cosyns B, Deaton C, Graham I, Hall MS, Hobbs FD, Lochen ML, Lollgen H, Marques-Vidal P, Perk J, Prescott E, Redon J, Richter DJ, Sattar N, Smulders Y, Tiberi M, van der Worp HB, van Dis I, Verschuren WM (2016) European Guidelines on cardiovascular disease prevention in clinical practice: the Sixth Joint Task Force of the European Society of Cardiology and other societies on cardiovascular disease prevention in clinical practice (constituted by representatives of 10 societies and by invited experts) Developed with the special contribution of the European Association for Cardiovascular Prevention & Rehabilitation (EACPR). Eur Heart J 37(29):2315–2381. https://doi.org/10.1093/eurheartj/ehw106
4. Ferguson JF, Allayee H, Gerszten RE, Ideraabdullah F, Kris-Etherton PM, Ordovas JM, Rimm EB, Wang TJ, Bennett BJ (2016) Nutrigenomics, the microbiome, and gene-environment interactions: new directions in cardiovascular disease research, prevention, and treatment: a scientific statement from the American Heart Association. Circ Cardiovasc Genet 9(3):291–313. https://doi.org/10.1161/hcg.0000000000000030
5. D'Agostino RB Sr, Vasan RS, Pencina MJ, Wolf PA, Cobain M, Massaro JM, Kannel WB (2008) General cardiovascular risk profile for use in primary care: the Framingham Heart Study. Circulation 117(6):743–753. https://doi.org/10.1161/circulationaha.107.699579
6. Conroy RM, Pyorala K, Fitzgerald AP, Sans S, Menotti A, De Backer G, De Bacquer D, Ducimetiere P, Jousilahti P, Keil U, Njolstad I, Oganov RG, Thomsen T, Tunstall-Pedoe H, Tverdal A, Wedel H, Whincup P, Wilhelmsen L, Graham IM (2003) Estimation of ten-year risk of fatal cardiovascular disease in Europe: the SCORE project. Eur Heart J 24(11):987–1003
7. Hippisley-Cox J, Coupland C, Robson J, Brindle P (2010) Derivation, validation, and evaluation of a new QRISK model to estimate lifetime risk of cardiovascular disease: cohort study using QResearch database. BMJ (Clinical research ed) 341:c6624. https://doi.org/10.1136/bmj.c6624
8. Damen JA, Hooft L, Schuit E, Debray TP, Collins GS, Tzoulaki I, Lassale CM, Siontis GC, Chiocchia V, Roberts C, Schlussel MM, Gerry S, Black JA, Heus P, van der Schouw YT, Peelen LM, Moons KG (2016) Prediction models for cardiovascular disease risk in the general population: systematic review. BMJ (Clinical research ed) 353:i2416. https://doi.org/10.1136/bmj.i2416
9. Goldstein BA, Navar AM, Carter RE (2017) Moving beyond regression techniques in cardiovascular risk prediction: applying machine learning to address analytic challenges. Eur Heart J 38(23):1805–1814. https://doi.org/10.1093/eurheartj/ehw302
10. Volzke H, Schmidt CO, Baumeister SE, Ittermann T, Fung G, Krafczyk-Korth J, Hoffmann W, Schwab M, Meyer zu Schwabedissen HE, Dorr M, Felix SB, Lieb W, Kroemer HK (2013) Personalized cardiovascular medicine: concepts and methodological considerations. Nat Rev Cardiol 10(6):308–316. https://doi.org/10.1038/nrcardio.2013.35
11. Ng K, Steinhubl SR, deFilippi C, Dey S, Stewart WF (2016) Early detection of heart failure using electronic health records: practical implications for time before diagnosis, data diversity, data quantity, and data density. Circ Cardiovasc Qual Outcomes 9(6):649–658. https://doi.org/10.1161/circoutcomes.116.002797

12. Karaolis MA, Moutiris JA, Hadjipanayi D, Pattichis CS (2010) Assessment of the risk factors of coronary heart events based on data mining with decision trees. IEEE Trans Inf Technol Biomed 14(3):559–566. https://doi.org/10.1109/TITB.2009.2038906
13. Nahar J, Imam T, Tickle KS, Chen Y-PP (2013) Association rule mining to detect factors which contribute to heart disease in males and females. Expert Syst Appl 40(4):1086–1093. https://doi.org/10.1016/j.eswa.2012.08.028
14. Austin PC, Tu JV, Ho JE, Levy D, Lee DS (2013) Using methods from the data-mining and machine-learning literature for disease classification and prediction: a case study examining classification of heart failure subtypes. J Clin Epidemiol 66(4):398–407. https://doi.org/10.1016/j.jclinepi.2012.11.008
15. Kurt I, Ture M, Kurum AT (2008) Comparing performances of logistic regression, classification and regression tree, and neural networks for predicting coronary artery disease. Expert Syst Appl 34(1):366–374. https://doi.org/10.1016/j.eswa.2006.09.004
16. Choi E, Schuetz A, Stewart WF, Sun J (2017) Using recurrent neural network models for early detection of heart failure onset. J Am Med Inform Assoc JAMIA 24(2):361–370. https://doi.org/10.1093/jamia/ocw112
17. Hassan N, Sayed OR, Khalil AM, Ghany MA (2016) Fuzzy soft expert system in prediction of coronary artery disease. Int J Fuzzy Syst. https://doi.org/10.1007/s40815-016-0255-0
18. Motwani M, Dey D, Berman DS, Germano G, Achenbach S, Al-Mallah MH, Andreini D, Budoff MJ, Cademartiri F, Callister TQ, Chang H-J, Chinnaiyan K, Chow BJW, Cury RC, Delago A, Gomez M, Gransar H, Hadamitzky M, Hausleiter J, Hindoyan N, Feuchtner G, Kaufmann PA, Kim Y-J, Leipsic J, Lin FY, Maffei E, Marques H, Pontone G, Raff G, Rubinshtein R, Shaw LJ, Stehli J, Villines TC, Dunning A, Min JK, Slomka PJ (2017) Machine learning for prediction of all-cause mortality in patients with suspected coronary artery disease: a 5-year multicentre prospective registry analysis. Eur Heart J 38(7):500–507. https://doi.org/10.1093/eurheartj/ehw188
19. Weng SF, Reps J, Kai J, Garibaldi JM, Qureshi N (2017) Can machine-learning improve cardiovascular risk prediction using routine clinical data? PLoS One 12(4):e0174944. https://doi.org/10.1371/journal.pone.0174944
20. Rao VSH, Kumar MN (2013) Novel approaches for predicting risk factors of atherosclerosis. IEEE J Biomed Health Inform 17(1):183–189. https://doi.org/10.1109/TITB.2012.2227271
21. Kukar M, Kononenko I, Grošelj C (2011) Modern parameterization and explanation techniques in diagnostic decision support system: a case study in diagnostics of coronary artery disease. Artif Intell Med 52(2):77–90. https://doi.org/10.1016/j.artmed.2011.04.009
22. Shouman M, Turner T, Stocker R (2012) Using data mining techniques in heart disease diagnosis and treatment. In: 2012 Japan-Egypt conference on electronics, communications and computers, 6–9 March 2012, pp 173–177. https://doi.org/10.1109/jec-ecc.2012.6186978
23. Melillo P, Izzo R, Orrico A, Scala P, Attanasio M, Mirra M, De Luca N, Pecchia L (2015) Automatic prediction of cardiovascular and cerebrovascular events using heart rate variability analysis. PLoS One 10(3):e0118504. https://doi.org/10.1371/journal.pone.0118504
24. Rumsfeld JS, Joynt KE, Maddox TM (2016) Big data analytics to improve cardiovascular care: promise and challenges. Nat Rev Cardiol 13(6):350–359. https://doi.org/10.1038/nrcardio.2016.42
25. Groeneveld PW, Rumsfeld JS (2016) Can big data fulfill its promise? Circ Cardiovasc Qual Outcomes 9(6):679–682. https://doi.org/10.1161/circoutcomes.116.003097
26. Tsipouras MG, Exarchos TP, Fotiadis DI, Kotsia AP, Vakalis KV, Naka KK, Michalis LK (2008) Automated diagnosis of coronary artery disease based on data mining and fuzzy modeling. IEEE Trans Inf Technol Biomed 12(4):447–458. https://doi.org/10.1109/TITB.2007.907985
27. Anooj PK (2012) Clinical decision support system: Risk level prediction of heart disease using weighted fuzzy rules. J King Saud Univ-Comput Inf Sci 24(1):27–40. https://doi.org/10.1016/j.jksuci.2011.09.002

28. Karabulut EM, Ibrikci T (2012) Effective diagnosis of coronary artery disease using the rotation forest ensemble method. J Med Syst 36(5):3011–3018. https://doi.org/10.1007/s10916-011-9778-y
29. Nahar J, Imam T, Tickle KS, Chen Y-PP (2013) Computational intelligence for heart disease diagnosis: a medical knowledge driven approach. Expert Syst Appl 40(1):96–104. https://doi.org/10.1016/j.eswa.2012.07.032
30. Alizadehsani R, Habibi J, Hosseini MJ, Mashayekhi H, Boghrati R, Ghandeharioun A, Bahadorian B, Sani ZA (2013) A data mining approach for diagnosis of coronary artery disease. Comput Methods Programs Biomed 111(1):52–61. https://doi.org/10.1016/j.cmpb.2013.03.004
31. Alizadehsani R, Zangooei MH, Hosseini MJ, Habibi J, Khosravi A, Roshanzamir M, Khozeimeh F, Sarrafzadegan N, Nahavandi S (2016) Coronary artery disease detection using computational intelligence methods. Knowl-Based Syst 109:187–197. https://doi.org/10.1016/j.knosys.2016.07.004
32. Verma L, Srivastava S, Negi PC (2016) A hybrid data mining model to predict coronary artery disease cases using non-invasive clinical data. J Med Syst 40(7):178. https://doi.org/10.1007/s10916-016-0536-z
33. Detrano R, Janosi A, Steinbrunn W, Pfisterer M, Schmid JJ, Sandhu S, Guppy KH, Lee S, Froelicher V (1989) International application of a new probability algorithm for the diagnosis of coronary artery disease. Am J Cardiol 64(5):304–310
34. Das R, Turkoglu I, Sengur A (2009) Effective diagnosis of heart disease through neural networks ensembles. Expert Syst Appl 36(4):7675–7680. https://doi.org/10.1016/j.eswa.2008.09.013
35. Exarchos KP, Carpegianni C, Rigas G, Exarchos TP, Vozzi F, Sakellarios A, Marraccini P, Naka K, Michalis L, Parodi O, Fotiadis DI (2015) A multiscale approach for modeling atherosclerosis progression. IEEE J Biomed Health Inform 19(2):709–719. https://doi.org/10.1109/jbhi.2014.2323935
36. Kennedy EH, Wiitala WL, Hayward RA, Sussman JB (2013) Improved cardiovascular risk prediction using nonparametric regression and electronic health record data. Med Care 51(3):251–258. https://doi.org/10.1097/MLR.0b013e31827da594
37. Orphanou K, Stassopoulou A, Keravnou E (2016) DBN-extended: a dynamic Bayesian network model extended with temporal abstractions for coronary heart disease prognosis. IEEE J Biomed Health Inform 20(3):944–952. https://doi.org/10.1109/jbhi.2015.2420534
38. Goff DC, Lloyd-Jones DM, Bennett G, Coady S, D'Agostino RB, Gibbons R, Greenland P, Lackland DT, Levy D, O'Donnell CJ, Robinson J, Schwartz JS, Shero ST, Smith SC, Sorlie P, Stone NJ, Wilson PWF (2013) 2013 ACC/AHA guideline on the assessment of cardiovascular risk. A report of the American College of Cardiology/American Heart Association Task Force on practice guidelines. https://doi.org/10.1161/01.cir.0000437741.48606.98
39. Goldstein BA, Navar AM, Pencina MJ, Ioannidis JP (2017) Opportunities and challenges in developing risk prediction models with electronic health records data: a systematic review. J Am Med Inform Assoc 24(1):198–208. https://doi.org/10.1093/jamia/ocw042
40. Batal I, Valizadegan H, Cooper GF, Hauskrecht M (2013) A temporal pattern mining approach for classifying electronic health record data. ACM Trans Intell Syst Technol 4(4). https://doi.org/10.1145/2508037.2508044
41. Batal I, Cooper GF, Fradkin D, Harrison J, Moerchen F, Hauskrecht M (2016) An efficient pattern mining approach for event detection in multivariate temporal data. Knowl Inf Syst 46(1):115–150. https://doi.org/10.1007/s10115-015-0819-6
42. Moskovitch R, Shahar Y (2015) Fast time intervals mining using the transitivity of temporal relations. Knowl Inf Syst 42(1):21–48. https://doi.org/10.1007/s10115-013-0707-x
43. Moskovitch R, Shahar Y (2009) Medical temporal-knowledge discovery via temporal abstraction. AMIA Annu Symp Proc 2009:452–456
44. Orphanou K, Stassopoulou A, Keravnou E (2014) Temporal abstraction and temporal Bayesian networks in clinical domains: a survey. Artif Intell Med 60(3):133–149. https://doi.org/10.1016/j.artmed.2013.12.007

45. Bellazzi R, Sacchi L, Concaro S (2009) Methods and tools for mining multivariate temporal data in clinical and biomedical applications. In: Conference proceedings: annual international conference of the IEEE engineering in medicine and biology society IEEE engineering in medicine and biology society annual conference 2009:5629–5632. https://doi.org/10.1109/iembs.2009.5333788
46. Miotto R, Li L, Kidd BA, Dudley JT (2016) Deep patient: an unsupervised representation to predict the future of patients from the electronic health records. Sci Rep 6:26094. https://doi.org/10.1038/srep26094

Title Cardiovascular Big Data Analytics

Ioanna Chouvarda and Nicos Maglaveras

Abstract The evolving pattern towards precision medicine is based on analytics at the—omics, physiology and eHealth domains. One of the main driving forces is the management and analytics of multi-level multi-scale and multi-source data containing different semantics and possibilities for the realization of personalized health through the precision medicine approach. In the case of cardiovascular big data analytics progress is evident especially at the levels of physiology and eHealth. Specifically there is progress in the ICU domain, where streaming data are the big data source comprising a paradigm for point-of-care (PoC) diagnostics helping the clinical decision support system (CDSS) for physiological assessment of the cardiorespiratory system, as well as in the eHealth domain through the uptake of advanced closed loop telemonitoring systems addressing connected health and coordinated care for multimorbid chronic disease patients. The quantification of specific data analytics, data management and computational needs for the realization of interfaces conveying from cloud to local level the necessary input to the medical users is a complex procedure, which calls for the optimal use of all the cloud, computing and machine learning and visualization tools, let alone the interoperability and data security standards and apps. In this chapter, we shall give an overview of the current state-of-the-art concerning cardiovascular big data analytics as a function of available information and communication technology, computational engineering, and user driven systems

I. Chouvarda (✉) · N. Maglaveras (✉)
Laboratory of Computing, Medical Informatics & Biomedical-Imaging Technologies, The Medical School, Aristotle University, Thessaloniki, Greece
e-mail: ioannach@auth.gr

N. Maglaveras
e-mail: nicmag@med.auth.gr

N. Maglaveras
Deptartment of Industrial Engineering & Management Sciences, Department of Electrical Engineering & Computer Science, McCormick School of Engineering and Applied Sciences, Northwestern University, Evanston, IL, USA

I. Chouvarda · N. Maglaveras
Center for Research and Technology Hellas, Institute of Applied Biosciences, Thessaloniki, Greece

S. Golemati and K. S. Nikita (eds.), *Cardiovascular Computing—Methodologies and Clinical Applications*, Series in BioEngineering,
https://doi.org/10.1007/978-981-10-5092-3_15

platforms for use in connected health and integrated care environments, as well as one basic example related to big data analytics as a result of streaming data at a PoC from a clinically controlled environment such as the Intensive Care Unit (ICU). The output from the application of advanced machine learning and multiparametric analytics methodology conveyed as a CDSS to the users is considered and viewed as perhaps the most important function for the success of the big data analytics and management platforms.

Keywords Cardiorespiratory systems · Big data analytics · Machine learning Intensive care unit · Ineffective efforts · COPD multi-morbid patients Connected health · CDSS

1 Introduction

During the last decade, the generation of biomedical and connected health data is increasingly machine accelerated. This availability of structured and unstructured health data (covering genomics, proteomics, metabolomics, as well as imaging, clinical diagnosis, and long-term continuous physiological sensing of an individual) facilitates value creation via biomedical informatics applications via new data driven approaches for translational research and generation of new knowledge and new insights into human health. Big data analytics can be successfully combined with VPH technologies to test hypotheses and produce robust and effective in silico medicine solutions towards personalized medicine [1]. A step further, big data in health are expected to leverage the healthcare services, as regards support in decision making in health systems and public health [2].

In turn, along with the new opportunities, new challenges arise for data management, and data integration in the era of big data. In [3] an overview of recent developments in big data in the context of biomedical and health informatics is presented, outlining also some of the key underlying issues that need to be tackled. The key characteristics initially defined for big data were Volume, Velocity, and Variety. Later, more factors were considered, including Variability, Veracity, and Value. These factors are summarized in Table 1.

Table 1 Big data properties

Volume	Continuous monitoring of vital signs, High throughput technologies
Velocity	Fast data generation, Need for fast or realtime response and decision making
Variety	Heterogeneous and unstructured data
Variability	Consistency of data over time, evolution
Veracity	trustworthiness of the data obtained, different levels of data quality
Value	Clinically relevant and actionable data

A major point as regards the last factor, value, is the necessary paradigm shift inherent in big data health research. Health research has been traditionally built on small and clean data, with carefully designed cleaned trials and extrapolation of their findings. A shift from hypothesis driven to data driven research is foreseen, based on machine learning techniques that mine patterns, clusters and associations from big (e.g. population representative) volumes of unclean data. To increase medical credibility, the produced knowledge and hypotheses can then be confirmed in smaller and cleaner datasets.

In [4], the big data sources defined as relevant improvement of cardiovascular care are structured data including administrative data, clinical registries and electronic health records, as well as unstructured data such as biometric data, patient reports and medical imaging data. Respectively, based on integration of these data, eight areas of application of big data analytics to improve cardiovascular care are highlighted, including predictive modelling for risk and resource use, population management, drug and medical device safety surveillance, disease and treatment heterogeneity, precision medicine and clinical decision support, quality of care and performance measurement, and public health and research applications.

2 Big Data Technologies

In [5] it is suggested that a big data system can be conceptually decomposed into a layered structure of three layers, i.e., the infrastructure layer, the computing layer, and the application layer, from bottom to top.

The *infrastructure layer* is typically a cloud based infrastructure, with virtualization and scalability capabilities, although high computational resources can be available also in the local-private space, which is especially relevant when data privacy issues are of concern.

The *computing layer* includes data integration, data management, and the programming model. As regards data integration from disparate sources into a unified form, semantics play a key role and also can facilitate querying of information [6]. I2b2 (Informatics for Integrating Biology and the Bedside), based on semantics, relational databases, as well as a flexible query tool and numerous analysis plugins, has been a widely adopted framework for integrating distributed clinical and genetic data for clinical research [7, 8]. Recently NoSQL-based extensions allowed more efficient management of high throughput data [9]. SQL clusters, NoSQL databases, and distributed file systems are favorable approaches for persistent data storage and highly efficient management of big data in health [10]. *The programming model* implements abstraction application logic and facilitates the data analysis applications. MapReduce is a common programming model [11].

The *application layer* implement various data analysis functions, including querying, and machine learning and enables domain specific combination of analytical methods.

2.1 Overview of Mainstream Tools

The Apache Hadoop[1] software library is a framework that allows for the distributed processing and storage of large data sets across clusters, supporting scalability from single servers to thousands of machines with local computation and storage. Some of the most important modules of this framework are:

(a) **The Hadoop Distributed File System (HDFS™)**: A distributed file system, accessible via APIs in different languages, that provides high-throughput access to application data, as it distributes large datasets across many data nodes as data blocks.
(b) **Hadoop YARN**: A job scheduling and cluster resource management framework.
(c) **Hadoop MapReduce**: A programming model for parallel processing of large data sets in large-scale distributed systems, by dividing tasks to multiple *workers* for better performance. There are two distinct stages: *mapping* and *reducing*.
(d) **Cassandra**: A scalable and fault tolerant database oriented to columnar data.
(e) **Hbase**: A scalable, distributed database that supports structured data storage for large tables.

Apache Spark™[2] is a fast and general engine for large-scale data processing (stream and batch), regarding cluster-based computing. It provides high-level APIs in many programming languages and tools for structured data processing, machine learning, graph processing, and streaming. It newer than Hadoop MAPREDUCE and seems to outperform it in terms of speed.

3 Big Data and Cardiovascular Applications

3.1 Translational Research for Cardiovascular Care

The advancement of cardiovascular proteomics and in cardiovascular systems medicine with big data technologies has been studied in [12, 13]. Mass spectrometry based large-scale analysis of cardiac proteins (in thousands), allows deeper studies of regulatory proteins, including membrane receptors and more. The increase in data size and analysis complexity leveraged computational proteomics, including clustering for co-expressed proteins, machine learning for disease signatures, network analysis for functional clustering, etc., and gain insights around spatial distributions of cardiac proteins, protein–protein interaction networks, or synthesis rates of proteins (e.g. in heart failure). Computational tools for proteomics data analysis, including opensource tools, have been developed and can be deployed at cloud level [2, 4–8, 10, 12–26]. High throughput techniques, supported by big data analytic

[1] http://hadoop.apache.org/.

[2] http://spark.apache.org/.

pipelines have allowed whole genome and exome sequencing for the identification of genes and genetic variations implicated in cardiomyopathies [22] and arrhythmias [19]. In parallel high performance computing allows for investigations at cellular, tissue and organ level [27, 28], as integrative modelling and translational research spanning across multiple spatial and temporal levels could be of immense value in personalized medicine.

3.2 Analysis of Clinical Records for Cardiac Care

In [29], the information encoded in EHRs regarding implicit or explicit interactions between heart failure patients and providers was considered and network analysis was applied. This analysis provided evidence on the widely shared record access, which can be the basis for optimising care coordination for cardiac patients. This is a characteristic example of the impact big data analytics may have on health related policies, although leveraging approaches from descriptive to predictive and eventually to prescriptive analytics still needs more efforts to mature. Analysis of clinical notes, i.e. unstructured data residing in EHRs, is of special interest and challenge, for the extraction of valuable information from reports [21].

3.3 Biosignal Analysis and Telecardiology Frameworks

ECG screening is a cost-effective and efficient means for screening and diagnosis, and its use can nowadays be extended by the wide presence of internet-connected phones, which can lead to huge volumes of home-based ECG data sources, provided that adequate quality is ensured. In [15], wireless smartphone ECG was assessed as regards its ability to support large-scale screening in diverse populations, comparing the standard 12-lead ECG to the smartphone ECG. Both ECGs detected atrial rate and rhythm, AV block, and QRS delay with equal accuracy, concluding that smartphone ECG enables screening in diverse populations, and can be furthermore enhanced by automated ECG analysis and notifications. Up to now, mhealth approaches for capturing and telemonitoring electrocardiograph (ECG), echocardiography (ECHO) and relevant medical images via smart phones have been proposed for remote monitoring, emergency detection and reduction of hospitalization. Current trends combine mobile computing with cloud computing for better storage, delivery, retrieval, and management [30], practically supporting tele-diagnosis of ECG and images, provided that data confidentiality, interoperability, and communication issues are resolved [16].

The WELCOME cloud data management and analytics system is presented in Fig. 1. Although the specific system is designed for telemonitoring of chronic patients with COPD, Heart Failure and other common conditions, it could be regarded as a general chronic telemedicine system heavily based on biosignals like ECG, respiration, wheezes, crackles etc. In order to support multiple sources of data and informa-

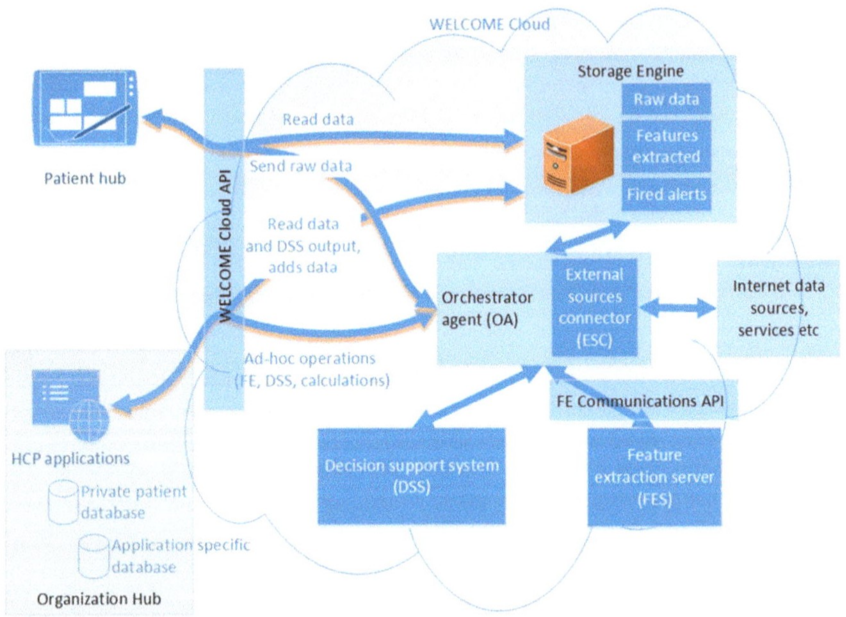

Fig. 1 The WELCOME cloud system for data management

tion, multiple access points, and different computational workflows, the main parts of this cloud system are: Restful web services communication, NoSQL RDF TRIPLE STORE Persistent Storage for big data management, a semantic data model based on HL7 FHIR [31], a scalable feature extraction server, a clinical DSS (CDSS) for comorbidity management and an orchestrator agent and workflow management.

The potential, pitfalls and issues to be addressed for wide adoption of telecardiology approaches are discussed by the Task Force of the e-Cardiology Working Group of European Society of Cardiology [32].

As regards platforms dedicated to big cardiovascular data processing, NeuroPigPen is described in [25], aiming to support large-scale electrophysiological signal processing (EEG, ECG, SpO_2). This framework uses Apache Hadoop, a distributed storage model and Pig data flow language. Cloudwave platform [24] incorporates optimized implementations (with MapReduce) of cardiac analysis algorithms for real-time analysis, visualization and querying of large volumes of electrophysiological signals, enhanced by semantic annotations. Fast computation of single and multichannel ECG (e.g., QRS complexes, RR intervals, and instantaneous heart rate) is then used for research related to sudden unexplained death in epilepsy. With respect to performance, a framework for real-time analytics and arrhythmia detection based on R programming language and Apache Storm is presented in [33].

3.4 Intensive Care Unit Analytics

Intensive care is a characteristic case where big bio-data are produced and a domain that can benefit from leveraging big data analytics, towards prediction of adverse events, and understanding of the highly dynamic and multidimensional phenomena of acute care. To highlight the volume problem in an ICU, the ICU ECG monitor with 1 kHz produces 86.4 million ECG samples a day per patient, besides the heart rate and respiration rate, chest wall movement which are usually sampled at lower rates. Among the pioneering studies that inspired ICU analytics was the MIMIC II database [23], made available in Physionet (Goldberger AL, Amaral LAN, Glass L, Hausdorff JM, Ivanov PCh, Mark RG, Mietus JE, Moody GB, Peng C-K [34], and later upgraded to MIMIC III database [17], including ICU clinical records of many thousands patients, along with biosignals for a percentage of them. Recently, a web based tool for visualization and exploration of MIMIC II data was proposed [18], while the need for complementing it with web based analytics was recognized.

The ICU domain, intensively data-driven and closely coupled with medical devices, has attracted the attention of industry. A big data analytics platform for neonatal intensive care has been implemented in [20] offering new research opportunities towards earlier detection and prevention of a wide range of deadly medical conditions. Artemis [35] is a real-time online analysis platform that enables concurrent analysis multiple patients' data streams to detect medically significant conditions that precede the onset of medical complications.

The scientific community also raised the need for connecting medical devices and clinical applications, based on standards [36], and alleviating the barriers posed by each company's proprietary system. OpenICE initiative[3] aims to provide a framework for the integration of devices and apps into the broader Medical Internet of Things. This has the potential to make available enormous volumes of ICU data.

In AEGLE project,[4] big ICU data analytics platform is based on integration of clinical data, monitor streaming data, and ventilation data, based on medical standards (LOINC,[5] ATC, ICD). Data quality is an important issue and preprocessing steps are introduced for each type of data. Analytics methods are based on optimized (via Hadoop and Spark) opensource code in R and Python, which is executed in a cloud based cluster. A semantic annotation of data and analytics tools allows the generation of analysis pipelines, and the flexible exploration of data and results. Web-based visualisation and exploratory analysis constitute a crucial step towards exposing data driven research and new features to domain experts and incorporating their feedback [37]. An example is presented in Fig. 2 for assisted ventilation analysis, as exposed via an AEGLE prototype to the domain expert. In assisted ventilation, there is need for patient-ventilator coupling; when patient's effort doesn't trigger the ventilator, and the assisted ventilation event is lost, an ineffective effort (IE) event takes place. The assisted ventilation study investigated the role of ineffective effort clusters on the

[3] https://www.openice.info/index.html.

[4] http://www.aegle-uhealth.eu/en/.

[5] https://loinc.org/.

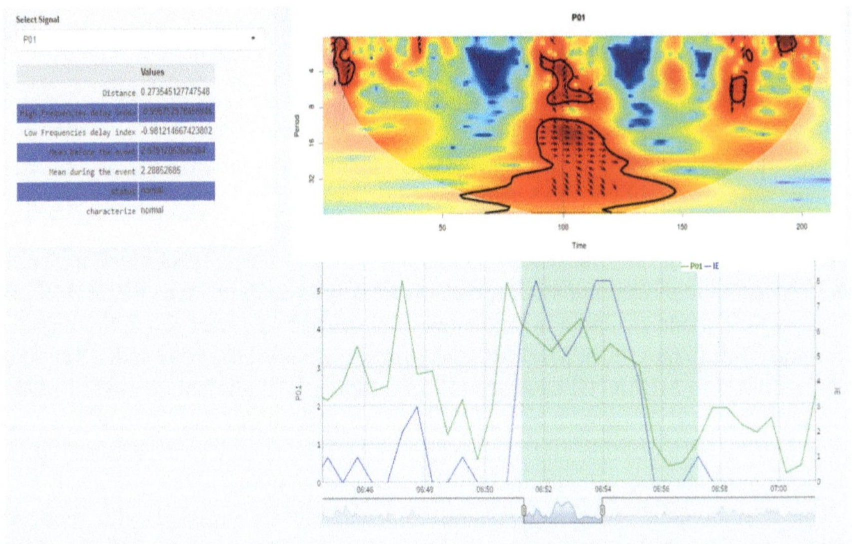

Fig. 2 A view of AEGLE's prototype for the analysis of ineffective efforts in assisted ventilation and exploration of the causality of IE clusters via cross wavelet phase. In this example at the upper graph we can see the cross-spectrum, and at the lower the IE signal and the P01, a measure of respiratory drive. Phases analysis suggests that changes in the patient's stimuli for respiration are leading the changes of the IE signal, and therefore it can be considered a possible cause

outcome of critically ill patients (prolonged mechanical ventilation and increased mortality). Vaporidi et al. [38] proposed a definition for serious IE clusters. This analysis now continues with generation of predictive models for serious ICU events.

In conclusion, as the ICU environment is basically seeking real-time responses, big data ICU analytics can be implemented as cloud based analytics of big ICU data used for offline analysis. In this case, multisite data can be used for enhanced analytics, and incorporation of new knowledge (e.g. prediction models) back at the local environment can take place, but the generation-application of new knowledge is not synchronous. The analytics can also be implemented at a local rather than cloud environment, provided that the necessary HPC is inplace. In this case, learning and applying patterns in the ICU system can be more synchronized.

4 Discussion

The evolution of technology in the medical device, computer science, electrical & computing engineering as well as in (bio)medical informatics and eHealth has produced more advanced and multi-purpose systems capable of enabling connected health and integrated care such as is the case of the EU WELCOME project. These systems' overall architecture as depicted in Fig. 1, show the capacity and the potential these systems have for generating big bio-data stemming from various sources (e.g. MDD, body area networks, environmental sources, social networks, electronic and personal health records etc.) as well as the need to efficiently and timely manage and analyze the resulting data and information creating a clinical decision support ecosystem residing both in the cloud and locally which can be self-adopting according to the users' queries. On the other hand it makes very clear the gap related to big bio-data analytics and calls for the development of solutions, where our basic pool of mainstream tools are referred to, and of course the accelerators such as GPUs/CUDA and other analogous technologies form the current computational state-of-the-art.

The ICU case presented here addresses the problem of patient to ventilator interaction (PVI), which is one of the unresolved problems in the ICU. This leads to time consumption due to the heuristic nature of the patient's weaning process from the respirator, as well as to complications in the cardiorespiratory system when weaning efforts are not successful due to the ineffective efforts from the patient, which overload the patients' already weak cardiorespiratory capacity. Thus, the nature of the data (streaming data) as well as the need for the time efficient optimization of the multiparametric model of ineffective efforts having as input over 200 vectors of parameters over hours and days, makes the clinical decision support system (CDSS) an ideal case of big biodata at point of care (PoC) diagnostics. Taking into account the effort from the scientific community lead by Physionet and the MIMIC databases developed over the past 20 years the actual clinical application of the AEGLE platform in the clustering of the ineffective efforts in the ICU coming from PVI, shows clearly the pathway the big biodata management and analytics need to follow in the near future so as to develop useable and user acceptable modules for everyday clinical practice [38].

Acknowledgements This work was supported in part by the EC projects AEGLE (Grant agreement 644906) and WELCOME (611223).

References

1. Viceconti M, Hunter P, Hose R (2015) Big data, big knowledge: big data for personalized healthcare. IEEE J. Biomed. Health Informat. 19(4):1209–1215
2. Martin-Sanchez F, Verspoor K (2014) Big data in medicine is driving big changes. Yearbook Med Informat 9(1):14–20
3. Andreu-Perez J et al (2015) Big Data for Health. IEEE Journal of Biomedical and Health Informatics 19(4):1193–1208
4. Rumsfeld JS, Joynt KE, Maddox TM (2016) Big data analytics to improve cardiovascular care: promise and challenges. Nat Rev Cardiol 13(6):350–359. http://www.ncbi.nlm.nih.gov/pubmed/27009423
5. Hu H et al (2014) Toward scalable systems for big data analytics: a technology tutorial. IEEE Access 2:652–687
6. Kokkinaki A, Chouvarda I, Maglaveras N (2012) Searching biosignal databases by content and context: research oriented integration system for ECG signals (ROISES). Comput Methods Prog Biomed 108(2):453–466

7. Natter MD et al (2013) An i2b2-based, generalizable, open source, self-scaling chronic disease registry. J Am Med Informat Assoc 20(1):172–179. http://jamia.oxfordjournals.org/content/20/1/172
8. Segagni D et al (2012) CARDIO-i2b2: integrating arrhythmogenic disease data in i2b2. Stud Health Technol Informat 1126–1128
9. Gabetta M et al (2015) BigQ: a NoSQL based framework to handle genomic variants in i2b2. BMC Bioinformat 16(1):415. http://www.biomedcentral.com/1471-2105/16/415
10. Krishnan K (2013) Data warehousing in the age of big data
11. Dean J, Ghemawat S (2010) MapReduce. Commun ACM 53(1):72
12. Lam MPY et al (2016) Cardiovascular proteomics in the era of big data: experimental and computational advances. Clin Proteom 13:23
13. Lindsey ML et al (2015) Transformative impact of proteomics on cardiovascular health and disease: a scientific statement from the American heart association. Circulation 132(9):852–872
14. Goloborodko AA et al (2013) Pyteomics—a python framework for exploratory data analysis and rapid software prototyping in proteomics. J Am Soc Mass Spectr 24(2):301–304
15. Haberman ZC et al (2015) Wireless smartphone ECG enables large-scale screening in diverse populations. J Cardiovasc Electrophysiol 26(5):520–526
16. Hsieh JC, Li AH, Yang CC (2013) Mobile, cloud, and big data computing: Contributions, challenges, and new directions in telecardiology. Int J Environ Res Public Health 10(11):6131–6153
17. Johnson AEW et al (2016) MIMIC-III, a freely accessible critical care database. Scientif Data 3:160035
18. Lee J, Ribey E, Wallace JR (2016) A web-based data visualization tool for the MIMIC-II database. BMC Med Informat Decision Making 16:15. http://www.ncbi.nlm.nih.gov/pubmed/26846781%5Cnhttp://www.pubmedcentral.nih.gov/articlerender.fcgi?artid=PMC4743095
19. Lubitz SA, Ellinor PT (2015) Next-generation sequencing for the diagnosis of cardiac arrhythmia syndromes. Heart Rhythm Official J Heart Rhythm Soc 12(5):1062–1070. http://www.sciencedirect.com/science/article/pii/S1547527115000405
20. McGregor C (2013) Big Data in neonatal intensive care. Computer 46(6):54–59
21. Nath C, Albaghdadi MS, Jonnalagadda SR (2016) A natural language processing tool for large-scale data extraction from echocardiography reports. PLoS One 11(4)
22. Nouhravesh N et al (2016) Analyses of more than 60,000 exomes questions the role of numerous genes previously associated with dilated cardiomyopathy. Mol Genetic Genom Med 4(6):617–623
23. Saeed M et al (2011) Multiparameter intelligent monitoring in intensive care II (MIMIC-II): A public-access intensive care unit database. Crit Care Med 39(5):952–960
24. Sahoo SS et al (2014) Heart beats in the cloud: distributed analysis of electrophysiological "Big Data" using cloud computing for epilepsy clinical research. J Am Med Informat Assoc JAMIA 21(2):263–271. http://jamia.oxfordjournals.org/content/21/2/263.abstract
25. Sahoo SS et al (2016) NeuroPigPen: a scalable toolkit for processing electrophysiological signal data in neuroscience applications using apache pig. Front Neuroinformat 10:18. http://journal.frontiersin.org/article/10.3389/fninf.2016.00018
26. Sheynkman GM et al (2014) Using Galaxy-P to leverage RNA-Seq for the discovery of novel protein variations. BMC Genom 15(1):703. http://www.pubmedcentral.nih.gov/articlerender.fcgi?artid=4158061&tool=pmcentrez&rendertype=abstract
27. Bernabeu MO et al (2009) CHASTE: incorporating a novel multi-scale spatial and temporal algorithm into a large-scale open source library. Philos Trans Ser A Math Phys Eng Sci 367(1895):1907–30. http://www.ncbi.nlm.nih.gov/pubmed/19380318
28. Cooper J, Scharm M, Mirams GR (2016) The cardiac electrophysiology web lab. Biophys J 110(2):292–300
29. Soulakis ND et al (2015) Visualizing collaborative electronic health record usage for hospitalized patients with heart failure. J Am Med Inform Assoc 22(2):299–311
30. Chouvarda I et al (2016) Clinical flows and decision support systems for coordinated and integrated care in COPD. In: 3rd IEEE EMBS international conference on biomedical and health informatics, BHI, pp 477–480

31. Beredimas N et al (2015) A reusable ontology for primitive and complex HL7 FHIR data types. In: 2015 37th annual international conference of the IEEE engineering in medicine and biology society (EMBC). IEEE, pp 2547–2550. http://ieeexplore.ieee.org/lpdocs/epic03/wrapper.htm?arnumber=7318911. Accessed 11 Dec 2015
32. Bruining N et al (2014) Acquisition and analysis of cardiovascular signals on smartphones: potential, pitfalls and perspectives by the task force of the e-Cardiology working group of European society of cardiology. European J Prevent Cardiol 21(2 suppl):4–13. http://cpr.sagepub.com/content/21/2_suppl/4%5Cnhttp://cpr.sagepub.com/content/21/2_suppl/4.full.pdf%5Cnhttp://cpr.sagepub.com/content/21/2_suppl/4.short%5Cnhttp://www.ncbi.nlm.nih.gov/pubmed/25354948
33. Agneeswaran VS et al (2013) Real-time analytics for the healthcare industry: arrhythmia detection. Big Data 1(3) 176–182. http://online.liebertpub.com/doi/abs/10.1089/big.2013.0018
34. Goldberger AL, Amaral LAN, Glass L, Hausdorff JM, Ivanov PCh, Mark RG, Mietus JE, Moody GB, Peng C-K, SH (2000) PhysioBank, PhysioToolkit, and PhysioNet components of a new research resource for complex physiologic signals. Circulation 101(23):215–220
35. Blount M et al (2010) Real-time analysis for intensive care: development and deployment of the artemis analytic system. IEEE Eng Med Biol Mag Quarter Mag Eng Med Biol Soc 29(2):110–118. http://www.ncbi.nlm.nih.gov/pubmed/20659848
36. Arney D et al (2012) Simulation of medical device network performance and requirements for an integrated clinical environment. Biomedical Instrumentation & Technology/Association for the Advancement of Medical Instrumentation 46(4). https://doi.org/10.2345/0899-8205-46.4.308. http://www.ncbi.nlm.nih.gov/pmc/articles/PMC3810397/
37. Chytas A et al (2016). Ineffective efforts in ICU assisted ventilation: feature extraction and analysis platform. In: Iliadis L, Maglogiannis I (eds.) Artificial intelligence applications and innovations: 12th IFIP WG 12.5 international conference and workshops, AIAI 2016, Thessaloniki, Greece, September 16–18, 2016, Proceedings. Cham: Springer International Publishing, pp. 642–650. http://dx.doi.org/10.1007/978-3-319-44944-9_57
38. Vaporidi K et al (2016) Clusters of ineffective efforts during mechanical ventilation: impact on outcome. Intensiv Care Med 1–8. http://dx.doi.org/10.1007/s00134-016-4593-z

Part VI
Specific Clinical Applications

Ultrasound Asymptomatic Carotid Plaque Image Analysis for the Prediction of the Risk of Stroke

Christos P. Loizou and Efthivoulos Kyriacou

1 Introduction

High-resolution vascular B-mode and Doppler ultrasound provide information not only on the degree of carotid artery stenosis but also on the characteristics of the arterial wall including the size and consistency of atherosclerotic plaques [1]. Carotid stenosis alone has limitations in predicting risk and does not show plaque vulnerability and instability, thus other ultrasonographic plaque morphologic characteristics have been studied for better prediction of the risk stroke. Plaque echogenicity as assessed by B-mode ultrasound has been found to reliably predict the content of soft tissue and the amount of calcification in carotid plaques. Additionally, it has been reported that subjects with echolucent atherosclerotic plaques have increased risk of ischemic cerebrovascular events [2]. More recent studies by Nicolaides et al. [3] Topakian et al. [4] and Kyriacou et al. [5], showed that plaque echolucency and plaque morphology can be used to predict stroke. Other studies have reported that plaques that are more echolucent and heterogeneous are often associated with higher cerebrovascular risk and the development of ipsilateral neurological symptoms [3, 6–10]. In contrast, homogeneous hypoechoic and hyperechoic plaques without evidence of ulceration usually remain asymptomatic.

Prediction of risk is important as it will aid clinicians in the selection of asymptomatic cases at higher risk. Equally important is the establishment of a method that

C. P. Loizou (✉)
Department of Electrical Engineering, Computer Engineering and Informatics, Cyprus University of Technology, Limassol, Cyprus
e-mail: christos.loizou@cut.ac.cy

E. Kyriacou
Department of Computer Science and Engineering, Frederick University, Nicosia, Cyprus
e-mail: e.kyriacou@frederick.ac.cy

S. Golemati and K. S. Nikita (eds.), *Cardiovascular Computing—Methodologies and Clinical Applications*, Series in BioEngineering,
https://doi.org/10.1007/978-981-10-5092-3_16

will allow for objective and quantitative evaluation of high risk cases, that are the ones that would most benefit from endarterectomy.

Atherosclerosis of the internal carotid artery (ICA) is known to be an important risk factor for stroke. Using the NASCET [11] method for the determination of stenosis the risk of stroke has been shown to range between 0.1–1.6% per year for asymptomatic individuals with ICA stenosis<75–80%. The risk rises to 2–3% per year for individuals with higher grades of stenosis. In the past two decades, carotid endarterectomy was extensively used for the reduction of stroke risk. This is because two randomized controlled trials, almost a decade apart, the ACAS in 1995 [12] and the ACST in 2004 [13] reported that in patients with asymptomatic ICA stenosis>60–70% (using the NASCET method) carotid endarterectomy reduced the risk of stroke from 2 to 1% per year. However, in these trials carotid endarterectomy was associated with a 2–3% perioperative rate of stroke or death making it marginally effective for asymptomatic patients.

This chapter presents methods that can be used for evaluation of high cerebrovascular risk using image normalization, despeckling, segmentation, texture and morphological appearance of plaques in combination with a number of clinical factors for the estimation of the stroke risk. Images and results presented are based on the analysis of images that were collected through a multicentre cohort study of patients with asymptomatic ICA called Asymptomatic Carotid Stenosis and Risk of Stroke (ACSRS) [3].

2 Collected Data

The data (ultrasound scans as shown in Fig. 1a, b and clinical data) were collected from patients based on a predefined protocol as follows: Patients were assessed as asymptomatic and included in the monitored group based on the following criteria/characteristics. Newly referred (<3 months) patients with 50–99% ICA stenosis in relation to the carotid bulb diameter (ECST method) without previous ipsilateral cerebral or retinal ischemic (CORI) symptoms and without neurological abnormalities were recruited to the study after written informed consent. Patients who had contralateral cerebral hemispheric/retinal or vertebrobasilar symptoms or signs of stroke/TIA were included if asymptomatic for at least 6 months prior to recruitment. For patients with bilateral carotid atherosclerosis the side with the more severe stenosis was considered ipsilateral (the study artery) [3].

At baseline, when all patients were asymptomatic; clinical and duplex ultrasound scanning data were collected. This procedure was repeated at 6 months intervals until a primary endpoint or the end of the study was reached. Exit points (i.e. when follow-up was stopped) were any of the above endpoints, death from any cause, carotid endarterectomy, stenting or loss to follow-up. Thus, patients that died, had carotid endarterectomy or had an ipsilateral ischemic event (often followed by a carotid endarterectomy) have been followed up to the event only. Apart from the ipsilateral fatal strokes there was no overlap between these events. Clinical data

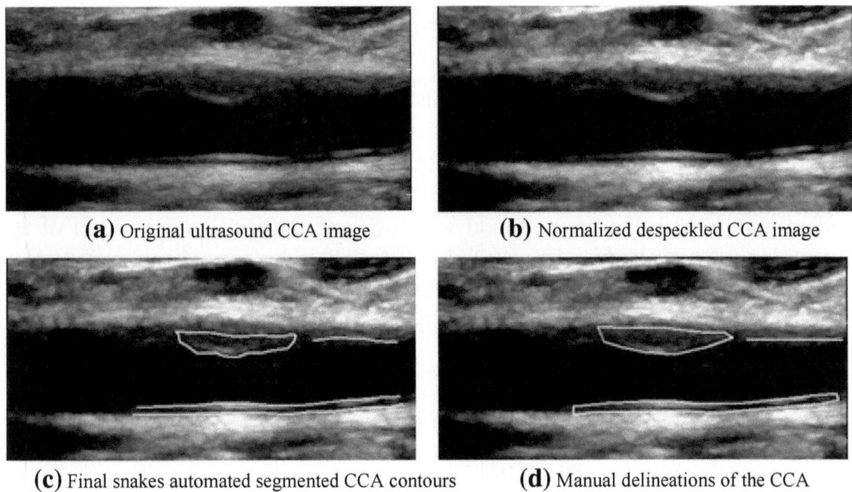

Fig. 1 **a** Original ultrasound CCA image, **b** normalized despeckled image with *DsFlsmv* filter (1 iterations, window 5 × 5), **c** final snakes automated contours after snakes deformation, and **d** manual complete delineations of the CCA performed by a cardiovascular surgeon

Table 1 Number of asymptomatic and stroke (including TIA's) cases, separated into subgroups according to ECST stenosis and NASCET stenosis. Follow-up 6 months to 8 years (mean, 48 months) [3]. Groups of years of event are for ≤3 years group1 and >3 years group 2

ECST st (%)	NASCET st (%)	No	Asymp (%)	Stroke (%)	Group 1/2
All		1121	991(88.4)	108(9.6)	65–27
50–69	<50	198	182(92)	12(6.1)	13–5
70–89	50–82	598	533(89.1)	56(9.4)	28–11
90–99	83–99	325	276(84.9)	40(12.3)	24–11

TIAs Transient Ischemic Attacks; *ECST* European Carotid Surgery Trial; *NASCET* North American Symptomatic Carotid Endarter. Trial

included parameters like total cholesterol, LDL cholesterol, HDL cholesterol, Kreatinine, Triglycerides etc. as published in [3]. Duplex ultrasound scanning data were performed using a protocol and standard procedure specified during the study. These included artery stenosis and plaque characteristics based on image analysis algorithms as described in the following paragraphs and published in [3, 5].

The total number of patients collected through the study was 1121 out of which 108 strokes or TIAs were recorded. The data characteristics of the different groups are shown in Table 1. Stroke and TIA subjects are used in this chapter. These can be further divided into group1 short term period (event happened in ≤3 years from baseline) and group2-long term period (event happened in >3 years from baseline). In case we want to further divide the risk groups.

3 Image Normalization and Despeckle Filtering

The collected ultrasound images were also intensity normalized, as described in [14], where a manual selection of blood and adventitia performed by the user of the system is required. The gray-scale-intensity normalized image was obtained through algebraic (linear) scaling of the image by linearly adjusting the image so that the median-gray-level value of the blood was 0–5, and the median gray level of the adventitia (artery wall) was 180–190 [14, 15]. Following normalization despeckle filtering was applied to the image using the local statistics DsFlsmv despeckle filter [16]. The filter was applied once to the image using a 5×5 pixel sliding window (see also Fig. 1a, b).

4 Plaque Image Segmentation

Following normalization and despeckle filtering, a snakes' based segmentation procedure initially proposed in [17, 18], was applied. The procedure was further applied using the integrated system for the complete segmentation of the common carotid artery as proposed in [17]. The atherosclerotic carotid plaque, intima media complex and wall borders were segmented and saved (see also Fig. 1).

5 Imaging Feature Sets

Several image analysis features can been used from the segmented plaque, in the statistical analysis and automated classification models as described in [5, 9, 19, 20]. These features presented in this chapter were also presented in previous published studies and can be computed using the "Plaque Texture Analysis software" by LifeQ medical (http://www.lifeqmedical.com/). The standardization of images was done using an image normalization protocol as documented in [3]. The image analysis algorithms used for this chapter are described in the following subsections (Table 2).

5.1 Statistical Features (SF)

The SF features extracted from the plaque area, are based on the first order statistical analysis and they are resolution independent [5, 15, 16, 21]. The following SF features were computed: (i) *Mean value*, (ii) *Median value*, (iii) *Standard Deviation*, (iv) *Skewness*, (v) *Kurtosis*.

Table 2 List of risk factors—feature sets investigated for the data sets given in Table 2 for the asymptomatic and stroke (including TIAs) plaques. For the continuous variables, mean ± standard deviation, and for categorical variables the frequency of yes/no are tabulated. Univariate analysis (ttest) was carried out for the continuous parameters and the P value is given, and chi-square test for the categorical parameters. Features that are significantly different at P < 0.001 were used for the risk modelling as given in the last column

	Asymptomatic (N = 991)	Stroke (inc. TIAs) (N = 108)	P value	Used in clasiff.
FS 1: ACSRS Clinical and plaque features [3]				
Stenosis (%ECST)	77.64 ± 12.830	81.52 ± 11.673	0.002	Yes
Log (GSM + 40)	4.301 ± 0.313	4.058 ± 0.250	0.000	Yes
(Plaque Area)$^{1/3}$	3.40 ± 0.676	3.987 ± 0.794	0.000	Yes
DWAs (#of Yes cases) [3]	614	88	0.000	Yes
History of contr. TIAs and/or Stroke (#of Yes cases)	139	34	0.000	Yes
FS 2: Texture Features—SGLDM [19]				
SGLDM_ASM_mean	4.42 ± .738	3.92 ± 0.838	0.000	Yes
SGLDM_con_mean	0.026 ± 0.0802	0.0676 ± 0.1150	0.000	Yes
ln (SGLDM_con_mean)	−5.813 ± 1.8080	−4.018 ± 1.7830	0.000	Yes
SGLDM_SAV_range	0.306 ± .1341	0.412 ± 0.1482	0.000	Yes
SGLDM_SVAR_mean	94.692 ± 49.2841	61.211± 33.3339	0.000	Yes
SGLDM_ent_mean	5.018 ± 0.8032	4.512 ± 0.9301	0.000	Yes
ln (SGLDM_ent_mean)	2.245 ± .1992	2.114 ± 0.2382	0.000	Yes
SGLDM_diffvar_mean	7.0951 ± 1.2341	6.220 ± 1.3939	0.000	Yes
FS 3: Texture Features—Morphology [20]				
L image cdf for n = 1	0.0438 ± 0.0451	0.019 ± 0.0218	0.000	Yes
L image cdf for n = 2	0.120 ± 0.1063	0.057 ± 0.0611	0.000	Yes
L image cdf for n = 3	0.208 ± 0.1641	0.103 ± 0.1054	0.000	Yes
L image cdf for n = 4	0.294 ± 0.2110	0.148 ± 0.1358	0.000	Yes
L image cdf for n = 5	0.374 ± 0.2491	0.193 ± 0.1628	0.000	Yes
L image pdf for n = 1	0.0438 ± 0.0451	0.019 ± 0.0218	0.000	Yes
L image pdf for n = 2	0.076 ± 0.0646	0.037 ± 0.0100	0.000	Yes
L image pdf for n = 3	0.088 ± 0.0662	0.047 ± 0.0475	0.000	Yes
L image pdf for n = 4	0.086 ± 0.0609	0.044 ± 0.0330	0.000	Yes
L image pdf for n = 5	0.080 ± 0.0563	0.045 ± 0.0331	0.000	Yes

TIAs Transient Ischemic Attacks; *ECST* European Carotid Surgery Trial; *GSM* Grey Scale Median; *DWA* Discrete White Areas (Present or Absent) [3]; *SGLDM* Spatial Gray Level Dependence Matrices; *ASM* Angular Second Moment, *CON* Contrast, *SAV* Sum Average; *SVAR* Sum Variance, ENT Entropy; *Diffvar* Difference Variance

5.2 *Spatial Gray Level Dependence Matrices (SGLDM)*

The spatial gray level dependence matrices [21, 22] are based on the estimation of the second-order joint conditional probability density functions, $f(i, j, d, \theta)$. The $f(i, j, d, \theta)$ is the probability that two pixels (k, l) and (m, n) with distance d in direction specified by the angle θ, have intensities of gray level i and gray level j. The estimated values for these probability density functions will be denoted by $P(i, j, d, \theta)$. In a $N_x \times N_y$ image, let $L_x = \{1, 2, \ldots, N_x\}$ be the horizontal spatial domain, $L_y = \{1, 2, \ldots, N_y\}$ be the vertical spatial domain and $I(x, y)$ be the image intensity at pixel (x, y). Formally, for angles quantized at 45° intervals the unnormalized probability density functions are given in [21–23].

Haralick et al. [22], also proposed a number of texture measures, which can be extracted from the spatial gray level dependence matrices as follows:
(i) *Angular second moment*, (ii) *Contrast*, (iii) *Correlation*, (iv) *Sum of squares: variance*, (v) *Inverse difference moment*, (vi) *Sum average*, (vii) *Sum variance*, (viii) *Sum entropy*, (ix) *Entropy* (x) *Difference variance*, (xi) *Difference entropy and* (xii) (xiii) *Information measures of correlation 1 and 2*.

For a chosen distance d (in this work $d = 1$ was used) we have four angular gray level dependence matrices, i.e. we obtain four values for each of the above 13 texture measures. The mean and the range of the four values of each of the 13 texture measures comprise a set of 26 texture features which can be used for classification. Some of the 26 features are strongly correlated with each other, and a feature selection procedure may be applied in order to select a subset or linear combinations of them. In this work, the mean values and the range of values were computed for each feature for $d = 1$ and they were used as two different feature sets.

5.3 *Morphological Analysis*

Morphological features associated with plaque composition as described in [20] were also considered. This leads to the consideration of morphological features that come from: (i) dark regions associated with lipid, thrombus, blood, or haemorrhage, (ii) bright regions associated with collagen and calcified components, and (iii) medium-brightness regions that fall between them. As discussed in [20], the most promising results were given by morphological analysis of the dark image components. Following image normalization, the binary L images are generated using:

$$L = \{(i, j) : \text{such that } I(i, j) < 25\} \quad (1)$$

where I denotes the normalized image. A multiscale morphological decomposition of each binary image is generated using the difference images.

$$
\begin{aligned}
d_0(L; B) &= L - L \circ B, \\
d_1(L;\ B) &= L \circ B - L \circ 2B \\
&\vdots \\
d_{n-1}(L;\ B) &= L \circ (n-1)B - L \circ nB,
\end{aligned}
\tag{2}
$$

where B denotes the '+' structural element, $\circ$ denotes the morphological open operation, and d_n denotes the binary difference image. The binary difference images are then used to generate the morphological pdf using

$$
pdf_K(n, B) = A(d_n(L; B))/A(L). \tag{3}
$$

where $A(L)$ represents the number of pixels in the image, and n was allowed to vary from 1 to 70. The cdf was defined in terms of the pdf using:

$$
cdf_L(n, B) = \begin{cases} 0, & n = 0, \\ \sum\limits_{r=0}^{n-1} pdf_L(r, B), & n > 0. \end{cases} \tag{4}
$$

images that gave significant differences in the classification of symptomatic versus asymptomatic cases were used as texture features. This led to the use of

$$
pdf_L(r, B),\ cdf(p, B), \quad r, p = 1, \ldots, 5. \tag{5}
$$

as explained in [20].

6 Risk Modeling

6.1 Classifiers

Risk modeling was carried out using the Support Vector Machine (SVM) (and the LibSVM [24] library for Matlab®) and the Probabilistic Neural Networks classifiers. The classifier was trained to classify the feature sets investigated into two classes: (i) asymptomatic plaques or (ii) stroke (including TIA's) (or symptomatic) plaques, i.e. unstable plaques.

The Support Vector Machine (SVM) method [24] is initially based on a nonlinear mapping of the initial data set using a function $\varphi(.)$ and then the identification of a hyperplane which is able to achieve the separation of two categories of data. The vectors defining the hyperplanes can be chosen to be linear combinations with parameters α_i of images of feature vectors that occur in the data base. With this choice of a hyperplane, the points x in the feature space that are mapped into the hyperplane are defined by the relation:

$$\sum \alpha_i K(x_i, x) = constant\,() \tag{6}$$

If $K(x, y)$ becomes small as y grows further from x, each element in the sum measures the degree of closeness of the test point x to the corresponding data base point x_i. In this way, the sum of kernels above can be used to measure the relative nearness of each test point to the data points originating in one or the other of the sets to be discriminated.

Details about the implementation of the SVM algorithm used can be found In [24]. The SVM network was investigated using Gaussian Radial Basis Function (RBF) kernels; this was decided as the rest of the kernel functions could not achieve satisfactory results. The SVM with RBF kernel was investigated using 10-fold cross validation in order to identify the best parameters such as the spread of.

The Probabilistic Neural Network (PNN) [25] classifier was used for developing classification models for the problem under study. The PNN falls within the category of nearest-neighbour classifiers. For a given vector $\mathbf{w}$ to be classified, an activation a_i is computed for each of the two classes of plaques ($i = 1, \ldots, 2$). The activation a_i is defined to be the total distance of $\mathbf{w}$ from each of the M_i prototype feature vectors $\mathbf{x}_j^{(i)}$ that belong to the i-th class:

$$a_i = \sum_{j=1}^{M_i} \exp\left[-\beta\left(\mathbf{w} - \mathbf{x}_j^{(i)}\right)^T\left(\mathbf{w} - \mathbf{x}_j^{(i)}\right)\right], \tag{7}$$

where β is a smoothing factor. This classifier was investigated for several spread radii in order to identify the best radius for the current problem.

6.2 *Evaluation*

The performances of the classifier systems were measured using the following parameters: (i) true positives (TP) when the system correctly classifies plaques as symptomatic, (ii) false positives (FP) where the system wrongly classifies plaques symptomatic while they are asymptomatic, (iii) false negatives (FN) when the system wrongly classifies plaques as asymptomatic while they are symptomatic, and (iv) true negatives (TN) when the system correctly classifies plaques as asymptomatic. To evaluate the ability of the classifiers to predict high risk cases the Sensitivity (SE), which is the likelihood that a symptomatic plaque will be detected given that it is symptomatic, and Specificity (SP) which is the likelihood that a plaque will be classified as asymptomatic given that it is asymptomatic, were also evaluated.

For the overall performance, the correct classification (CC) rate, which gives the percentage of correctly classified plaques, is also provided [26] (see Table 3).

Table 3 High risk modelling prediction results of asymptomatic versus stroke (including TIAs), measures (mean ± standard deviation) are given for 2000 runs (10 bootstrapping sets of 100 asymptomatic and 100 stroke (including TIAs) cases drawn at random from the corresponding 991 asymptomatic, and 108 stroke cases; and the leave one out method was then run on each of the 200 set)

FS 1: ACSRS	FS 2: SGLDM	FS 3: Morphology	Classifier	% Correct classifications	% Sensitivity	% Specificity	% False negatives	% False positives
+			S	74 ± 2.5	78 ± 3.8	71 ± 4.0	23 ± 3.8	30 ± 4.0
+			P	64 ± 4.2	64 ± 3.3	65 ± 5.3	36 ± 3.3	35 ± 5.3
	+		S	**77 ± 1.8**	82 ± 3.4	72 ± 1.2	**18 ± 3.4**	**28 ± 1.2**
	+		P	65 ± 4.8	65 ± 6	65 ± 4.6	35 ± 6	35 ± 4.6
		+	S	72 ± 1.8	82 ± 4.3	63 ± 3.2	18 ± 4.3	37 ± 3.2
		+	P	63 ± 2.2	70 ± 3.6	56 ± 4.6	30 ± 3.6	44 ± 4.6
+	+		S	**76 ± 2.4**	79 ± 3.5	72 ± 3.0	**21 ± 3.5**	**28 ± 3.0**
+	+		P	64 ± 2.9	63 ± 4.9	66 ± 3.2	37 ± 4.9	34 ± 3.2
+		+	S	**76 ± 2.6**	80 ± 5	71 ± 6.3	**20 ± 5**	**29 ± 6.3**
+		+	P	67 ± 2.9	69 ± 3.9	64 ± 3.2	31 ± 3.9	36 ± 3.2
	+	+	S	74 ± 3.5	78 ± 4.7	70 ± 9.7	22 ± 4.7	30 ± 9.7
	+	+	P	65 ± 3.9	65 ± 5.9	65 ± 3.2	35 ± 5.9	35 ± 3.2
+	+	+	S	75 ± 4.2	78 ± 5.0	73 ± 6.9	22 ± 5.0	27 ± 6.9
+	+	+	P	64 ± 3.5	63 ± 4.2	66 ± 4.2	37 ± 4.2	34 ± 4.2

Features sets used as tabulated in Table 2; *FS 1* ACSRS Clinical and plaque features; *FS 2* Texture Features—SGLDM; *FS 3* Texture Features—Morphology. Risk modelling was carried out using the Probabilistic Neural Networks (P) and the Support Vector Machines (S) classification models

7 Results

A total of 1121 patients between 39 and 89 years (mean age 70.0 ± SD 7.7, 61% male) were recruited during 1998–2002 with a follow-up of 6–96 months (mean 48 months) in the context of the ACSRS study (see Table 2). A total of 130 first ipsilateral CORI events occurred (59 strokes of which 12 were fatal, 49 TIAs and 22 amaurosis fugax). There were 49 first contralateral CORI events (18 ischemic strokes of which 7 were fatal, 22 TIAs and 9 amaurosis fugax). There were 2 vertebrobasilar strokes. AF cases were excluded from the study thus having 1099 cases.

Features with significant difference at $P < 0.001$ were used in the prediction models. Figure 2 shows examples of normalised gray scale and color contoured images of segmented plaques with selected plaque features for both asymptomatic, and symptomatic plaques.

It is noted that as documented in the ACSRS study [3], comorbid conditions such as LDL, diabetes, etc. were not associated with the development of stroke in this population because they were high or present in the majority of patients. Also, the population of patients is with >50% carotid stenosis and are all high risk arteriopaths. Compared to the clinical features, it is interesting to note that the mean values for

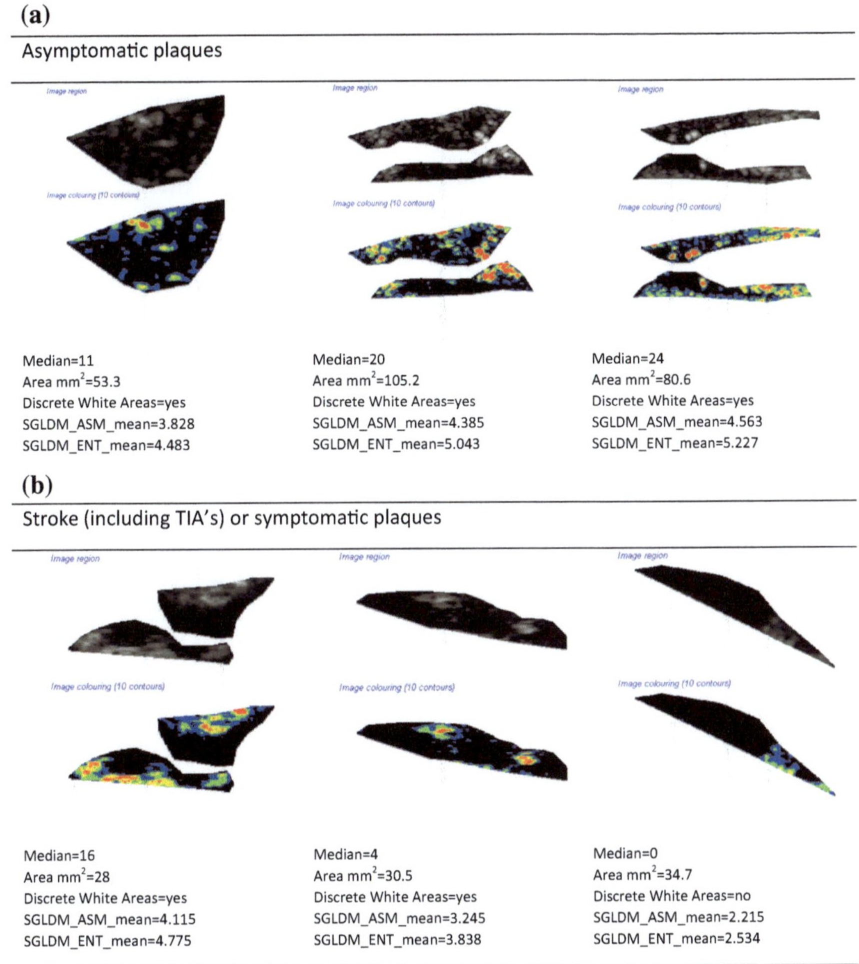

Fig. 2 Examples of normalised gray scale and color contoured images of segmented plaques with selected plaque features: **a** asymptomatic, and **b** stroke (including TIA's) or symptomatic (see Table 2 for feature description)

the different texture features give relatively large differences between asymptomatic and stroke cases. Unfortunately, texture features also exhibit higher variations than clinical features.

Table 3 tabulates the results from several runs using the SVM and PNN classifiers. The best correct classification in combination with high sensitivity and hi specificity was achieved using the SVM classifier and the SGLDM features. High risk modelling using the prediction results of asymptomatic vs stroke (including TIAs) are given in Table 3 based on the feature sets tabulated in Table 3: FS 1: ACSRS Clinical and plaque features; FS 2: Texture Features—SGLDM; FS 3: Texture Features—Mor-

Table 4 Confusion matrices for the best SVM prediction model and of the corresponding PNN model based on FS2 Texture—SGLDM features

	Prediction			
Observed	a		b	
	SVM		PNN	
	Sym	Asym	Sym	Asym
Sym. 108	89 (82%)	19 (18%)	71 (65%)	37 (35%)
Asym. 991	277 (28%)	714 (72%)	346 (35%)	645 (65%)
Total 1099	366	733	417	682

Sym. represents high risk cases that ended up having a stroke (including TIA's), whereas Asym. represents asymptomatic cases. AF cases were excluded from the study; Positive Predictive Value PPV = 24% (SVM), 17% (PNN
Negative Predictive value NPV = 97% (SVM), 94.5% (PNN)
Correct Classifications = 73% (SVM), 65% (PNN)

phology. Risk modelling was carried out using the Probabilistic Neural Networks (P) and the Support Vector Machines (S) classification models. The results are the average of 2000 runs, where 10 bootstrapping sets of 100 asymptomatic and 100 stroke (including TIAs) cases were drawn at random from the corresponding 991 asymptomatic, and 108 stroke cases.

Table 4 tabulates the results of the best risk prediction model based on SVM using the SGLDM plaque texture features. It can be seen that for this model, for the 1099 cases from the ACSRS dataset, the SVM model could correctly predict at baseline 89 out of the 108 cases that were symptomatic.

8 Conclusions

This chapter demonstrates how image texture and morphology analysis algorithms are used in order to classify ultrasound images of carotid plaques. Until now the results using different classifiers are very promising and have the potential for computer assisted identification of patients with asymptomatic carotid stenosis at increased risk of stroke. The results using image texture analysis algorithms presented in this chapter [5] are comparable with previous work carried out with different datasets [20, 21]. The Haralick SGLDM texture features gave best results in all studies whereas the statistical feature gray scale median (GSM) proved again a good and simple descriptor for plaque instability.

Morphological features help us understand the inter-relations among different intensity regions. We have examined morphological results from dark, mid-range, and high intensity regions. We have found that there was significant overlap between the pattern spectra coming from symptomatic and asymptomatic plaques. Furthermore, as we expected, probability density function (*pdf*) estimates were visually verified to be noisier than cumulative distribution function estimates. For larger morphological components, the *pdf* started to decrease, and the variance in the estimates increased significantly. Thus, most of the discriminating power was concentrated in the smaller components for lower scales.

The application of these techniques in combination with analysis of videos and motion of plaques is something that is still under research investigation and looks that is going to give some more promising results.

References

1. Reiter M, Horvat R, Puchner S, Rinner W, Polterauer P, Lammer J, Minar E, Bucek RA (2007) Plaque imaging of the internal carotid artery—correlation of b-flow imaging with histopathology. Am J Neuroradiol 28:122–126
2. Mathiesen E, Bonan K, Joakimsen O (2001) Echolucent plaques are associated with high risk of ischemic cerebrovascular events in carotid stenosis: the Tromso study. Circulation 103:2171–2175
3. Nicolaides A, Kakkos S, Kyriacou E, Griffin M et al (2010) Asymptomatic internal carotid artery stenosis and cerebrovascular risk stratification. J Vasc Surg 52(4):1486–1496
4. Topakian R, King A, Kwon S, Schaafsma A, Shipley M, Markus H (2011) Ultrasonic plaque echolucency and emboli signals predict stroke in asymptomatic carotid stenosis. Neurology 77:751–758
5. Kyriacou EC, Petroudi S, Pattichis CS, Pattichis MS, Griffin M, Kakkos S, Nicolaides A (2012) Prediction of high risk asymptomatic carotid plaques based on ultrasonic image features. IEEE Trans Inf Technol Biomed 16(5):966–973
6. AbuRahma A, Wulu J, Crotty B (2002) Carotid plaque ultrasonic heterogeneity and severity of stenosis. Stroke 33:1772–1775
7. Leahy AL, McCollum PT, Feeley TM et al (1998) Duplex ultrasonography and selection of patients for carotid endarterectomy: plaque morphology or luminal narrowing? J Vasc Surg 8:558–562
8. Langsfeld M, Gray-Weale AC, Lusby RJ (1989) The role of plaque morphology and diameter reduction in the development of new symptoms in asymptomatic carotid arteries. J Vasc Surg 9:548–557
9. Kakkos SK, Stevens JM, Nicolaides AN, Kyriacou E, Pattichis CS, Geroulakos G, Thomas D (2007) Texture analysis of ultrasonic images of symptomatic carotid plaques can identify those plaques associated with ipsilateral embolic brain infarction. Eur J Vas Endovasc Surg 33(4):422–429
10. Gray-Weale AC, Graham JC, Burnett JR et al (1988) Carotid artery atheroma: comparison of preoperative B-mode ultrasound appearance with carotid endarterectomy specimen pathology. J Cardiovasc Surg 29:676–681
11. Fox A (1993) How to measure carotid stenosis. Radiology 186:316–318
12. Executive Committee for the Asymptomatic Carotid Atherosclerosis Study (1995) Endarterectomy for asymptomatic carotid artery stenosis. J Am Med Assoc 273:1421–1428
13. MRC Asymptomatic Carotid Surgery Trial (ACST) Collaborative Group (2004) Prevention of disabling and fatal strokes by successful carotid endarterectomy in patients without recent neurological symptoms: randomized controlled trial. Lancet 363:1491–1502
14. Elatrozy T, Nicolaides AN, Tegos T, Zarka A, Griffin M, Sabetai M (1998) The effect of B-mode ultrasonic image standardization of the echodensity of symptomatic and asymptomatic carotid bifurcation plaque. Int Angiol 17(3):179–186
15. Loizou CP, Pattichis CS, Pantziaris MS, Tyllis T, Nicolaides AN (2006) Quantitative quality evaluation of ultrasound imaging in the carotid artery. Med Biol Eng Comput 44(5):414–426

16. Loizou CP, Theofanous C, Pantziaris M, Kasparis T (2014) Despeckle filtering software toolbox for ultrasound imaging of the common carotid artery. Comput Methods Programs Biomed 114(1):109–124
17. Loizou CP, Pattichis CS, Pantziaris M, Nicolaides A (2007) An integrated system for the segmentation of atherosclerotic carotid plaque. IEEE Trans Inf Technol Biomed 11(6):661–667
18. Loizou CP, Pantziaris M (2015) An integrated system for the complete segmentation of the common carotid artery bifurcation in ultrasound images. J Biomed Eng Inform 1(1):11–24
19. Christodoulou CI, Pattichis CS, Pantziaris M, Nicolaides A (2003) Texture based classification of atherosclerotic carotid plaques. IEEE Trans Med Imaging 22(7):902–912
20. Kyriacou E, Pattichis M, Pattichis CS, Mavrommatis A, Christodoulou CI, Kakkos S, Nicolaides A (2009) Classification of atherosclerotic carotid plaques using morphological analysis on ultrasound images. J Appl Intell 30(1):3–23
21. Kyriacou E, Pattichis M, Christodoulou C, Pattichis C, Kakkos S, Griffin M, Nicolaides A (2005) Ultrasound imaging in the analysis of carotid plaque morphology for the assessment of stroke, in plaque imaging: pixel to molecular level. In: Suri JS, Yuan C, Wilson DL, Laxminarayan S (eds) Studies in health technology and informatics, vol 113, IOS Press. pp 241–75. ISBN: 1-58603-516-9
22. Haralick RM, Shanmugam K, Dinstein I (1973) Texture features for image classification. IEEE Trans Syst Man Cybern SMC-3:610–621
23. Weszka JS, Dyer CR, Rosenfield A (1976) A comparative study of texture measures for terrain classification. IEEE Trans Syst Man Cybern SMC-6:269–285
24. Chang CC, Lin CJ (2011) LIBSVM: a library for support vector machines. ACM Trans Intell Syst Technol 2(3). http://www.csie.ntu.edu.tw/~cjlin/libsvm
25. Ross SM (2014) Introduction to probability and statistics for engineers and scientists, 3rd edn. Elsevier/Academic Press, Amsterdam
26. Ma H, Bandos AI, Rockette HE, Gur D (2013) On use of partial area under the ROC curve for evaluation of diagnostic performance. Stat Med 32(20):3449–3458

Signal Analysis in Atrial Fibrillation

Raúl Alcaraz and José J. Rieta

Abstract Recent advances and clinical applications of signal analysis in the characterization of the most common supra-ventricular arrhythmia, i.e. atrial fibrillation (AF), are summarized in this chapter. The analysis of invasive and non-invasive electrocardiographic signals has revealed useful clinical information in a broad variety of scenarios, thus opening new perspectives in the understanding of the currently unknown mechanisms triggering and maintaining the arrhythmia.

1 Introduction

Atrial fibrillation (AF) is the most frequent cardiac arrhythmia in clinical practice [1]. Its prevalence is close related to age, thus increasing significantly among old people. Indeed, whereas only about 0.15% of population under 50 years present AF, 17% of those older than 80 years suffer from this arrhythmia [2]. Moreover, although AF is not life-threatening in itself, it is associated with a five-fold risk of stroke and a three-fold incidence of congestive heart failure, such that AF patients present twice the risk of death than healthy people with the same age [3]. Hospitalizations are also very common in patients with this arrhythmia, thus leading to spend on the management of AF, at least, 15% of the healthcare budget in cardiac diseases [4]. These facts, along with the progressive growth of the elderly population, turn AF as a major health challenge in the developed world [5].

Despite the soaring research efforts in the last years, the pathophysiological mechanisms underlying AF are still not completely known [6]. During the fibrillation, the normal electrical activation degenerates into a chaotic pattern depolarizing

R. Alcaraz (✉)
Research Group in Electronic, Biomedical and Telecommunication Engineering,
University of Castilla-La Mancha, Cuenca, Spain
e-mail: raul.alcaraz@uclm.es

J. J. Rieta
BioMIT.org, Electronic Engineering Department,
Universidad Politécnica de Valencia, Valencia, Spain
e-mail: jjrieta@upv.es

S. Golemati and K. S. Nikita (eds.), *Cardiovascular Computing—Methodologies and Clinical Applications*, Series in BioEngineering,
https://doi.org/10.1007/978-981-10-5092-3_17

uncoordinatedly the atrial cells. However, it is undescribed yet how this chaotic pattern starts, maintains and sometimes finishes spontaneously [6]. A few theories to explain that behavior have been proposed in the last decades, including the existence of focal atrial activations (repetitive ectopic discharges), reentrant mechanisms (mother-waves, rotors, multiple wavelets) or longitudinal/transmural dissociated conduction between epicardial and endocardial heart layers, but any of them has been totally corroborated to date [6]. Hence, the lack of precise knowledge about the mechanisms triggering and maintaining AF renders its current diagnosis and treatment poorly effective [7].

To gain novel and helpful insights about the mechanisms supporting AF, signal processing techniques have been widely used to characterize invasive and noninvasive electrocardiographic (ECG) recordings in a broad variety of scenarios. The most useful clinical information obtained in this way is summarized in this chapter, without paying special attention to the mathematical description of the algorithms.

2 Some Basic Aspects About AF

2.1 Classification of AF

The duration of AF episodes has been commonly used to classify the arrhythmia [8]. Thus, its first stage is usually paroxysmal AF (PAF), which is featured by short episodes finishing spontaneously or with intervention in less than one week. In the next stage, named persistent AF (PEAF), the episodes persist for more than 7 days and normally require an intervention for their termination. When AF lasts for more than a year, it is called long-standing PEAF. It is worth noting that about 20% of PAF patients progress to PEAF in about four years [8]. Finally, when it is impossible to restore sinus rhythm (SR) and the patient and clinicians make a joint decision to avoid more rhythm-control strategies, the arrhythmia is labeled as permanent AF [8].

2.2 Current Management of AF Patients

Regardless of AF stage, three main objectives are pursued during its treatment, i.e.: (i) to prevent systemic or cerebral embolism; (ii) to control heart rate during AF (rate-control therapy) and (iii) to restore and maintain SR (rhythm-control therapy) [9]. To achieve the first goal, oral anticoagulants are usually prescribed in most AF patients. However, this treatment is unable to reduce common symptoms associated to the arrhythmia and, therefore, the patients have to be also treated with rate- and/or rhythm-control strategies. Although maintaining SR and preventing AF recurrences clearly improve the patient's quality of life, rate-control is an important objective for many AF patients. Both kinds of treatments are not mutually exclusive, however, recent studies have provided no improvement when they are combined with respect to rate-control alone [9]. Thus, current guidelines recommend an individualized decision regarding the choice of rate- versus rhythm-control with the primary goal of alleviating AF symptoms [10]. Therefore, rate-control by administration of β-blocker drugs is today applied to most patients with permanent AF, as well as to a few ones with PAF and PEAF [9].

The major obstacle to consider a rhythm-control strategy as the first-line treatment for AF is the high mid- or long-term recurrence of the arrhythmia [9]. Nonetheless, this kind of therapy is essential to reduce symptoms in many patients with PAF and PEAF. Thus, the main current options are electrical cardioversion (ECV), antiarrhythmic drugs, catheter ablation and MAZE surgery. However, given the low effectivity of ECV and antiarrhythmic drugs, catheter ablation is nowadays a very common procedure. Indeed, the isolation of pulmonary veins has proven to be an useful treatment to restore SR for long time in most patients with PAF, as well as in about half of the patients with PEAF [11]. To improve the success rate of the procedure in this later case, many experts have proposed to target atrial zones beyond pulmonary veins. However, no consensus has been reached yet about which additional atrial areas should be ablated [11]. Finally, the Cox-MAZE surgery is the most effective treatment to restore SR and prevent AF recurrence. In fact, several studies have reported long-term success rate higher than 85% for this procedure. Nonetheless, today the surgery is only applied to treat patients with permanent AF and other concomitant cardiac disorders [12].

2.3 *Invasive and Non-invasive ECG Recordings of AF*

Two kinds of recordings have been typically used to study AF, i.e., the surface ECG, and invasive intra-atrial electrograms (EGMs). The most relevant characteristics of these signals, as well as the main preprocessing steps used for their denoising and conditioning will be next described.

2.3.1 The Surface ECG Recording

The ECG signal is a noninvasive and widely used way to study AF, because the heart's electrical activity is recorded by using several leads placed on the patient's thorax. Compared with the invasive EGM, the ECG signal presents some interesting advantages, including its capability to acquire data for long periods of time, as well as the reduced costs and risks involved for the patient [13]. However, this recording is easily disturbed by noise and interferences and, therefore, it has to be cleaned before further analysis. To this respect, the signal is typically high-pass, low-pass and notch filtering to reduce baseline wandering, muscular noise and the powerline interference, respectively [14].

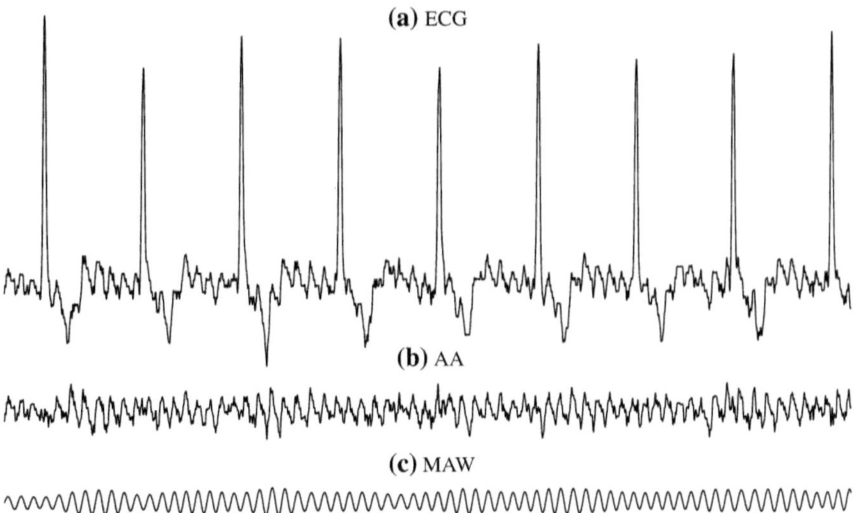

Fig. 1 Example of a common surface ECG (**a**), the extracted AA signal by the average QRST complex subtraction (**b**) and, finally, its MAW obtained by band-pass filtering (**c**)

Interestingly, the ECG is able to obtain simultaneously atrial and ventricular activities during each cardiac cycle, such that they can be separately analyzed. Nonetheless, for that purpose both activities have to be firstly detached, this task not being trivial. Although the P-wave is easily discerned from the QRST complex in patients with SR, this is not the case for patients with AF. Indeed, the P-wave is replaced by fibrillatory waves with variable timing, shape and morphology, which are moreover overlapped with QRST complexes both in time and frequency domains [13]. In last years, a variety of algorithms to separate atrial and ventricular activities have been proposed. Some of them exploit multi-lead ECG spatial diversity by using tools as principal component analysis or blind source separation. In contrast, other methods are based on cancelling every individual QRST complex by subtracting a temple obtained from the average of all beats [15]. These techniques are able to work even with single-lead ECG signals, which are common in contexts where very long periods of time have to be recorded [15]. Regardless of how the atrial activity (AA) was obtained, it is worth noting that its main atrial wave (MAW) has been widely analyzed in previous works [16]. This signal is computed from the AA by applying a bandwidth filtering centered on its dominant atrial frequency (DAF) to reduce noise and ventricular residua from the QRST cancellation [16]. A representative example of a common ECG recording and its AA and MAW signals is shown Fig. 1.

A strong feature of AF is that patients often present a fast and irregular ventricular response [17]. This behavior has been broadly studied by characterizing the heart rate variability (HRV) in time, frequency and complexity domains, such that this analysis is nowadays a clinically accepted tool to assess the role of autonomic nervous system (ANS) in AF [18]. However, its result hardly depends on a robust detection of the

R-peaks, thus existing a wide variety of algorithms for that purpose [19], as well as for correcting wrong locations due to the presence of artifacts and abnormal beats [20].

2.3.2 The Intra-atrial EGM Recording

For a thorough study of AF, different invasive EGMs are captured along with the ECG, including bipolar and unipolar signals from endocardial and epicardial electrodes, optical as well as non-contact recording systems [21]. Although to lesser extent than the ECG, these recordings are also contaminated by common noise and nuisance signals, thus also requiring to be filtered [22]. Additionally, whereas unipolar signals are commonly characterized by a notable far-field contamination of ventricular activity, bipolar signals mainly record local atrial activations from the regions where electrodes are located. Nonetheless, bipolar recordings from some atrial areas close to the ventricles, such as the coronary sinus, often also present ventricular contamination. In contrast to the ECG, in this case only a few algorithms have been proposed to separate atrial and ventricular activities [23, 24]. Nonetheless, the resulting signal has been widely featured with a variety of signal processing tools.

To this last respect, the automatic identification of local activation waves (LAWs), such as Fig. 2 shows for an example, is a very interesting challenge. Indeed, from the detected points, different map-based representations can be reconstructed for different atrial structures, thus locating successfully areas with delayed or blocked conduction, fibrosis and other electrophysiological alterations [25]. Nowadays, a few algorithms to detect LAWs, both from unipolar and bipolar EGMs, can be found in the literature [26, 27], but most of them fail to work robustly with highly complex and fractionated signals [28].

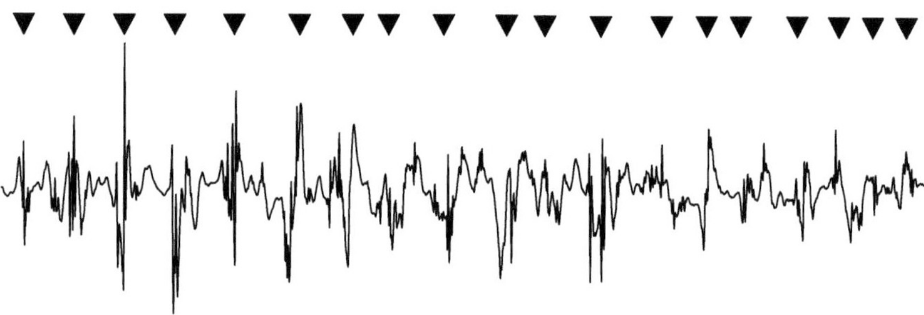

Fig. 2 Illustrative example of a fractionated bipolar EGM signal, where its LAWs have been automatically detected by the algorithm proposed by Osorio et al. [28]

3 Analysis of the Surface ECG Recording

3.1 Characterization of the Atrial Activity

The AA signal extracted from the ECG recording has been characterized from a broad variety of facets, the most relevant ones being described next.

3.1.1 Spectral Analysis of the AA Signal

The DAF is nowadays a clinically accepted marker of the atrial substrate status [29]. The most common approach for its computation is based on estimating the AA spectral distribution and, then, determining the frequency with the largest peak [30]. Although different alternatives have been proposed to compute the AA spectral content, the most used one is the Welch periodogram. In this approach Fourier transform is applied to short and overlapped AA segments and the resulting signals are then averaged to reduce the variance in the spectral estimation. An key aspect to obtain accurate DAF measures is to consider, at least, two second-length AA intervals [15].

This frequency index has been analyzed in a broad variety of clinical scenarios, thus providing very relevant and useful information. Indeed, it has proven to be sufficiently sensitivity to quantify changes in atrial electrophysiology during natural evolution of PAF, e.g., in the electrical atrial remodeling as well as in the autonomic tone [6]. For instance, higher values of DAF has been associated with longer PAF episodes during a follow-up of about 12 months [31]. Within each PAF episode, the time course of DAF has also been analyzed. Thus, an increase of this frequency has been noticed during the first minutes after the onset of PAF, such as Fig. 3a displays. Contrarily, a decrease has also been seen some seconds before the spontaneous termination of the arrhythmia (see Fig. 3b) [32, 33].

On the other hand, the DAF has also been used to monitor the effect of different AF treatments, as well as to predict a priori their mid- and long-term outcome. To this respect, the index has proven to be highly predictive of the spontaneous termination of PAF [34]. In a similar way, considering only patients with new-onset AF, the DAF has also been able to identify those patients where the arrhythmia terminates spontaneously with a sensitivity of 89% and a specificity of 71% [35]. Regarding the use of pharmacological treatments to restore SR in the patient, the DAF has shown a promising ability to identify suitable candidates for some drugs. Indeed, DAF values lower than 6 Hz have been able to detect accurately AF termination in patients under intravenous ibutilide and oral flecainide [30]. Similarly, higher values of DAF have also been observed in patients responding negatively to internal [36] and external electrical cardioversions [37]. Additionally, the combination of DAF with some echocardiographic parameters has also reported an improved ability to anticipate the ECV outcome [37].

Finally, changes in the DAF as a response to catheter ablation have been recently assessed. Thus, most works have identified a DAF decrease during the procedure,

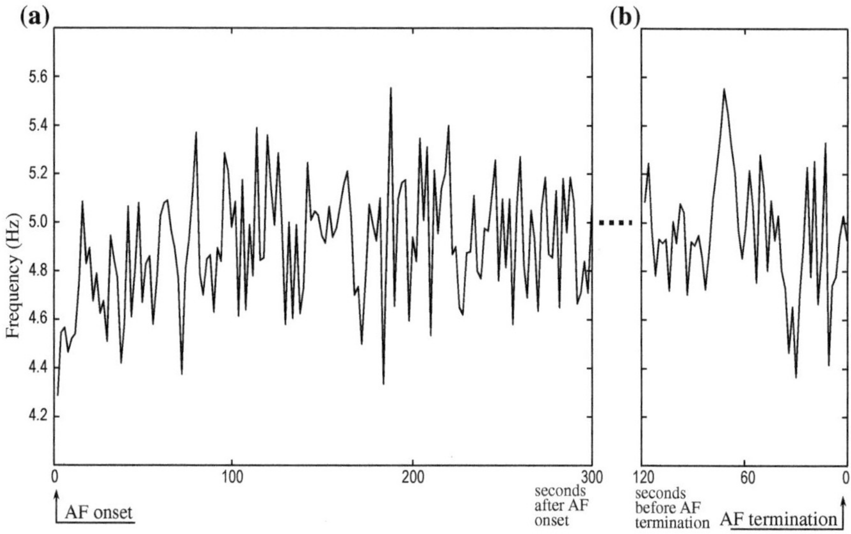

Fig. 3 Time course of the DAF for the first five minutes after the onset of PAF (**a**), as well as for the last two minutes before its spontaneous termination (**b**). This plot was obtained as an average from a set of 45 patients [32]

but no consensus has still been reached about the role of this aspect to anticipate its long-term outcome. In fact, whereas some authors have suggested that a DAF decrease about 5–10% is associated with a long-term maintenance of postoperative SR [38, 39], others have been unable to notice a similar observation [40, 41]. Maybe, the different ablation protocols used for the studies could explain this inconclusive situation. More recently, some AA spectral parameters beyond the DAF have been analyzed to improve its predictive ability [42]. Thus, some single metrics have shown to be better predictors than the DAF, such as the amplitude of its first harmonic and the AA harmonic structure for PAF and PEAF, respectively. Nonetheless, the combination of several of these parameters has achieved accuracy values higher than 80% to predict the ablation outcome for both types of AF.

3.1.2 Time-Frequency Analysis of the AA Signal

A relevant limitation of the described spectral analysis is its inability to estimate with high precision how the DAF evolves along the time. In fact, atrial electrophysiological features quickly progress during AF and, therefore, the AA can be considered as a strong time-dependent signal [43]. Hence, to track accurately long-term DAF variations, different time–frequency transformations have been proposed. The simplest method for that purpose is the short-term Fourier transform, which has been successfully used to anticipate spontaneous termination of PAF in more than 90% of patients [44]. However, despite this positive result, some authors have proven that

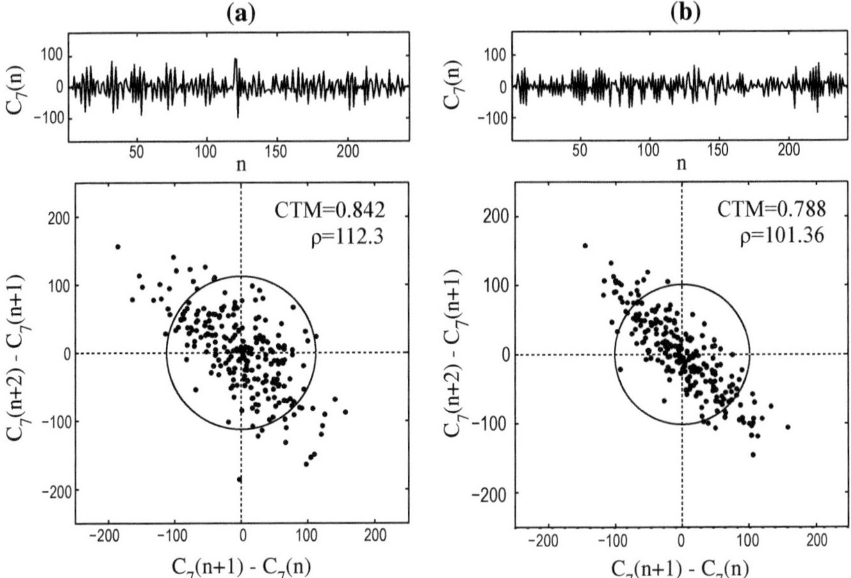

Fig. 4 Typical examples of the seventh time scale ($C_7(n)$) of the AA signal together with its dispersion plot for PEAF patients responding positively (**a**) and negatively (**b**) to ECV after a follow-up of one month. Regularity of the time series was estimated from the dispersion graphs through the central tendency measure (CTM)

this time-frequency method is unable to track very quick DAF changes, thus proposing the use of more complex algorithms [45]. As an example, using Wigner-Ville distribution to estimate the phase time course of short ECG signals, an increased ability to discern between different stage of AF has been recently found [46].

A pioneering time-frequency transformation to track evolution of DAF and its harmonics has also been introduced by Stridh et al. [45]. The inclusion of harmonics in the DAF tracking not only improves its estimation, but the harmonic pattern contains information of clinical significance in several scenarios, as previously mentioned for catheter ablation. Finally, note that Wavelet transform has also been widely used to estimate how some time-frequency properties of fibrillatory waves evolve along the time. To this respect, decomposing the AA signal into several time scales and analyzing the regularity from some of these new time series, useful information has been obtained to predict spontaneous termination of PAF, as well as to anticipate the ECV outcome in patients with PEAF [47, 48]. As an example, Fig. 4 shows the seventh time scale ($C_7(n)$) of the AA signal, together with its dispersion graph, for typical patients with positive and negative responses to ECV. From the dispersion plot, the central tendency measure (CTM) was estimated as the rate of points within a circle of radio ρ centered on the origen [47].

3.1.3 Regularity Analysis of the AA Signal

The organization presented by the AA signal has also been widely analyzed in the last years, thus revealing significant clinical information in multiple scenarios. Although a standard definition for the AA organization cannot be found in the literature, this aspect refers to the level of repetitive patterns presented by fibrillatory waves. Indeed, this kind of measurement is able to reflect heterogeneity in atrial conduction, because some previous works have proven the presence of well-defined and repetitive fibrillatory waves during organized atrial rhythms and, contrarily, highly fragmented and irregular waves during disorganized episodes of AF [49]. To estimate AA organization in the described way, different signal processing tools have been applied to the surface fibrillatory waves. However, the most widely used algorithm is based on computing regularity of the MAW signal by using the well-known sample entropy [16]. This methodology has revealed an interesting ability to predict a broad variety of AF organization-dependent events [16]. In fact, it has been able to anticipate spontaneous termination of PAF with a high accuracy (about 95%), as well as to predict the ECV outcome in more than 90% of PEAF patients [16]. Additionally, analyzing the AA organization with this method after each electrical shocks, a relevant decrease only for the patients who finally reverted to SR and maintained this rhythm for a long time has also been noticed [50].

In addition to sample entropy, other nonlinear indices have also been used to estimate AA organization. To this respect, classical information theory metrics, such as the correlation dimension, the largest Lyapunov exponent and the Lempel-Ziv complexity, have been able to discern successfully between episodes of AF and atrial flutter [51]. As expected, more irregular and disorganized fibrillatory waves were observed for AF than both for typical and atypical flutters. In a similar line, Sun & Wang have also reported a promising ability to anticipate spontaneous termination of PAF by analyzing the AA temporal structure in terms of recurrent plots [52]. More recently, the spatial organization of the fibrillatory waves has been analyzed by representing their variation from two orthogonal leads in a single plane [53]. In this way several minutes before the conversion of AF to an atrial tachyarrhythmia during catheter ablation have been analyzed and the expected progression towards more organized fibrillatory waves has been successfully quantified.

3.2 Characterization of the Ventricular Activity

3.2.1 Analysis During SR

AF is usually characterized by an irregular ventricular response with a higher average rate than for SR. This is the result of bombarding the atrioventricular (AV) node with many irregular and quick impulses, of which only a few ones can be conducted to the ventricles. Thus, heart rate variability (HRV) analysis has provided very useful information from the inherent conduction properties of that atrial structure [54]. Moreover, today it is also clinically accepted that HRV analysis is able to quantify successfully changes in the ANS, which plays a key role in the triggering of PAF [55]. This fact has motivated a huge number of works analyzing HRV before the arrhythmia onset [56]. In fact, according with the enhanced parasympathetic activity noticed by different authors just before the onset of AF [57], some nonlinear indices, including scale exponents for the detrended fluctuation analysis and some entropies, have reported a significant complexity decrease [58, 59]. In a similar way, a very recent study has found a progressive decrease in typical HRV spectral parameters just after the termination of PAF, thus suggesting that the ANS could also contribute extensively in that event [60].

On the other hand, HRV analysis has also proven a promising prognostic value about the effectivity of different AF treatments. To this respect, the preoperatively computed mean value of the RR-interval series as well as its low-frequency spectral energy have been associated with early and late recurrences of AF after successful ECV [61]. These metrics have suggested an increased sympathetic and reduced vagal modulation before the procedure only for those patients with a high risk of AF recurrence. Contrarily, in internal electrical cardioversion under general anesthesia AF recurrence has been associated with an increase in vagal modulation [62]. Regarding catheter ablation, HRV before and one year after irrigated-tip, contact-force sensing-guided and cryoballoon procedures have been compared making use of several time and frequency parameter [63]. In the three cases a similar increase in the parasympathetic activity for patients with AF recurrence have been reported. A similar result has also been observed for the common ablation procedure based on the isolation of pulmonary veins [64].

Finally, note that HRV has been analyzed after coronary artery bypass grafting and aortic surgery to anticipate the onset of postoperative AF. More precisely, the use of nonlinear indices to compute HRV complexity has been able to predict the development of AF after on-pump coronary artery bypass grafting, but not after off-pump one [65]. Additionally, a similar analysis of the RR-interval series after aortic surgery has provided no alteration between patients developing or not postoperative AF [66]. This result suggests that transection of ascending aorta for repair of an aortic aneurysm does not prevent AF compared to patients with intact ascending aorta. In a more general context, low HRV complexity during surgical procedures has also been associated with an increased mortality risk for a postoperative period of 48 h [67].

3.2.2 Analysis During AF

Because an organized AA usually precedes termination of induced and PAF [16], Lombardi et al. [68] have analyzed whether a similar finding is also applicable to the ventricular activity. However, any significant change in mean and variance of RR-interval series during initial, central and final parts of PAF episodes has been observed. Contrarily, nonlinear HRV characterization through Lorenz plots and entropy-based metrics has identified several promising harbingers of spontaneous termination of PAF [69]. In view of these contradictory findings, further studies are required to clarify the ANS role in the arrhythmia maintenance and termination.

On the other hand, HRV has also been analyzed to stratify several risks associated with AF. To this respect, Stein et al. [70] have reported that energy concentrated on ultra-low- and high-frequency in HRV is able to identify the combined risk of mortality or requirement for mitral valve surgery in AF patients with chronic severe mitral regurgitation. Similarly, some time and frequency HRV parameters have also provided an interesting ability to predict survival in patients with permanent AF and advanced heart failure [71]. In contrast to these works, Platonov and Holmqvist [72] have not find a significant link between HRV complexity and mortality in patients with mild to moderate chronic heart failure, enrolled in the *Muerte Súbita en Insuficiencia Cardiaca* (MUSIC) study. Hence, more investigation in this field seems to be required yet.

As previously mentioned, the main conduction features of the AV node have also been explored through the HRV analysis. To this respect, the functional refractory period of this atrial structure and its conduction rate of atrial impulses have been widely estimated through the lower envelope for a Poincaré plot-based representation of the RR-interval series [73]. Interestingly, the analysis of 24-h Holter recordings from 48 permanent AF patients has revealed that these two conduction properties of the AV node also present a circadian rhythm [73]. Additionally, the study of long-term ECG recordings has allowed to discern two clearly differentiated sections in histograms of RR-interval series for most PEAF patients [74]. This result suggests the existence of two predominant conduction routes throughout the AV node, the functional refractoriness being more pronounced for the fastest one [74]. A similar result has also been observed by using three dimensional Poincaré plots. It is worth noting that in this later work a statistically significant link between the RR-interval series regularity for the predominant pathway and the AA organization has also been found [75].

In last years the AV node behavior under different drugs has also been characterized by studying mainly HRV complexity and variability. To this respect, the ventricular response of patients with PAF has been analyzed under the administration of quinidine, thus reporting different RR-interval series distributions as a function of DAF, which decreased in the course of drug's infusion [76]. Some other studies have also reported that the modification of the AV node conduction properties under rate-control drugs (e.g. diltiazem, verapamil, metoprolol, and carvedilol) increases variability of the RR-interval series, but not its irregularity [77]. Contrarily, the use of β-blockers has only shown an alteration in the RR-interval series irregularity [78].

3.3 Synchronization Between Atrial and Ventricular Activities

Some of the aforementioned works have suggested that the rate and organization of the atrial activations bombarding the AV may play a key role in the ventricular response during AF [75, 76, 79]. However, in these works the relationship between atrial and ventricular activations has been globally analyzed by characterizing separately the time series resulting from both activities [75, 79]. Indeed, both data series have been mainly featured through statistical variables, estimated from their probabilistic density function [79], or via indirect estimators obtained from several second-length ECG recordings [80]. Contrarily, instantaneous interdependency between atrial and ventricular anctivations has been recently quantified by using estimators of synchronization between time series [81, 82].

To this respect, coupling between atrial and ventricular time series has been assessed through cross sample entropy [81], as well as via the stroboscopic observation of the ventricular phase at times triggered by the atrial activation [82]. In both cases, beat-to-beat atrial and ventricular coupling is evaluated, thus allowing instantaneous tracking of AV conduction properties. Precisely, in this way a strong dependence between the synchronization of atrial and ventricular activities and the degree of AA organization has been corroborated, according to previous works [81]. Moreover, the effect of an increase in atrial rate on the synchronization of atrial and ventricular activations has also been analyzed, thus revealing that the shortening of atrial intervals determines higher instability in the AV node conduction [83]. Another more recent finding is that the variability and irregularity of the ventricular response is influenced both by atrial rate and conduction parameters of the AV node [54].

4 Study of Intra-atrial EGM Recordings

4.1 Analysis of Single-Lead EGM Signals

As an alternative to the surface ECG analysis, the main dynamics reflected on single-lead EGMs have also been assessed to obtain precise estimates of AF organization. In fact, as for the ECG, temporal AF organization has been quantified by computing similar and repetitive patterns in the signal. Thus, according to the facility for discerning atrial activations in the EGM, Wells et al. discerned three kinds of AF, named types I, II and III [84], and numerous algorithms have been proposed for their automatic identification. This aspect is highly interesting, because these types of AF have been associated with atrial regions showing different conduction properties [85]. Note that one of the first attempts was proposed by Hoekstra et al. [86], who used nonlinear indices to discern type I from types II and III AF signals. Several years later, Mainardi et al. proposed the application of conditional entropy to the single-lead EGM for an improved discrimination of these kinds of AF [87].

Interestingly, these two algorithms have been used to quantify the effect of different drugs on AF organization. Precisely, they have been able to identify subtle variations of organization in different atrial sites after the administration of cibenzoline [88] and isoproterenol [89].

More recently, the automatic identification of complex and fractionated atrial EGMs (CFAEs) has gained great interest. This kind of signal is very similar to the type III AF and, in the last decade, has become a potential target for ablation, because it has been strongly associated with atrial zones supporting AF [11]. Given that detection of CFAEs by visual inspection is time-consuming and subjective, a variety of algorithms for their automatic identification have been recently proposed. Most of them are based on quantifying morphological irregularity in the signal through entropy-based metrics and other specific indices estimating multifractality [90, 91].

Individual analysis of each single-lead EGM captured from a basket catheter has also provided organization differences between relatively close atrial areas. Thus, Pitschner et al. [92] have found that the region anterior to the tricuspid valve shows the most chaotic activity during permanent AF. In a similar line, Cervigón et al. [93] have also reported statistically significant organization differences in the left atrium between PAF and PEAF. Finally, some authors have only reported an organization increase in right atrium under the administration of antiarrhythmic [94] and anesthetic [95] drugs.

4.2 Analysis of Multiple and Simultaneous EGM Recordings

In the last decade the mutual analysis of simultaneous EGM signals acquired from different atrial regions has been proposed to provide spatiotemporal estimates of AF organization. Briefly, the AA generated in an atrial region is evaluated in relation to the activity obtained in another zone. In this way, interesting complementary information to the one obtained by the analysis of single-lead EGMs has been revealed. In fact, linear and nonlinear estimates of the coupling between pairs of EGMs have reached a very high accuracy in the automatic identification of types I, II, and III AF episodes [87, 96]. Moreover, the synchronization analysis between atrial areas has also been useful to quantify the underlying effect of adrenergic stimulation [97] and different antiarrhythmic drugs [98] on AF organization. More recently, stronger causal links have been noticed among areas located in the right than in the left atrium during PAF, thus supporting the hypothesis that high-frequency periodic sources in the left atrium may maintain the arrhythmia [93]. Contrarily, similar relationships have been observed among zones of both cameras in patients with PEAF [93].

On the other hand, the joint interpretation of simultaneous EGM signals covering a specific area has resulted in the concept of atrial mapping. Nowadays, the most commonly used approach is isochronal or activation mapping, which is aimed at creating a spatial model of the excitation sequence [99]. In this representation the LAWs have to be firstly detected and, then, the delays regarding an origen are color-coded. Other representations, including propagation, voltage, frequency or geometric maps, are also able to provide useful clinical information for the treatment of AF [100]. However, phase mapping is the most used one in the last years, because it is able to represent more clearly propagation of electrical waveforms. Indeed, the EGM phase transformation allows to enhance the relative timing of the events, rather than the simply instantaneous activity. Moreover, the application of this kind of analysis, together with other undescribed mathematical operations, to the EGMs acquired by a panoramic catheter with 64 poles has proven to be able to identify time and spatial stable rotors in PAF and PEAF patients [101].

Finally, it is interesting to remark that these maps were initially designed to cover a small atrial region, but nowadays the construction of 3D maps representing completely the atria is possible by the sequential acquisition of EGM recordings on the whole endocardial surface [100]. This approach is time-consuming and presents some problems associated to the sequential reconstruction of the map, however it has achieved to improve and facilitate significantly the current procedures of catheter ablation of AF [100].

4.3 *Simultaneous Analysis of Surface and Invasive Recordings*

With the aim of identifying noninvasively those sources responsible for the maintenance of AF before the ablation procedure, some authors have compared information obtained from intra-atrial recordings with the one collected from body surface potential maps (BSPM) [102, 103]. Among the main results, it has been revealed that BSPM systems are able to replicate noninvasively the endocardial distribution of DAFs and, moreover, can also identify small areas supporting the high-frequency sources suspected to maintain AF [104]. Additionally, this kind of analysis has also been able to estimate a similar frequency gradient between both atria to the one obtained from intra-cardiac EGMs for patients responding negatively to catheter ablation [103]. Interestingly, the phase analysis of these surface ECG recordings has also shown reentrant patterns with spatiotemporal stability in the atrial conduction of AF patients [105]. However, to achieve this result, the recordings have had to be previously band-pass filtered to reduce the effect of the atrial electrical activity occurring at different frequencies and this kind of aggressive processing has been recently proven to generate artificial and non-realistic rotors [106]. Therefore, the noninvasive location of rotors from BSPM deserves further investigation.

Finally, it is also worth noting that a commercial system has been recently introduced to reconstruct cardiac surface potentials by applying non-described mathematical algorithms to 252 signals acquired on the patient's torso [102]. The system also requires a non-contrast thoracic CT scan to obtain high-resolution images of the biatrial geometry and the relative electrode positions. Although its use to terminate with AF has been proven in a considerable number of patients with PAF and PEAF, no prospective multicenter studies have been published yet to confirm its real value in the context of catheter ablation of AF [107]. Nonetheless, they are certainly coming in a close future.

5 Conclusions

Recent advances in the analysis of surface and intra-cardiac ECG recordings have provided powerful solutions for the enhanced knowledge of the mechanisms triggering and maintaining AF. Moreover, spectral, morphological and organization analyses of that single- and multi-lead signals have also revealed clinically useful information to improve current diagnosis and therapy of this cardiac arrhythmia.

Acknowledgements This work has been supported by grants DPI2017–83952–C3 MINECO/AEI/FEDER, UE and SBPLY/17/180501/000411 from Junta de Comunidades de Castilla-La Mancha.

References

1. Chugh SS, Roth GA, Gillum RF et al (2014) Global burden of atrial fibrillation in developed and developing nations. Glob Heart 9(1):113–9
2. Zoni-Berisso M, Lercari F, Carazza T et al (2014) Epidemiology of atrial fibrillation: European perspective. Clin Epidemiol 6:213–20
3. Khoo CW, Krishnamoorthy S, Lim HS et al (2012) Atrial fibrillation, arrhythmia burden and thrombogenesis. Int J Cardiol 157(3):318–23
4. Wodchis WP, Bhatia RS, Leblanc K et al (2012) A review of the cost of atrial fibrillation. Value Health 15(2):240–8
5. Van Wagoner DR, Piccini JP (2013) Albert CM (2015) Progress toward the prevention and treatment of atrial fibrillation: a summary of the heart rhythm society research forum on the treatment and prevention of atrial fibrillation, Washington, DC, December 9–10. Heart Rhythm 12(1):e5–e29
6. Schotten U, Dobrev D, Platonov PG et al (2016) Current controversies in determining the main mechanisms of atrial fibrillation. J Intern Med 279(5):428–38
7. Fabritz L, Guasch E, Antoniades C (2016) Expert consensus document: defining the major health modifiers causing atrial fibrillation: a roadmap to underpin personalized prevention and treatment. Nat Rev Cardiol 13(4):230–7
8. January CT, Wann LS, Alpert JS et al (2014) 2014 AHA/ACC/HRS guideline for the management of patients with atrial fibrillation: a report of the American College of Cardiology/American Heart Association Task Force on Practice Guidelines and the Heart Rhythm Society. J Am Coll Cardiol 64(21):e1–76
9. Margulescu AD, Mont L (2017) Persistent atrial fibrillation vs paroxysmal atrial fibrillation: differences in management. Expert Rev Cardiovasc Ther 15(8):601–618
10. Kirchhof P, Benussi S, Kotecha D et al (2016) 2016 ESC guidelines for the management of atrial fibrillation developed in collaboration with EACTS. Eur Heart J 37(38):2893–2962
11. Bond R, Olshansky B, Kirchhof P (2017) Recent advances in rhythm control for atrial fibrillation. F1000Res 6:1796
12. Albåge A, Johansson B, Kennebäck G et al (2016) Long-term follow-up of cardiac rhythm in 320 patients after the Cox-Maze III procedure for atrial fibrillation. Ann Thorac Surg 101(4):1443–9

13. Petrutiu S, Ng J, Nijm GM et al (2006) Atrial fibrillation and waveform characterization. a time domain perspective in the surface ECG. IEEE Eng Med Biol Mag 25:24–30
14. Sörnmo L, Laguna P (2005) Bioelectrical signal processing in cardiac and neurological applications. Elsevier Academic Press
15. Sörnmo L, Stridh M, Husser D et al (2009) (1887) Analysis of atrial fibrillation: from electrocardiogram signal processing to clinical management. Philos Trans A Math Phys Eng Sci 367:235–53
16. Alcaraz R, Rieta JJ (2010) A review on sample entropy applications for the non-invasive analysis of atrial fibrillation electrocardiograms. Biomed Signal Process Control 5:1–14
17. Zhang Y, Mazgalev TN (2004) Ventricular rate control during atrial fibrillation and AV node modifications: past, present, and future. Pacing Clin Electrophysiol 27(3):382–93
18. Sassi R, Cerutti S, Lombardi F et al (2015) Advances in heart rate variability signal analysis: joint position statement by the e-Cardiology ESC working group and the European heart rhythm association co-endorsed by the Asia Pacific heart rhythm society. Europace 17(9):1341–53
19. Merah M, Abdelmalik TA, Larbi BH (2015) R-peaks detection based on stationary wavelet transform. Comput Methods Programs Biomed 121(3):149–60
20. Nabil D, Reguig F (2015) Ectopic beats detection and correction methods: a review. Biomed Signal Process Control 18:228–244
21. Stevenson WG, Soejima K (2005) Recording techniques for clinical electrophysiology. J Cardiovasc Electrophysiol 16(9):1017–22
22. Martínez-Iniesta M, Ródenas J, Alcaraz R et al (2017) Waveform integrity in atrial fibrillation: The forgotten issue of cardiac electrophysiology. Ann Biomed Eng 45(8):1890–1907
23. Rieta JJ, Hornero F (2007) Comparative study of methods for ventricular activity cancellation in atrial electrograms of atrial fibrillation. Physiol Meas 28(8):925–36
24. Corino VDA, Rivolta MW, Sassi R et al (2013) Ventricular activity cancellation in electrograms during atrial fibrillation with constraints on residuals' power. Med Eng Phys 35(12):1770–7
25. Verheule S, Tuyls E, van Hunnik A et al (2010) Fibrillatory conduction in the atrial free walls of goats in persistent and permanent atrial fibrillation. Circ Arrhythm Electrophysiol 3(6):590–9
26. Ng J, Sehgal V, Ng JK et al (2014) Iterative method to detect atrial activations and measure cycle length from electrograms during atrial fibrillation. IEEE Trans Biomed Eng 61(2):273–8
27. Cantwell CD, Roney CH, Ng FS et al (2015) Techniques for automated local activation time annotation and conduction velocity estimation in cardiac mapping. Comput Biol Med 65:229–42
28. Osorio D, Alcaraz R, Rieta J (2017) A fractionation-based local activation wave detector for atrial electrograms of atrial fibrillation. In: Computing in Cardiology, vol 44, pp 1–4
29. Gadenz L, Hashemi J, Shariat M et al (2017) Clinical role of dominant frequency measurements in atrial fibrillation ablation–a systematic review. J. Atr. Fibrillation 9(6):1–7
30. Bollmann A, Kanuru NK, McTeague KK et al (1998) Frequency analysis of human atrial fibrillation using the surface electrocardiogram and its response to ibutilide. Am J Cardiol 81(12):1439–1445
31. Niwano S, Fukaya H, Sasaki T et al (2007) Effect of oral l-type calcium channel blocker on repetitive paroxysmal atrial fibrillation: spectral analysis of fibrillation waves in the holter monitoring. Europace 9(12):1209–15
32. Alcaraz R, Rieta JJ (2009) Non-invasive organization variation assessment in the onset and termination of paroxysmal atrial fibrillation. Comput Methods Progr Biomed 93(2):148–154
33. Petrutiu S, Sahakian AV, Swiryn S (2007) Abrupt changes in fibrillatory wave characteristics at the termination of paroxysmal atrial fibrillation in humans. Europace 9(7):466–70
34. Nilsson F, Stridh M, Bollmann A et al (2006) Predicting spontaneous termination of atrial fibrillation using the surface ECG. Med Eng Phys 28(8):802–8
35. Husser D, Cannom DS, Bhandari AK et al (2007) Electrocardiographic characteristics of fibrillatory waves in new-onset atrial fibrillation. Europace 9(8):638–42

36. Bollmann A, Mende M, Neugebauer A et al (2002) Atrial fibrillatory frequency predicts atrial defibrillation threshold and early arrhythmia recurrence in patients undergoing internal cardioversion of persistent atrial fibrillation. Pacing Clin Electrophysiol 25(8):1179–84
37. Bollmann A, Husser D, Steinert R et al (2003) Echocardiographic and electrocardiographic predictors for atrial fibrillation recurrence following cardioversion. J Cardiovasc Electrophysiol 14(10 Suppl):S162–S165
38. Yoshida K, Chugh A, Good E et al (2010) A critical decrease in dominant frequency and clinical outcome after catheter ablation of persistent atrial fibrillation. Heart Rhythm 7(3):295–302
39. Matsuo S, Lellouche N, Wright M et al (2009) Clinical predictors of termination and clinical outcome of catheter ablation for persistent atrial fibrillation. J Am Coll Cardiol 54(9):788–95
40. Raine D, Langley P, Murray A et al (2005) Surface atrial frequency analysis in patients with atrial fibrillation: assessing the effects of linear left atrial ablation. J Cardiovasc Electrophysiol 16(8):838–44
41. Garibaldi M, Zarzoso V, Latcu DG et al (2012) Predicting catheter ablation outcome in persistent atrial fibrillation using atrial dominant frequency and related spectral features. Conf Proc IEEE Eng Med Biol Soc 2012:613–6
42. Alcaraz R, Hornero F, Rieta JJ (2016) Electrocardiographic spectral features for long-term outcome prognosis of atrial fibrillation catheter ablation. Ann Biomed Eng 44(11):3307–3318
43. Al Abed A, Guo T, Lovell NH et al (2013) Optimisation of ionic models to fit tissue action potentials: application to 3D atrial modelling. Comput Math Methods Med 2013:951234
44. Vayá C, Rieta JJ (2009) Time and frequency series combination for non-invasive regularity analysis of atrial fibrillation. Med Biol Eng Comput 47(7):687–96
45. Stridh M, Sörnmo L, Meurling CJ et al (2004) Sequential characterization of atrial tachyarrhythmias based on ECG time-frequency analysis. IEEE Trans Biomed Eng 51(1):100–14
46. Ortigosa N, Fernández C, Galbis A et al (2016) Classification of persistent and long-standing persistent atrial fibrillation by means of surface electrocardiograms. Biomed Tech (Berl) 61(1):19–27
47. Alcaraz R, Rieta JJ (2012) Central tendency measure and wavelet transform combined in the non-invasive analysis of atrial fibrillation recordings. Biomed Eng Online 11:46
48. Sterling M, Huang DT, Ghoraani B (2014) Developing time-frequency features for prediction of the recurrence of atrial fibrillation after electrical cardioversion therapy. Conf Proc IEEE Eng Med Biol Soc 2014:5498–501
49. Alcaraz R, Hornero F, Martínez A et al (2012) Short-time regularity assessment of fibrillatory waves from the surface ECG in atrial fibrillation. Physiol Meas 33(6):969–84
50. Alcaraz R, Rieta JJ, Hornero F (2009) Non-invasive atrial fibrillation organization follow-up under successive attempts of electrical cardioversion. Med Biol Eng Comput 47(12):1247–55
51. Kao T, Su Y, Lu C et al (2005) Differentiation of atrial flutter and atrial fibrillation from surface electrocardiogram using nonlinear analysis. J Med Biolog Eng 25(3):117–122
52. Sun R, Wang Y (2008) Predicting termination of atrial fibrillation based on the structure and quantification of the recurrence plot. Med Eng Phys 30(9):1105–11
53. Baykaner T, Trikha R, Zaman JAB et al (2017) Electrocardiographic spatial loops indicate organization of atrial fibrillation minutes before ablation-related transitions to atrial tachycardia. J Electrocardiol 50(3):307–315
54. Masè M, Disertori M, Marini M et al (2017) Characterization of rate and regularity of ventricular response during atrial tachyarrhythmias insight on atrial and nodal determinants. Physiol Meas 38(5):800–818
55. Shaffer F, Ginsberg JP (2017) An overview of heart rate variability metrics and norms. Front Public Health 5:258
56. Boon K, Khalil-Hani M, Malarvili M (2018) Paroxysmal atrial fibrillation prediction based on HRV analysis and non-dominated sorting genetic algorithm. Comput Methods Progr Biomed 153:171–184
57. Bollmann A, Lombardi F (2006) Electrocardiology of atrial fibrillation. Current knowledge and future challenges. IEEE Eng Med Biol Mag 25(6):15–23

58. Tuzcu V, Nas S, Börklü T et al (2006) Decrease in the heart rate complexity prior to the onset of atrial fibrillation. Europace 8(6):398–402
59. Shin DG, Yoo CS, Yi SH et al (2006) Prediction of paroxysmal atrial fibrillation using nonlinear analysis of the R-R interval dynamics before the spontaneous onset of atrial fibrillation. Circ J 70(1):94–9
60. Huang JH, Lin YK, Hsieh MH et al (2017) Modulation of autonomic nervous activity in the termination of paroxysmal atrial fibrillation. Pacing Clin Electrophysiol 40(4):401–408
61. Choi W, Choi E, Piccirillo G et al (2014) Pre-cardioversion heart rate variability predicts recurrence of atrial fibrillation after electrical cardioversion. Exp Clin Cardiol 20(8):4419–4431
62. Bertaglia E, Zoppo F, Bonanno C et al (2005) Autonomic modulation of the sinus node following electrical cardioversion of persistent atrial fibrillation: relation with early recurrence. Int J Cardiol 102(2):219–23
63. Mori H, Kato R, Ikeda Y, et al (2017) Analysis of the heart rate variability during cryoballoon ablation of atrial fibrillation. Europace
64. Seaborn GEJ, Todd K, Michael KA et al (2014) Heart rate variability and procedural outcome in catheter ablation for atrial fibrillation. Ann Noninvasive Electrocardiol 19(1):23–33
65. Wongcharoen W, Kiatkumpol C, Phromminitikul A et al (2014) The predictive effort of heart rate variability on atrial fibrillation after coronary artery bypass grafting. Exp Clinical Cardiol 20(64):145–159
66. Compostella L, Russo N, D'Onofrio A et al (2015) Abnormal heart rate variability and atrial fibrillation after aortic surgery. Rev Bras Cir Cardiovasc 30(1):55–62
67. Mandel-Portnoy Y, Levin MA, Bansilal S et al (2016) Low intraoperative heart rate volatility is associated with early postoperative mortality in general surgical patients: a retrospective case-control study. J Clin Monit Comput 30(6):911–918
68. Lombardi F, Tarricone D, Tundo F et al (2004) Autonomic nervous system and paroxysmal atrial fibrillation: a study based on the analysis of RR interval changes before, during and after paroxysmal atrial fibrillation. Eur Heart J 25(14):1242–8
69. Sun RR, Wang YY (2009) Predicting spontaneous termination of atrial fibrillation based on the RR interval. Proc Inst Mech Eng H 223(6):713–26
70. Stein KM, Borer JS, Hochreiter C et al (1994) Variability of the ventricular response in atrial fibrillation and prognosis in chronic nonischemic mitral regurgitation. Am J Cardiol 74(9):906–11
71. Frey B, Heinz G, Binder T et al (1995) Diurnal variation of ventricular response to atrial fibrillation in patients with advanced heart failure. Am Heart J 129(1):58–65
72. Platonov PG, Holmqvist F (2011) Atrial fibrillatory rate and irregularity of ventricular response as predictors of clinical outcome in patients with atrial fibrillation. J Electrocardiol 44(6):673–7
73. Hayano J, Ishihara S, Fukuta H et al (2002) Circadian rhythm of atrioventricular conduction predicts long-term survival in patients with chronic atrial fibrillation. Chronobiol Int 19(3):633–48
74. Oka T, Nakatsu T, Kusachi S et al (1998) Double-sector Lorenz plot scattering in an R-R interval analysis of patients with chronic atrial fibrillation: incidence and characteristics of vertices of the double-sector scattering. J Electrocardiol 31(3):227–35
75. Climent AM, Guillem MS, Husser D et al (2009) Poincaré surface profiles of RR intervals: a novel noninvasive method for the evaluation of preferential AV nodal conduction during atrial fibrillation. IEEE Trans Biomed Eng 56(2):433–42
76. Gelzer AR, Moïse NS, Vaidya D et al (2000) Temporal organization of atrial activity and irregular ventricular rhythm during spontaneous atrial fibrillation: an in vivo study in the horse. J Cardiovasc Electrophysiol 11(7):773–84
77. Corino VDA, Ulimoen SR, Enger S et al (2015) Rate-control drugs affect variability and irregularity measures of RR intervals in patients with permanent atrial fibrillation. J Cardiovasc Electrophysiol 26(2):137–41

78. Corino VDA, Holmqvist F, Mainardi LT et al (2014) Beta-blockade and A1-adenosine receptor agonist effects on atrial fibrillatory rate and atrioventricular conduction in patients with atrial fibrillation. Europace 16:587–94
79. Climent AM, Atienza F, Millet J et al (2011) Generation of realistic atrial to atrial interval series during atrial fibrillation. Med Biol Eng Comput 49(11):1261–8
80. Corino VDA, Sandberg F, Mainardi LT et al (2011) An atrioventricular node model for analysis of the ventricular response during atrial fibrillation. IEEE Trans Biomed Eng 58(12):3386–95
81. Alcaraz R, Rieta JJ (2013) Nonlinear synchronization assessment between atrial and ventricular activations series from the surface ECG in atrial fibrillation. Biomed Signal Process Control 8(6)
82. Mase M, Glass L, Disertori M et al (2013) The AV shynchrogram: a novel approacth to quantify atrioventricular couplin during atrial arrhythmias. Biomed Signal Process Control 8(6):1008–1016
83. Masè M, Marini M, Disertori M et al (2015) Dynamics of AV coupling during human atrial fibrillation: role of atrial rate. Am J Physiol Heart Circ Physiol 309(1):H198–205
84. Wells JL Jr, Karp RB, Kouchoukos NT et al (1978) Characterization of atrial fibrillation in man: studies following open heart surgery. Pacing Clin Electrophysiol 1:426–38
85. Gaita F, Calò L, Riccardi R et al (2001) Different patterns of atrial activation in idiopathic atrial fibrillation: simultaneous multisite atrial mapping in patients with paroxysmal and chronic atrial fibrillation. J Am Coll Cardiol 37(2):534–41
86. Hoekstra BP, Diks CG, Allessie MA et al (1995) Nonlinear analysis of epicardial atrial electrograms of electrically induced atrial fibrillation in man. J Cardiovasc Electrophysiol 6(6):419–40
87. Mainardi LT, Porta A, Calcagnini G et al (2001) Linear and non-linear analysis of atrial signals and local activation period series during atrial-fibrillation episodes. Med Biol Eng Comput 39(2):249–54
88. Hoekstra BPT, Diks CGH, Allessie MA et al (1997) Nonlinear analysis of the pharmacological conversion of sustained atrial fibrillation in conscious goats by the class Ic drug cibenzoline. Chaos 7(3):430–446
89. Mainardi LT, Corino VDA, Lombardi L et al (2004) Assessment of the dynamics of atrial signals and local atrial period series during atrial fibrillation: effects of isoproterenol administration. Biomed Eng Online 3(1):37
90. Cirugeda-Rodán E, Novak D, Kremen V et al (2015) Caracterization of complex fractionated atrial electrograms by sample entropy: an international multi-center study. Entropy 17(11):7493–7509
91. Orozco-Duque A, Novak D, Kremen V et al (2015) Multifractal analysis for grading complex fractionated electrograms in atrial fibrillation. Physiol Meas 36(11):2269–84
92. Pitschner HF, Berkovic A, Grumbrecht S et al (1998) Multielectrode basket catheter mapping for human atrial fibrillation. J Cardiovasc Electrophysiol 9(8 Suppl):S48–56
93. Cervigón R, Moreno J, Reilly RB et al (2010) Entropy measurements in paroxysmal and persistent atrial fibrillation. Physiol Meas 31(7):1011–20
94. Berkowitsch A, Carlsson J, Erdogan A et al (2000) Electrophysiological heterogeneity of atrial fibrillation and local effect of propafenone in the human right atrium: analysis based on symbolic dynamics. J Interv Card Electrophysiol 4(2):383–94
95. Cervigón R, Moreno J, Sánchez C et al (2009) Atrial fibrillation organization: quantification of propofol effects. Med Biol Eng Comput 47(3):333–41
96. Masè M, Faes L, Antolini R et al (2005) Quantification of synchronization during atrial fibrillation by Shannon entropy: validation in patients and computer model of atrial arrhythmias. Physiol Meas 26(6):911–23
97. Mainardi LT, Corino VDA, Lombardi L et al (2006) Linear and nonlinear coupling between atrial signals. Three methods for the analysis of the relationships among atrial electrical activities in different sites. IEEE Eng Med Biol Mag 25(6):63–70
98. Corino VDA, Mantica M, Lombardi F et al (2006) Assessment of spatial organization in the atria during paroxysmal atrial fibrillation and adrenergic stimulation. Biomed Tech (Berl) 51(4):260–3

99. Yaksh A, Kik C, Knops P et al (2014) Atrial fibrillation: to map or not to map? Neth Heart J 22(6):259–66
100. Kim D, Ahn H (2012) Current stuatus and future cardiac mapping in atrial fibrillation. In: Choi PJI (ed) Atrial fibrillation—basic research and clinical applications, chap. 6. InTech, pp. 93–124
101. Narayan SM, Vishwanathan MN, Kowalewski CAB, et al (2017) The continuous challenge of af ablation: From foci to rotational activity. Rev Port Cardiol 36(Suppl 1):9–17
102. Haissaguerre M, Hocini M, Denis A et al (2014) Driver domains in persistent atrial fibrillation. Circulation 130(7):530–8
103. Atienza F, Climent AM, Guillem MS (2015) Frontiers in non-invasive cardiac mapping: rotors in atrial fibrillation-body surface frequency-phase mapping. Card Electrophysiol Clin 7(1):59–69
104. Zhou Z, Jin Q, Chen LY et al (2016) Noninvasive imaging of high-frequency drivers and reconstruction of global dominant frequency maps in patients with paroxysmal and persistent atrial fibrillation. IEEE Trans Biomed Eng 63(6):1333–1340
105. Rodrigo M, Guillem MS, Climent AM et al (2014) Body surface localization of left and right atrial high-frequency rotors in atrial fibrillation patients: a clinical-computational study. Heart Rhythm 11(9):1584–91
106. King B, Porta-Sánchez A, Massé S et al (2017) Effect of spatial resolution and filtering on mapping cardiac fibrillation. Heart Rhythm 14(4):608–615
107. Nattel S, Xiong F, Aguilar M (2017) Demystifying rotors and their place in clinical translation of atrial fibrillation mechanisms. Nat Rev Cardiol 14(9):509–520

Cardiovascular Computing in the Intensive Care Unit

Spyretta Golemati

Abstract Clinical practice in the intensive care unit (ICU) faces a number of challenges, including accurate and early detection of pathological processes, and the related decision-making often relies on haemodynamic monitoring. In this chapter, applications are presented of computerised approaches for analysing data obtained from haemodynamic monitoring in the ICU. Haemodynamic monitoring is primarily concerned with assessing the performance of the cardiovascular system and conventionally relies on blood pressure measurements and echocardiography, for estimating cardiac output and other physiological variables. In addition to haemodynamic monitoring, less common techniques in the ICU (applanation tonometry, carotid and venous ultrasound), can also be used in cardiovascular computing applications. Such applications span a wide range of clinically relevant issues, including organisation and archiving of data into structured databases, data analytics, decision making and prediction, as well as estimation of arterial stiffness. Large, comprehensive, publicly available databases facilitate benchmarking of machine learning algorithms using real-world data. Such algorithms can in turn contribute to improving sepsis prediction in the ICU through (a) the identification of new features useful for prediction and (b) the processing of large data amounts, so as to consider combined contributions of individual features. The evidence produced so far indicates that cardiovascular data archiving and analysis using advanced computing methodologies is promising for addressing crucial issues in the ICU, and highlights the role that clinical data analysis will increasingly play in both knowledge generation and medical practice.

S. Golemati (✉)
First Intensive Care Unit, Medical School, National Kapodistrian University of Athens, Athens, Greece
e-mail: sgolemati@med.uoa.gr

S. Golemati and K. S. Nikita (eds.), *Cardiovascular Computing—Methodologies and Clinical Applications*, Series in BioEngineering,
https://doi.org/10.1007/978-981-10-5092-3_18

1 Introduction

The intensive care unit (ICU) has been called the hallmark of the modern hospital, where teams of dedicated professionals, using the latest technology, strive to save lives that in the past would almost surely be lost. In addition to deciding about admitting or discharging patients, ICU operational procedures include a number of safety practices used during the provision of direct patient care at the bedside and elsewhere. The major challenges faced by intensive care clinicians include accurate and early detection of pathological processes, which often remain hidden until they are well along their course, as well as rapid identification of proper treatments and verification that those treatments are working properly [1].

Decision making in the ICU is a particularly stressful and difficult operation for the physician, and presents substantial challenges, including increased complexity and variety of cases, interpretation of vast amounts of heterogeneous data and limited time available. Intensive care practice is characterised by a very close temporal relationship between monitoring, decision-making and treatment. As an example, management of sepsis, a condition resulting when the body's response to infection causes life-threatening organ dysfunction, is a complicated clinical challenge requiring early recognition and management of infection, haemodynamic issues, and other organ dysfunctions [2].

To stabilise ICU patients, bedside monitoring is essential, and allows the acquisition of large amounts of data, which are used for decision making. Among different types of ICU monitoring, haemodynamic monitoring is a key component in the effective management of the critically ill patient, i.e. the patient at high risk of death. Haemodynamic monitoring is primarily concerned with assessing the performance of the cardiovascular system and determining the correct therapeutic intervention to optimise end-organ oxygen delivery. The spectrum of haemodynamic monitoring ranges from simple clinical assessment and routine bedside monitoring to point-of-care ultrasonography and various invasive monitoring devices. Functional haemodynamic monitoring is that aspect of the measure of cardiovascular variables, either alone or in response to a physiologic perturbation, that defines a pathophysiological state, drives therapy or identifies cardiovascular insufficiency more accurately and often earlier than possible by analysis of static haemodynamic variables. Haemodynamic monitoring is crucial for assessing haemodynamic status in shocked patients and for guiding fluid treatment and administration of vasoactive drugs. Appropriate and early application of diagnostic information from haemodynamic monitoring has been shown to reduce mortality in septic shock.

It is useful to recognise that bedside data must be extracted and organised to become information, and that an expert should then interpret this information before it becomes knowledge for diagnostic and/or therapeutic purposes. As is the case with other types of monitoring, haemodynamic monitoring produces large amounts of data, which are now available electronically. Such availability allows further processing of the produced data, towards extracting information useful for facilitating decision-making.

The purpose of this chapter is to provide an overview of computerised approaches for analysing data obtained from haemodynamic monitoring in the ICU. In this context, the basic principles of haemodynamic monitoring are presented, a variety of recently developed computerised methods are described, and their potential for clinical applications in the ICU is discussed.

2 Cardiovascular Data in the ICU

In this section, brief descriptions are provided for cardiovascular data acquisition methods which have been used in applications of cardiovascular computing in the ICU. These include conventional haemodynamic monitoring, including blood pressure monitoring and echocardiography, as well as less commonly encountered techniques, including applanation tonometry, and carotid and venous ultrasound.

2.1 Haemodynamic Monitoring in the ICU

Currently available methods for assessing haemodynamic status include clinical assessment, serial biomarker interpretation, blood pressure monitoring, ultrasonography, bioreactance monitoring, pulse oximetry to estimate oxygen saturation, central venous pressure assessment, and the pulmonary artery (Swan-Ganz) catheter [3]. Over the last few decades, haemodynamic monitoring has evolved from basic monitoring of cardiac output to sophisticated devices allowing assessment of a large number of physiological variables [4]. The accuracy, reliability, validity and applicability vary with each of these devices and methods. The choice of monitoring technique should be individualised and depends on the underlying patient pathology, whether the patient is fully ventilated, the invasiveness of the monitoring technique, clinician experience and whether dynamic (continuous) or static monitoring is required.

2.2 Blood Pressure Monitoring

Mean blood pressure is measured with intensive care monitors via the calculation of the integral of the blood pressure wave. Blood pressure fluctuates around its mean value, following a complex mechanism, and reaching a systolic (maximal) and a diastolic (minimal) value. The difference of the two last values is the pulse pressure. Figure 1 shows an example of blood pressure waveform and derived static indices. Interpretation of these static blood pressure indices allows assessment of a patient's haemodynamic status [5]. Blood pressure measurement is achieved through the insertion of catheters in an artery in the wrist.

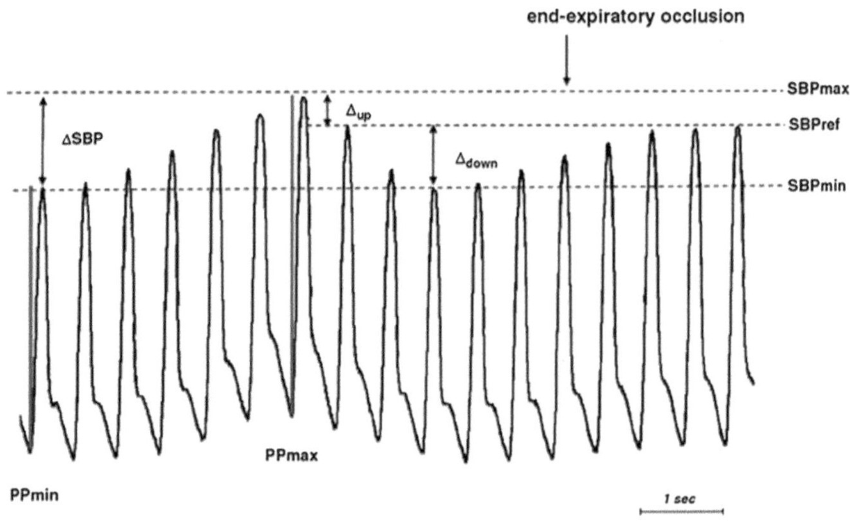

Fig. 1 Dynamic indexes of preload-dependence derived from the blood pressure curve. SBP: systolic blood pressure, SBPmax: maximal systolic blood pressure, SBPmin: minimal systolic blood pressure, SBPref: reference systolic blood pressure, PPmax: maximal pulse pressure, PPmin: minimal pulse pressure (Reprinted by permission from Springer Customer Service Centre GmbH: Springer Nature Intensive Care Medicine [5], 2010)

2.3 *Echocardiography*

Echocadiography is an appealing tool for haemodynamic monitoring due to its advantages, including non-invasiveness, safety, non-ionising radiation and bedside availability [6]. It allows real-time anatomical and functional cardiac assessment in very different situations, as in sepsis or acute respiratory distress syndrome (ARDS). However, it is operator dependent and is associated with a steep learning curve. Some pioneers started to use echocardiography in the ICU in the 1980s, especially in sepsis where it was able to detect profound cardiac failure. After many years of development and clinical studies in critically ill patients, scientific societies defined critical care echocardiography as echocardiography performed by intensivists themselves at the bedside for diagnosis of cardiac failure and haemodynamic monitoring.

Transthoracic echocardiography (TTE) is often used as a first-line approach as it is especially suitable for basic assessment, where intensivists perform a quick and focused examination to diagnose or exclude 'gross' cardiac abnormalities [6]. Transoesophageal echocardiography (TEE) is especially accurate in mechanically ventilated patients with ARDS or septic shock, where advanced critical care echocardiography is required. Whereas TTE is totally non-invasive, TEE is considered as

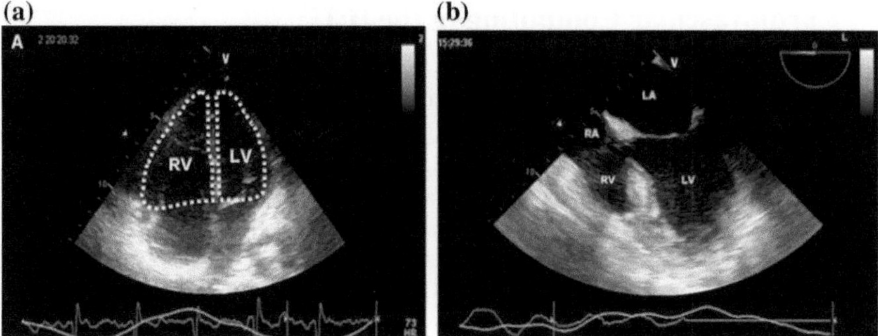

Fig. 2 **a** Apical four-chamber view by a transthoracic approach: RV dilatation in a patient with acute cor pulmonale. **b** Transoesophageal 4-chamber view in a ventilated patient. The probe is introduced into the esophagus 30 cm from the dental arch. Note that the right ventricle appears normally triangular. RA: right atrium, RV: right ventricle, LA: left atrium, LV: left ventricle (Reprinted by permission from Springer Customer Service Centre GmbH: Springer Nature Journal of Clinical Monitoring and Computing [6], 2012)

semi-invasive because of esophageal intubation [6]. Figure 2 shows examples of TTE and TEE images.

Over the last few years, a new approach to haemodynamic evaluation called functional haemodynamic monitoring has been developed [7]. It is less based on numbers and invasive tools, and more on qualitative and "functional" assessment, and on prediction of treatment effect. Echocardiography is perfectly adapted to this new approach.

2.4 *Less Common Techniques in the ICU*

In an attempt to address the potential adverse effects associated with arterial catheter placement, applanation tonometry has been shown promising for non-invasive beat-to-beat blood pressure monitoring [8].

Point of care ultrasound of the common carotid artery has been demonstrated to be accurate and feasible, and can be a noninvasive alternative for measuring cardiac output in the critically ill [9]. More recently, ultrasound imaging of the jugular vein has allowed the extraction of waveforms of cardiac variation in this vascular area, which can be used to estimate haemodynamic parameters, including stroke volume and central venous pressure, as well as intravascular dehydration [10].

3 Cardiovascular Computing in the ICU

Data derived from haemodynamic monitoring and other cardiovascular-related measurements can be used in several computing applications towards improving clinical practice in the ICU. Such applications span a wide range of clinically relevant issues, including archiving and organisation of data into structured databases, data analytics, decision making and prediction, as well as estimation of arterial stiffness.

3.1 ICU Databases

The huge amounts of data generated in the hospital ICU offer great opportunities to understand and improve care, but this is not fully realised nor exploited due to limitations in integration and reproducibility of data. The traditional approach to create evidence needs to be re-considered so as to take advantage of technological advancements in software and hardware allowing creation and maintenance of comprehensive databases with highly detailed ICU data [11]. These databases can motivate clinical investigations, facilitate the development of clinical decision support tools, and permit the benchmarking of algorithms with the use of real-world data. They are also useful in clinical research when prospective randomised clinical trial results are absent, as is the case with several ICU issues.

A number of commercial and non-commercial ICU databases have been suggested, archiving patient demographic and disease-related information such as underlying disease, severity of illness, and unit- and hospital-specific information (e.g., length of stay, mortality, and readmission). Such databases aim mainly to assess and compare the severity of ICU patient conditions and outcomes, as well as treatment costs, across participating ICUs, relying on relatively few selected pieces of information. For example, the non-commercial database maintained by the Australian and New Zealand Intensive Care Society now contains data from more than 900,000 ICU stays. Examples of commercial ICU databases include APACHE Outcomes, with data from approximately 150,000 ICU stays since 2010, and Philips eICU, a telemedicine intensive care support provider, including data from participating ICUs. Philips eICU is estimated to maintain a database of over 1.5 million ICU stays, and is expanding by 400,000 patient records yearly from over 180 subscribing hospitals. This tightly controlled database is made available to selected researchers via the eICU Research Institute [12].

The Medical Information Mart for Intensive Care (MIMIC-III) database (Fig. 3) allows free access to a large critical care database, enabling clinical research and education [13]. MIMIC-III is the evolution of Multiparameter Intelligent Monitoring in the Intensive care (MIMIC-II), and is a single-centre database comprising information relating to patients admitted to critical care units at a large tertiary care hospital. Data include haemodynamic recordings as well as additional clinical features, and as opposed to other databases, includes waveform data. MIMIC-III contains data associated with 53,423 distinct hospital admissions for adult patients (aged 16 years or

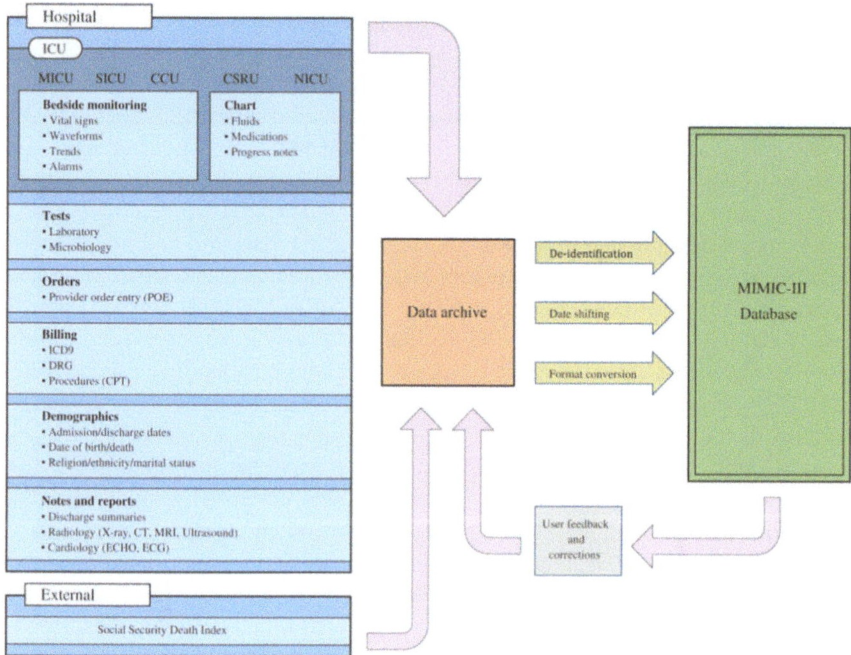

Fig. 3 Overview of the MIMIC-III database (Reprinted from [13]; license: https://creativecommons.org/licenses/by/4.0/)

above) admitted to critical care units between 2001 and 2012. In addition, it contains data for 7870 neonates admitted between 2001 and 2008. The data covers 38,597 distinct adult patients and 49,785 hospital admissions. Data available in the MIMIC-III database ranges from time-stamped, nurse-verified physiological measurements made at the bedside to free-text interpretations of imaging studies provided by the radiology department.

3.2 *ICU Data Analytics, Decision Making and Prediction*

The data generated in the ICU are used to make decisions about the patient treatment. To make decisions, ICU clinicians currently use two types of information, including (a) parameters derived from bedside physiological measurements (e.g. mean arterial pressure), and (b) quantitative metrics of level of severity (e.g. the Acute Physiology and Chronic Health Evaluation (APACHE) score) [14]. The application of statistical methods, and in more advanced stages, of machine learning techniques can yield interesting information about ICU events. Statistical methods allow the investigation of associations between physiological parameters and clinical endpoints. Machine learning methodologies go beyond statistical analysis and provide further insight into the fundamental mechanisms of disease, towards prediction. They are data-driven approaches, based on large and comprehensive collections of patient records with known diagnosis, therapies and course [14]. A large number of such data-analytics-based investigations have relied on the publicly available MIMIC databases, but some studies have used data from different ICUs. The major issues highlighted in such applications include prediction, namely which patients will survive/die/progress to a worse state, and the identification of the optimal parameters for valid prediction.

A commonly encountered issue in the ICU regards detection and prediction of mortality in sepsis, and various levels of sepsis, including severe sepsis and septic shock. This issue has been investigated in a number of machine learning applications in the ICU. The use of feature selection and multivariate regression analysis in the MIMIC-II database identified dynamic variables surrounding a hypotensive event, including difference values before and after the event, as better predictors of mortality than the APACHE-IV score, thus highlighting them as not commonly used potential markers [15]. An improved classification approach for sepsis prediction, superior to other similar methods, was presented in [16], based on haemodynamic and other parameters from a publicly available database containing data of patients with abdominal septic shock. Haemodynamic parameters, along with clinical and laboratory data, in two subject subgroups of the MIMIC-II database were subjected to uni- and multivariate analysis, and an association was found between nonsurvivors and low values of blood pressure, cardiac output, and blood pH and oxygenation [17]. Mean arterial pressure levels and heart rate, along with respiratory rate, derived from the MIMIC-II database, were used to extract sequential patterns utilised by coupled hidden Markov models to predict septic shock in ICU patients [18]. This novel approach, which relies on sequence-based physiological pattern markers to learn dynamic physiological behaviour, allows building of powerful risk stratification models for septic shock patients. In a more recent work, prolonged elevated heart rate was associated with decreased survival in a large and heterogeneous cohort of ICU patients from the MIMIC-III database, using multivariable weighted logistic regression analysis [19]. Based on the previously outlined studies, computerised methods can contribute to improving sepsis prediction in the ICU through (a) the identification of new features useful for prediction and (b) the processing of large data amounts, so as to consider contributions of individual data to sepsis prediction.

Other ICU issues that have been investigated using computerised approaches include the management of hypotension and the identification of delirium. Using regression analysis and measurements of mean arterial pressure of more than 2,000 subjects of the MIMIC-II database, Lee et al. found an inverse association between vasoactive agents and in-hospital mortality and length of stay [20]. This study has implications for the care of critically ill patients with hypotension and illustrates the utility of electronic medical records in research when randomised controlled trials are difficult to conduct. Delirium is an important syndrome found in patients in the ICU, however, it is usually under-recognised during treatment. Oh et al showed that delirious patients can be successfully distinguished from non-delirious patients by using heart rate variability and machine learning [21].

3.3 Estimation of Arterial Stiffness

Arterial stiffness is an established risk factor for cardiovascular disease. Arterial stiffening, however, has adverse effects not only for subjects with cardiovascular disease, but also for the general population. In the ICU, the feasibility of measuring arterial stiffness and the effect of drug treatment has been the topic of a number of studies. Central arterial (aortic) stiffness has been mostly investigated [22–25], although the stiffness of the radial artery has also been reported [24].

Several different methods can be used to estimate arterial stiffness, some of which are more applicable in clinical practice than others. Some techniques provide information on systemic or regional arterial stiffness, while others provide information on local stiffness of the vessel being studied [26]. In ICU applications, methodologies include catheter- or tonometry-based measurement of blood pressure, and the use of ultrasound to estimate arterial diameter (and its changes during the cardiac cycle) or the stroke volume. Stiffness indices, including distensibility, compliance, pulse wave velocity, stroke-volume-to-pulse-pressure ratio can then be calculated from these measurements, using appropriate formulae [26]. In the ICU setting, invasive measurements are possible, which allow access to, and therefore assessment of arterial stiffness in, arterial beds for which noninvasive estimation is not possible, for example central arteries.

The application of the previous methodologies has yielded interesting findings about arterial stiffness in the ICU setting. The feasibility of measuring local arterial stiffness has been demonstrated for the descending aorta, while similar measurements were proven more challenging in the ascending aorta [22]. In this case, aortic elastic properties were calculated using simultaneous acquisitions of catheter-derived pressure and transoesophageal-ultrasound-based area indices, to which a biomechanical model was fitted (Fig. 4). Aortic distensibility and compliance coefficients were found to increase with blood pressure reduction induced by infusion of sodium nitroprusside [22]. Arterial stiffness has been reported to be positively related to pulse pressure in critically ill patients, and especially in aged subjects with haemodynamic stability [23]. In this study, total arterial stiffness was estimated by coupling echocardiography and arterial tonometry; the latter was performed at the radial artery and translated to aortic pressure using a validated transfer function. Noninvasive determination of central artery stiffness obtained from peripheral radial artery tonometry has been demonstrated to be useful in clinical practice, as it was associated with invasive, catheter-based, measurements [24]. In the same study, an increase of arterial stiffness was observed with infusion of norepinephrine, both invasively and noninvasively. More recently, shear strains, an index partly representative of arterial stiffness, were estimated in the carotid artery of young and elderly subjects in the ICU from B-mode ultrasound [27].

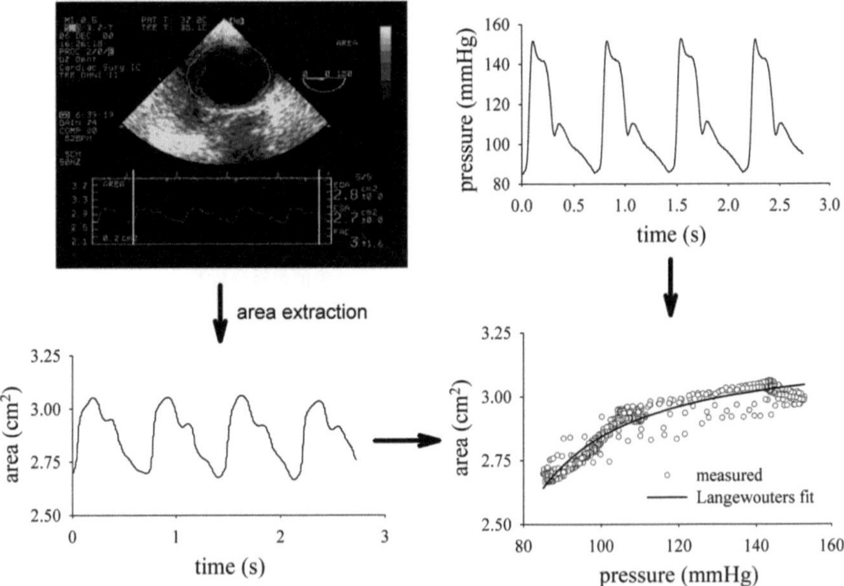

Fig. 4 Area data extracted from the acoustic quantification image with use of customised software. Area and pressure data are aligned in time, area is plotted as a function of pressure, and the arctangent model of Langewouters is fitted through the data (Reprinted, with permission, from [22])

4 Summary, Future Perspectives and Concluding Remarks

Cardiovascular data generated in the ICU setting can be used in computing applications to produce new knowledge about crucial pathophysiological phenomena, towards enhancing decision making and improving current practices. Data acquired in the context of conventional haemodynamic monitoring as well as with less common techniques in the ICU (applanation tonometry, carotid and venous ultrasound) can be organised in structured databases and analysed by means of advanced computerised methods towards improving outcome prediction in clinical practice. Data organisation in databases is useful for the evaluation of machine learning algorithms allowing the systematic investigation of physiological patterns. Analysis of data using statistical and machine learning methodologies provides insight into disease mechanisms and is promising for improving prediction of mortality in sepsis, a crucial issue in the ICU.

Advances in engineering, and electronic and computing technology allow the acquisition and storage of huge amounts of data, representing information from heterogeneous sources (e.g. several physiological parameters) recorded over long periods of time. Valuable knowledge is contained in these data, but only a small portion of it is currently utilised. The systematic application of computing methodologies in the data is promising towards exhaustive exploitation and extraction of useful hidden information.

Thorough cardiovascular data organisation and analysis will allow the generation of quantitative evidence, which is necessary for understanding and mapping treatment effects and for facilitating decision making. Personalisation is also possible and desired, towards improved risk stratification, i.e. identification of patient subgroups prone to specific states (survival, death, worsening). Evidence-based personalised practices will further allow to systematically address a number of ICU issues that remain open.

In conclusion, cardiovascular data organisation and analysis using advanced computing methodologies is promising for addressing crucial issues in the ICU, highlighting the role that clinical data mining will increasingly play in both knowledge generation and medical practice.

References

1. Angus DC (2007) Caring for the critically ill patient: challenges and opportunities. JAMA 298:456–458
2. Vincent JL (2006) Is the current management of severe sepsis and septic shock really evidence based? PLoS Med 3(9):e346
3. Laher AE, Watermeyer MJ, Buchanan SK, Dippenaar N, Simo NCT, Motara F, Moolla M (2017) A review of hemodynamic monitoring techniques, methods and devices for the emergency physician. Am J Emerg Med 35:1335–1347
4. Huygh J, Peeters Y, Bernards J, Malbrain MLNG (2016) Hemodynamic monitoring in the critically ill: an overview of current cardiac output monitoring methods. F1000Res 5: F1000Faculty Rev-2855
5. Augusto JF, Teboul JL, Radermacher P, Asfar P (2011) Interpretation of blood pressure signal: physiological bases, clinical relevance, and objectives during shock states. Intensiv Care Med 37(3):411–419
6. Au SM, Vieillard-Baron A (2012) Bedside echocardiography in critically ill patients: a true hemodynamic monitoring tool. J Clin Monit Comput 26(5):355–360
7. Pinsky MR, Payen D (2005) Functional hemodynamic monitoring. Crit Care 9(6):566–572
8. Meidert AS, Huber W, Müller JN et al (2014) Radial artery applanation tonometry for continuous non-invasive arterial pressure monitoring in intensive care unit patients: comparison with invasively assessed radial arterial pressure. Br J Anaesth 112(3):521–528
9. Gassner M, Killu K, Bauman Z, Coba V, Rosso K, Blyden D (2015) Feasibility of common carotid artery point of care ultrasound in cardiac output measurements compared to invasive methods. J Ultrasound 18(2):127–133
10. Nakamura K, Qian K, Ando T, Inokuchi R, Doi K, Kobayashi E, Sakuma I, Nakajima S, Yahagi N (2016) Cardiac variation of internal jugular vein for the evaluation of hemodynamics. Ultrasound Med Biol 42(8):1764–1770
11. Celi LA, Mark RG, Stone DJ, Montgomery RA (2013) "Big data" in the intensive care unit. closing the data loop. Am J Respir Crit Care 187(11):1157–1160
12. McShea M, Holl R, Badawi O, Riker RR, Silfen E (2010) The eICU research institute - a collaboration between industry, health-care providers, and academia. IEEE Eng Med Biol Mag 29:18–25
13. Johnson AEW, Pollard TJ, Shen L, Lehman LH, Feng M, Ghassemi M, Moody B, Szolovits P, Celi LA, Mark RG (2016) MIMIC-III: a freely accessible critical care database. Sci Data 3:160035

14. Pinsky MR, Dubrawski A (2014) Gleaning knowledge from data in the intensive care unit. Am J Respir Crit Care Med 190(6):606–610
15. Mayaud L, Lai PS, Clifford GD, Tarassenko L, Celi LA, Annane D (2013) Dynamic data during hypotensive episode improves mortality predictions among patients with sepsis and hypotension. Crit Care Med 41(4):954–962
16. Vieira SM, Mendona LF, Farinha GJ, Sousa JM (2013) Modified binary PSO for feature selection using SVM applied to mortality prediction of septic patients. Appl Soft Comput 13(8):3494–3504
17. Carrara M, Baselli G, Ferrario M (2015) Mortality prediction model of septic shock patients based on routinely recorded data. Comput Math Methods Med 2015:761435
18. Ghosh S, Li J, Cao L, Ramamohanarao K (2017) Septic shock prediction for ICU patients via coupled HMM walking on sequential contrast patterns. J Biomed Inform 66:19–31
19. Sandfort V, Johnson AEW, Kunz LW, Vargas JD, Rosing DR (2018) Prolonged elevated heart rate and 90-day survival in acutely ill patients: data from the MIMIC-III database. J Intensiv Care Med (in press)
20. Lee J, Kothari R, Ladapo JA, Scott DJ, Celi LA (2012) Interrogating a clinical database to study treatment of hypotension in the critically ill. BMJ Open 2:e000916
21. Oh J, Cho D, Park J et al (2018) Prediction and early detection of delirium in the intensive care unit by using heart rate variability and machine learning. Physiol Meas 39: 035004, 14
22. Heerman JR, Segers P, Roosens CD, Gasthuys F, Verdonck PR, Poelaert JI (2005) Echocardiographic assessment of aortic elastic properties with automated border detection in an ICU: in vivo application of the arctangent Langewouters model. Am J Physiol Heart Circ Physiol 288:H2504–H2511
23. Lamia B, Teboul JL, Monnet X, Osman D, Maizel J, Richard C, Chemla D (2007) Contribution of arterial stiffness and stroke volume to peripheral pulse pressure in ICU patients: an arterial tonometry study. Intensiv Care Med 33:1931–1937
24. Wittrock M, Scholze A, Compton F, Shaefer JH, Zidek W, Tepel M (2009) Noninvasive pulse wave analysis for the determination of central artery stiffness. Microvasc Res 77:109–112
25. Monge García MI, Cano AG, Romero MG (2011) Dynamic arterial elastance to predict arterial pressure response to volume loading in preload-dependent patients. Critic Care 15(R15):9
26. Mackenzie IS, Wilkinson IB, Cockroft JR (2002) Assessment of arterial stiffness in clinical practice. Q J Med 95:67–74
27. Golemati S, Cokkinos DD, Zakynthinos S (2018) Shear strain in the carotid artery of young and elderly subjects using B-mode ultrasound: a pilot study. In: World congress on biomechanics, Dublin, Ireland

MIX
Papier aus verantwortungsvollen Quellen
Paper from responsible sources
FSC® C105338

If you have any concerns about our products,
you can contact us on
ProductSafety@springernature.com

In case Publisher is established outside the EU,
the EU authorized representative is:
Springer Nature Customer Service Center GmbH
Europaplatz 3, 69115 Heidelberg, Germany

Printed by Libri Plureos GmbH
in Hamburg, Germany

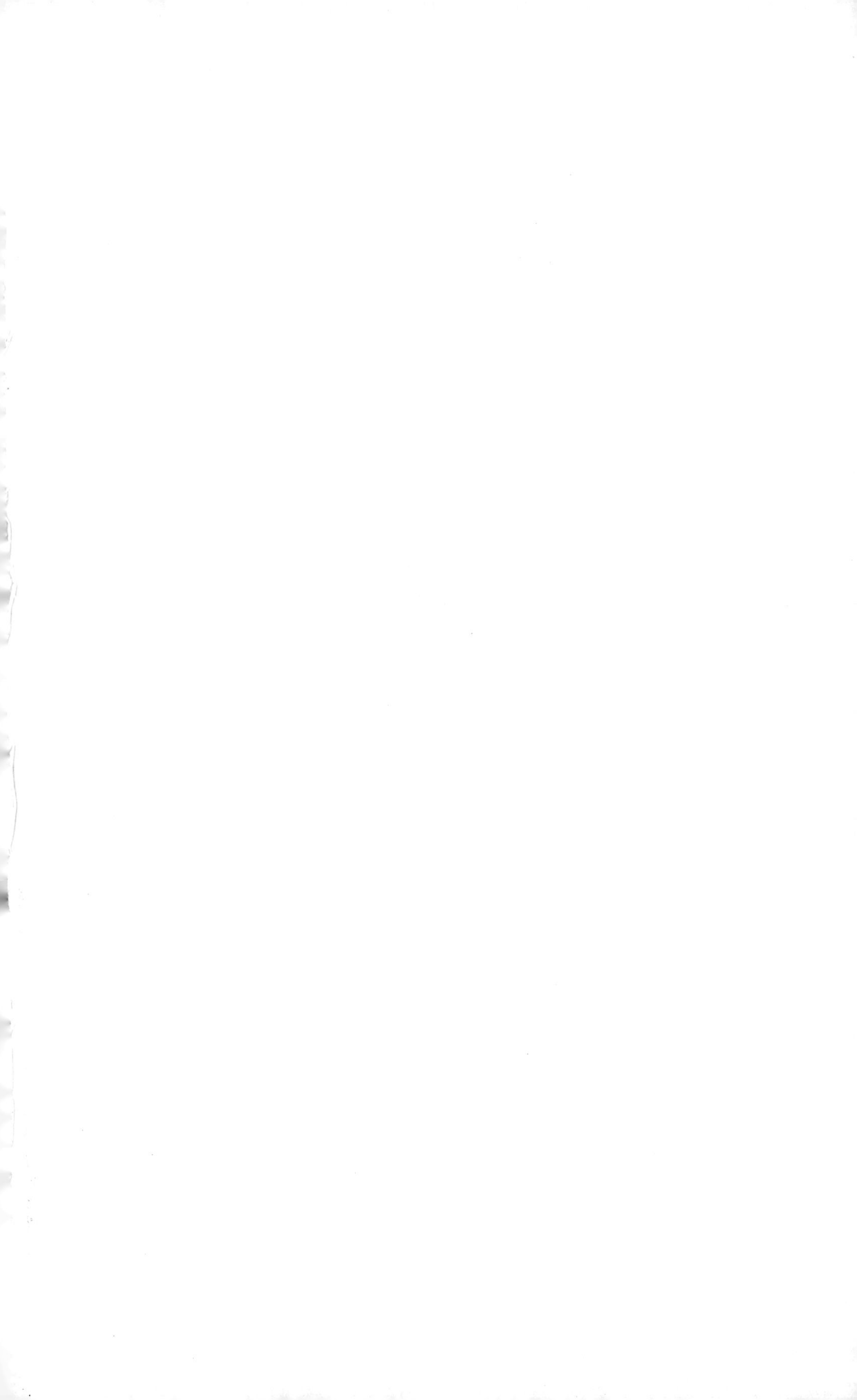